PROGRESS IN MALARIA RESEARCH

PROGRESS IN MALARIA RESEARCH

LEE O. KONING
EDITOR

Nova Biomedical Books
New York

For permission to use material from this book please contact us:
Telephone 631-231-7269; Fax 631-231-8175
Web Site: http://www.novapublishers.com

Library of Congress Cataloging-in-Publication Data

Progress in malaria research / editor, Lee O. Koning.
p. cm.
Includes bibliographical references and index..
ISBN-13: 978-1-60021-590-2 (hardcover)
ISBN-10: 1-60021-590-4 (hardcover)
1.Malaria—Research. 2. Malaria—Chemotherapy. I. Koning, Lee O.
[DNLM: 1. Malaria, Falciparum—drug therapy. 2. Antimalarials—pharmacokinetics. WC 770 P964 2007]
RC159.A5P7786 2007
616.9'3620072—dc22

2007003368

Published by Nova Science Publishers, Inc. ✢ New York

Contents

Preface

Malaria is an infectious disease that is widespread in tropical and subtropical regions. It infects between 300 and 500 million people every year and causes between one and three million deaths annually, mostly among young children in Sub-Saharan Africa. Malaria is not just a disease commonly associated with poverty, but is also a cause of poverty and a major hindrance to economic development. Malaria is one of the most common infectious diseases and an enormous public-health problem. Malaria is one of the most common infectious diseases and an enormous public-health problem. The disease is caused by protozoan parasites of the genus Plasmodium. The most serious forms of the disease are caused by Plasmodium falciparum and Plasmodium vivax, but other related species (Plasmodium ovale and Plasmodium malariae) can also infect humans. This group of human-pathogenic Plasmodium species are usually referred to as malaria parasites.

Malaria parasites are transmitted by female Anopheles mosquitoes. The parasites multiply within red blood cells, causing symptoms that include fever, anemia, chills, flu-like illness, and in severe cases, coma and death. Malaria transmission can be reduced by preventing mosquito bites with mosquito nets and insect repellents, or by mosquito control by spraying insecticides inside houses and draining standing water where mosquitoes lay their eggs.

One of the most important recent advances in malaria research is the mapping of the Plasmodium falciparum genome. For the next five to ten years, until an effective vaccine is developed, malaria control will largely be dependent on vector control measures such as improvements in housing construction, source reduction, impregnated bednets, and residual insecticide treatment.

This new book presents new research in this field from around the globe.

Chapter I - Artemisinin and its developed derivatives, dihydroartemisinin (DHA), artemether (AM), arteether (AE), artesunate (AS), and artelinate (AL), are highly effective against the erythrocytic stages of *P. falciparum* in vivo and in vitro. In the past two decades, toxicity studies have shown a dose-dependent neurotoxic effect in animal species administered intramuscularly or intragastrically with artemisinins, especially with oil-soluble AM and AE. In contrast, few neurotoxic effects are induced by water-soluble AS and AL, which have never produced any CNS side-effects in animal species after intravenous injection. Pharmacokinetic profiles demonstrate that drug exposure time plays a more important role in producing neurotoxicity than drug exposure level, production of the more active metabolite (DHA), or drug location in the CNS system. In addition, it has been demonstrated that at a below human therapeutic dose, injectable AS can cause fetal death due to a build up of high peak concentration of AS during the sensitive period of the early gestation days (GD) in animals. To date, however, the neurotoxicity and reprotoxicity have not been convincingly established in humans treated with any of artemisinins. Fatal neurotoxicity can be avoided by reducing the drug exposure time that varies greatly between the different artemisinin compounds. Also reproductive toxicity can be avoided by limiting the exposure of artemisinins during this sensitive period in fetal development (GD 9–14 in rats and GD 15 to week 6 in humans).

Pharmacokinetic/pharmacodynamic evaluations demonstrate that the rapid efficacy of artemisinins is principally due to the drug peak concentration (C_{max}) and their antimalarial potency. Other pharmacokinetic parameters, such as drug exposure level (AUC) and drug exposure time (half-life), tend to be of minor significance. The fundamental and reliable measures of efficacy in cure and mortality rates for uncomplicated and severe malaria show that current artemisinins (AS, AM, and DHA) have great role in artemisinin-based combination therapy (ACT) or monotherapy and provide a clear-cut advantage over other antimalarials currently in use. Most recently, a decrease in mortality (34.7%) has been demonstrated in a large study using intravenous AS, as opposed to the standard of care quinine injection. Artemisinins as a group are poorly efficacious at curing malaria as monotherapy. However, this shortfall has been overcome by using ACTs and AS injection in combination or in sequential administration with slower acting antimalarial drugs. When considering the demonstrated rapid parasite killing of parasites and variance between individual patients in both pharmacokinetics and pharmacodynamics, initial monotherapy and larger loading dose of AS injection may be needed to ensure that the maximum effect is obtained in all patients with severe and complicated malaria.

Chapter II - Transfer experiments of immunoglobulin from donors immune to *Plasmodium (P.) falciparum* malaria to patients symptomatic with *P. falciparum* malaria lead to a reduction in parasitemia and demonstrated the importance of immunoglobulines in anti-plasmodial immunity. Subsequent immunoepidemiological studies demonstrated that antibodies against *P. falciparum* bloodstage antigens are in addition to their antiparasitic effect essential in protection against complications of *P. falciparum* infection like severe anemia, placental malaria in pregnancy and possibly cerebral malaria which account for the majority of malaria related morbidity and mortality worldwide. Comparison of antibody levels between patients with complicated and uncomplicated *P. falciparum* malaria have shown that it is not the global quantity of antiplasmodial antibodies indicating previous exposure to the parasite which is associated with protecion from complications. Studies showed that antibodies against specific blood stage antigens on the surface of parasitized red blood cells and merozoites are most closely associated with protection from complications of *P. falciparum* malaria. Targets for antibodies which were found to be protective against complications of *P. falciparum* infection include in merozoites: merozoite surface proteins (MSP) 1 and 2, glutamate rich protein on the merozoite surface and apical merozoite antigen-1 and rhoptry protein-1. On the erythrocyte surface *P. falciparum* membrane protein-1, which is involved in cytoadherence, induces antibodies protective against complications. Antibodies against glycosylphosphatidylinositol (GPI) anchors of proteins on the merozoite surface, which may prevent cytoadherence promoting induction of endothelial adhesion molecules by tumor necrosis factor, have also been associated with clinical immunity.

Within the antigens mentioned only specific regions elicited protective antibodies like the C-terminal 19kDa fragment or block 2 of MSP-1 or the acylated phosphoinositol portion of GPI. Protective antibodies were found to be of the subclasses IgG-1 and IgG-3 for protein antigens involved. This may be partially due to their ability to bind to Fc receptors on monocytes promoting antibody dependent cellular inhibiton.

Future research needs to aim at a comprehensive analysis of antigens eliciting a protective antibody response. This could be achieved by using 2-dimensional immunoblotting of bloodstage antigens comparing immunoglobulin subclass responses to the full profile of parasite proteins identified by proteomics and mass spectrometry between patients with clinical immunity to *P. falciparum* and patients with complicated *P. falciparum* malaria. The relative importance of the various different antigens involved in inducing a protective response needs to be quantified.

Chapter III - Malaria represents a major health and socio-economic problem in Tanzania mainland (with a total population 35.6 million people) as in all of sub-Saharan Africa. Generally, malaria ranks number one in terms of morbidity and mortality. Malaria case-management has lately been hampered significantly by rapid development and spread of chloroquine parasite resistance in the mainland, like elsewhere, especially for *P. falciparum* malaria to the long-time established first line anti-malarial drug – chloroquine (CQ). The current recommended first and second line antimalarial drugs in the country are sulphadoxine – pyrimethamine (SP) and amodiaquine respectively. However, SP is reported to develop resistance rapidly and has necessitated changing the malaria treatment policy in most subs-Saharan Countries. Tanzania again will be moving (phasing out SP) to artemesinin fixed combination therapy by November, 2006.

Early diagnosis and prompt effective treatment represent the fundamental strategy of malaria control. National treatment guidelines are essential tools for health workers to exercise such a control. Following reports of increasing chloroquine (CQ) resistance the government on the Tanzanian mainland changed drug policy from chloroquine to sulphadoxine-pyrimethamine (SP) as first line drug for uncomplicated malaria. For example Zanzibar (Tanzania islands) as well as other countries in the region), the Ministries of Health has embarked directly to more efficacious artemesinin based fixed drug combination therapies a bit earlier than Tanzania mainland because of SP treatment failure mostly in East, central and southern Africa.

Fixed combination therapy, is a new strategy for malaria treatment, which is based on the hypothesis that two (or more) components of different mechanisms of action protect each other from development of resistance, simultaneously enhancing the efficacy and promoting compliance. Artemisinin as well as its two derivatives, e.g. artemether and artesunate, constitute a family of compounds with several attractive features for such a combination, due mainly to their rapid onset of effective action against multidrug-resistant P. falciparum and their gametocitocidal effect, which potentially reduces transmission of resistant strains. No cross-resistance with other known anti-malarials has been shown both in vivo and *in vitro*.

Chapter IV - The clinical utility of positron emission tomography (PET) is well documented, and high-resolution imaging of ^{18}F-fluorodeoxyglucose (FDG) has been used for many years to study glucose utilization in neoplasms and major organs such as the brain, heart and spleen. However, little attention was directed to the use of FDG-PET for parasitic diseases including malaria. Recently, to elucidate the clinical features of severe malaria, we performed whole-body FDG-PET of *Plasmodium coatneyi*-infected acute phase Japanese macaques (*Macaca fuscata*). Our previous studies demonstrated that the Japanese macaque is highly susceptible to *P. coatneyi* infection and that pathologic findings in infected monkeys are similar to those observed in human falciparum malaria. The *P. coatneyi*-infected Japanese macaque thus appears to be a useful model for pathological and pathophysiological studies of severe falciparum malaria. We present here direct evidence concerning glucose uptake by FDG-PET scanning in *P. coatneyi*-infected macaques, and demonstrate the relationship of such uptake to histopathological changes observed in the tissue.

We focused on the cerebral metabolic changes induced by severe malaria. We observed diffuse and heterogeneous reduction of metabolism in the cerebral cortex in the acute phase of malaria infection. Histopathological examination revealed preferential sequestration of parasitized red blood cells (PRBCs) in the cerebral microvasculature. However, neither hemorrhagic change nor necrosis was observed in HE- and Nissl-stained brain tissues. This suggests that reduction of cerebral metabolism occurs before parenchymal changes appear in the brain. This may be one reason why more than half of cerebral malaria patients have no neurological sequelae after recovery.

The current study revealed also distinct elevation of FDG up-take in the spleen of infected monkeys. The infected monkeys clearly exhibited increase in splenic FDG uptake indicating marked enhancement of glucose metabolism. The Standardized Uptake Values (SUVs) of the spleen in the infected monkeys were significantly higher than those in the uninfected monkey. At autopsy, splenomegaly was clearly present in all infected monkeys, and histopathologic findings included hyperplasia of lymphoid follicles in white pulp, a large number of activated macrophage, and congestion of PRBCs and malaria pigments in red pulp. Increase in splenic glucose uptake may thus be closely related to activation of splenic clearance system against blood-stage malarial parasites.

These findings will improve understanding of physiological alterations of the host in serious malarial infection. We believe that whole-body FDG-PET may be useful for evaluating and monitoring pathophysiological processes involved in severe malaria.

Chapter V - Transmission of malaria through the oral route is analyzed looking at the evolutionary origin of Apicomplexa, Coccidia, Haemosporidia, and *Plasmodium* parasites. Discussion is done on the two ways of oral transmission proposed: by ingesting the meat of an infected animal, or by ingestion of the infective form of a coccidian. This discussion is linked to experimental observations to sustain a theory that consider that the original coccidian from which *Plasmodium* evolved is an *Isospora* that did not disappear in the process of speciation and, it is still with us forming part of the cycle of a parasite that behave like plasmodium and/or coccidian, depending on the host they infect. The stage of the parasite that make connection between *Plasmodium* and coccidian, may be the sporozoite, although merozoites may be involved in infections transferred by blood forms.

Chapter VI - *Background:* Malaria has remained the major killer in Africa as a million children die of the disease every year. This problem is compounded by the emergence of resistance to the commonly used anti-malarial treatments. However, the collective action of the international community led to the establishment of the global fund which made more resources available for malaria control. WHO on view of an increasing resistance to chloroquine, recommended the use of artemisinin- based combination therapies for treatment of malaria. Every country or region in the same country has chosen its first and second lines of treatment. Northern Sudan has chosen artesunate/sulphadoxine-pyremethamine (AS/SP) and artemether/lumefantrine (ART/LUM) respectively as a first and second line treatment while southern Sudan has selected artesunate/amodiaquine (AS/AQ) as the first line of treatment. Central Sudan represents an area of seasonal unstable transmission of malaria where we have run two clinics to test the efficacies of these chosen lines of treatment for two consecutive years. Here we present the results of the second year.

Patients and methods: Sixty two patients with uncomplicated *P. falciparum* malaria were treated with AS/SP and 29 patients with ART/LUM in two different health centers. The patients were of all ages and did not have another cause of fever.

Results: All patients responded adequately to the first and the second lines of treatment without adverse side effects.

Conclusions: AS/SP and ART/LUM are efficacious for the treatment of malaria in an area of seasonal unstable transmission.

Chapter VII - The serum concentration of total lipids, β- / pre-β-lipoproteins and cholesterol were measured in fifty adult patients (25 males and females each), age range 18 – 35, presenting with acute, and uncomplicated *falciparum* malaria infection. Diagnosis was confirmed by microscopic examination of Giemsa-stained thin blood slides (parasite density = 1000 – 10,000 asexual forms / ml of blood). An age-matched group comprising of 20 healthy, malaria-negative adults were enrolled for comparative purposes. There was an insignificant increase in the serum concentration of total lipids in both the patient groups: (12.43 ± 4.61 g/l, males) and (13.77 ± 4.42 g/l, females) relative to the healthy individuals (9.84 ± 0.51 g/l) $p > 0.05$. β- and pre-β lipoprotein concentration was significantly elevated in the patients when compared to the healthy individuals: 7.58 ± 3.28 g/l (male patients), 7.60 ± 5.11 g/l (female patients) and 6.22 ± 2.40 g/l (healthy individuals), $p < 0.05$. Serum cholesterol was also significantly elevated in the malaria patients: 15.75 mmol/l (male patients), 12.08 ± 2.95 mmol/l (female patients) and 9.35 mmol/l (healthy individuals), $p < 0.05$. Uncontrolled haemolysis of both parasitized and unparasitized erythrocytes of all ages is one of the major determinants of the pathogenicity of human *falciparum* malaria infection. It leads to massive destruction of red blood cells, release of parasite-derived toxins and oxidant compounds responsible for the pathogenic outcomes observed in this endemic tropical disease. Since the erythrocyte membranes are predominantly lipid in composition, the release of such lipids following haemolysis can account for the observed perturbations in the serum lipid profile of patients presenting with this disease.

Chapter VIII - Most of deaths due to malaria occur in sub-Saharan region of Africa mainly children under five years who die in the 48 first hours of the illness. The necessity to have a quick diagnosis, a precocious, adequate and accessible treatment at all levels of society becomes mandatory to the endemic countries. The main objective of this document is to contribute to the reduction of the mortality and the morbidity related to malaria by proposing a better definition of the policies and strategies for fighting against malaria by using community based actions. Specifically, it is (i) to determine and to capitalize all community based management experiences for fighting against malaria, (ii) to determine the mechanisms of inter and into sector development of partnership for both mobilization of financial resource and the coordination of the community activities at all area of the medical pyramid of a country, (iii) to define ways to strengthen the social appropriation and the community participation for fighting against malaria, to create an impact and to perpetuate a long-term actions (iv) to provide to actors and community partners, orientations that imply or likely to be implied the Community based management of activities. To reach the Millennium Objectives for Development 2015, the endemic countries will have to overcome the challenge of malaria control at each level from family to community so that this disease does not represent any more neither, a major public health problem, nor a factor of impoverishment of the populations.

In: Progress in Malaria Research
Editor: Lee O. Koning, pp. 1-98

ISBN: 978-1-60021-590-2

Chapter I

Rapid Efficacy and Lethal Toxicity of the Artemisinin Derivatives Related to Drug Pharmacokinetic Profiles in Humans and in Animal Species

Qigui Li*, Wilbur K. Milhous and Peter J. Weina
Division of Experimental Therapeutics, Walter Reed Army Institute of Research, Silver Spring 20910, USA

1. Abstract

Artemisinin and its developed derivatives, dihydroartemisinin (DHA), artemether (AM), arteether (AE), artesunate (AS), and artelinate (AL), are highly effective against the erythrocytic stages of *P. falciparum* in vivo and in vitro. In the past two decades, toxicity studies have shown a dose-dependent neurotoxic effect in animal species administered intramuscularly or intragastrically with artemisinins, especially with oil-soluble AM and AE. In contrast, few neurotoxic effects are induced by water-soluble AS and AL, which have never produced any CNS side-effects in animal species after intravenous injection. Pharmacokinetic profiles demonstrate that drug exposure time plays a more important role in producing neurotoxicity than drug exposure level, production of the more active metabolite (DHA), or drug location in the CNS system. In addition, it has been demonstrated that at a below human therapeutic dose, injectable AS can cause fetal death due to a build up of high peak concentration of AS during the sensitive period of the early gestation days (GD) in animals. To date, however, the neurotoxicity and reprotoxicity have not been convincingly established in humans treated with any of artemisinins. Fatal neurotoxicity can be avoided by reducing the drug exposure time that varies greatly between the different artemisinin compounds. Also

* The corresponding author should be addressed: Qigui Li, PhD. Chief of Pharmacokinetics/Pharmacodynamics; Department of Pharmacology; Division of Experimental Therapeutics; Walter Reed Army Institute of Research; 503 Robert Grant Avenue; Silver Spring, MD 20307-5100, USA; Tel: (301) 319-9351; Fax: (301) 319-7360; E-mail: qigui.li@na.amedd.army.mil

reproductive toxicity can be avoided by limiting the exposure of artemisinins during this sensitive period in fetal development (GD 9–14 in rats and GD 15 to week 6 in humans).

Pharmacokinetic/pharmacodynamic evaluations demonstrate that the rapid efficacy of artemisinins is principally due to the drug peak concentration (C_{max}) and their antimalarial potency. Other pharmacokinetic parameters, such as drug exposure level (AUC) and drug exposure time (half-life), tend to be of minor significance. The fundamental and reliable measures of efficacy in cure and mortality rates for uncomplicated and severe malaria show that current artemisinins (AS, AM, and DHA) have great role in artemisinin-based combination therapy (ACT) or monotherapy and provide a clear-cut advantage over other antimalarials currently in use. Most recently, a decrease in mortality (34.7%) has been demonstrated in a large study using intravenous AS, as opposed to the standard of care quinine injection. Artemisinins as a group are poorly efficacious at curing malaria as monotherapy. However, this shortfall has been overcome by using ACTs and AS injection in combination or in sequential administration with slower acting antimalarial drugs. When considering the demonstrated rapid parasite killing of parasites and variance between individual patients in both pharmacokinetics and pharmacodynamics, initial monotherapy and larger loading dose of AS injection may be needed to ensure that the maximum effect is obtained in all patients with severe and complicated malaria.

2. Introduction

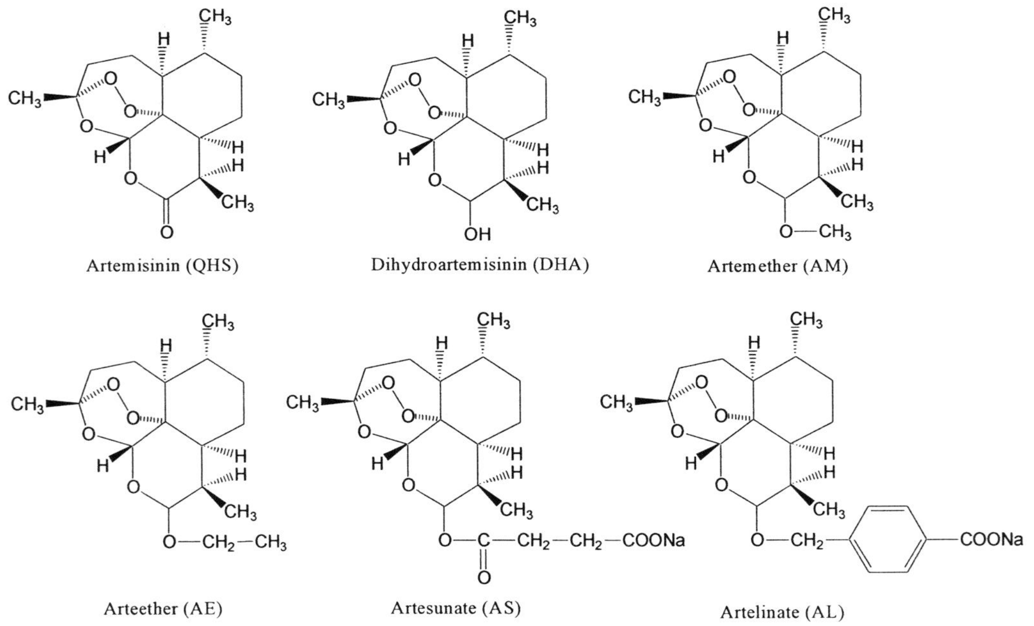

Figure1. Structures of artemisinin (QHS) and its five derivatives, dihydroartemisinin (DHA), artemether (AM), arteether (AE), artesunate (AS) and artelinate (AL).

Artemisinin (QHS) has been identified as the active antimalarial principle of *qinghao*, a plant used for centuries to treat malaria in China. QHS and its developed derivatives, dihydroartemisinin (DHA), artemether (AM), arteether (AE), and artesunate (AS), are in use for the treatment of uncomplicated, complicated or severe malarias, including multidrug resistant *falciparum* malaria. Another derivative of QHS, artelinate (AL), is in the development of pre-clinical stage. These compounds have several advantages including the more rapid clearance of parasites in the periphery, more rapid resolution of fever, less toxicity and reduction in the transmission potential of *falciparum* malaria. Also, there have been no reports of parasite resistance to date. The chemical structures of the five-artemisinin derivatives and their parent, QHS, are presented in figure 1.

2.1. Efficacy Potency of Five Artemisinin Analogues *In Vitro* and *In Vivo*

Our *in vitro* testing [1] recently reported the relative antimalarial potency of artemisinin and control compounds against W-2 (chloroquine-resistant clone of *P. falciparum*) parasites are 0.004 (chloroquine) < 0.29 (mefloquine) < 0.72 (AL) < 1.0 (QHS) < 1.84 (AM) < 2.41 (AE) < 3.01 (AS) < 3.59 (DHA), and against D-6 (mefloquine-resistant clone of *P. falciparum*) parasites are 0.12 (mefloquine) < 0.16 (chloroquine) < 0.32 (AL) < 1.0 (QHS) < 1.22 (AM) < 1.87 (AE) < 2.48 (AS) < 2.99 (DHA). Artemisinin drugs were also evaluated against Chinese, Philippine and African isolates and clones of *P. falciparum*, and data showed a very similar order of antimalarial potency for the artemisinin derivatives (table 1) [2-4].

Table 1. In *vitro* sensitivity profile with 50% inhibitory concentration (IC_{50}) of artemisinin derivatives and positive control drugs against chloroquine-resistant clone of *P. falciparum* from Indochina (W2), mefloquine-resistant clone of *P. falciparum* from Sierra Leone (D6), Philippine and African isolators of *P. falciparum* by an isotopic microdilution drug sensitivity test using tritium-labeled hypoxanthine [1-3]

Compounds	W2 [1] ng/ml (n = 6)	D6 [1] ng/ml (n = 6)	Philippine [2] nM (n = 23-38)	Africa [3] nM (Range)
Artemisinin	0.83 ± 0.10	1.49 ± 0.04	2.8 ± 1.4	9.31 - 58.2
Dihydroartemisinin	0.28 ± 0.06	0.30 ± 0.09		
Artemether	0.48 ± 0.07	0.73 ± 0.24	1.4 ± 1.3	5.97 - 22.7
Arteether	0.37 ± 0.09	0.48 ± 0.14	0.9 ± 0.5	5.71 – 24.8
rtesunate	0.35 ± 0.12	0.36 ± 0.05	0.9 ± 0.5	
Artelinic acid	1.24 ± 0.15	2.78 ± 0.76		4.66 – 22.5
Chloroquine	202.7 ± 38.1	5.75 ± 1.23	43 ± 17	34.9 – 1670
Mefloquine	3.08 ± 0.90	7.24 ± 2.40	2 ± 0.5	20.8 – 97.1

Values are mean ± SD; W-2: Indochina clone, resistant to chloroquine, sensitive to mefloquine. D-6: Sierra Leone clone, sensitive to chloroquine, resistant to mefloquine.

Results indicated that DHA and AS were shown to be more highly effective than other artemisinin derivatives. Stage-specific activity of the five-artemisinin analogues differed from that of quinine-type antimalarials, and each derivative displayed a unique stage-specific profile. DHA was highly effective against all parasite stages of *P. falciparum* isolates and clones, in most cases achieving 100% growth inhibition within 2-4 h of exposure [5]. QHS, and to a lesser extent AM, were most active against rings and schizonts, demonstrating relatively little activity against trophozoites stage of *Plasmodium falciparum* [5-7]. AE, AS, and AL were most effective against the late-stage ring parasites and trophozoites stages of *P. falciparum, P. cynomolgi, P. vinckei petteri and P. berghei* [8-15]. Compared with DHA, other artemisinin drugs including artemisinin itself only achieve 60-80% growth inhibition that lasted 3-10 hours longer (table 2).

Table 2. Stage-specific sensitivity and growth inhibition of artemisinin derivatives with different isolates and clones of *Plasmodium falciparum* in vitro [5-15]

Drugs effects	Erythrocytic stages			Gametocyto-cidal effects	Parasite growth inhibitory with drug exposure time (hr)*		
	Ring	Tropho-zoites	Schizonts		100%	60-80%	30-50%
QHS	+	+	+	+	6-12	6-10	1-3
DHA	++	++	++	+	2-4		1-2
AM	++		+			8-10	1-6
AE	++	+		+			
AS	++	+		+			
AL	+	+		+		3-6	

*Drug concentration in the culture exposure tests was 10^{-5}-10^{-6} M. QHS = artemisinin, DHA = Dihydroartemisinin, AM = Artemether, AE = Arteether, AS = Artesunate, AL = Artelinate

In general, the stage dependency of drug effects decreased with increasing drug concentrations and exposure times. Stage specificity of drug effect was particularly dependent on exposure time for the artemisinin drugs [9]. The stage-specific sensitivities and growth inhibitions of the artemisinin drugs are summarized in table 2. Only DHA was rapidly effective against all stages of the parasite life cycle and completely inhibited the parasite growth within the shortest exposure time (2-4 hr). Since AS is prodrug of DHA in intro and in vivo [16], these results confirm the greater in vitro potency of DHA compared to the other artemisinin derivatives.

In vivo studies in animal species using the *P. berghei*-infected mouse model, the *P. falciparum*-infected Aotus monkey, and the *P. cynomolgi* infection in rhesus monkey have confirmed that artemisinin and derivatives are highly effective antimalarial compounds. In the mouse model (table 3), the dose of AM and AE curing 50% of infected mice (CD_{50}) had a mean value of 55 mg/kg following single subcutaneous injection [17]. The mean dose for AS and AL was 421 and 211 mg/kg, respectively, after daily for 3 consecutive days subcutaneously [18], suggesting that AL showed two-fold greater antimalarial activity than AS in mice via this route of administration. In the Aotus monkey model, the ED_{50} were 7.1 mg/kg for AM and 11.8 mg/kg for AE during 3 days treatments [17]. In addition, AE is curative at a dose of 5 mg/kg for 3 days after intramuscular administration against blood-induced *P. cynomolgi* infection in rhesus monkey [19]. The curative dose of AS is 3.3 mg/kg initially and then 1.7 mg/kg at 8 and 24 hr after the first intravenous dose in rhesus monkeys infected with *P. coatneyi* [20].

The comparison of the therapeutic potential in monotherapy of artemisinin drugs in humans for 3-5 days treatments is summarized in table 4 [21-43]. The rates of recrudescence, fever, and parasite clearances are traditional parameters for the efficacy of the antimalarial drugs in humans. These three parameters exhibit the therapeutic potential of intramuscular AE with sesame oil (Artemotil), which has much less efficacy [21, 22] compared to that of intramuscular AM [23-32], oral and intravenous AS [33, 34], and the oral DHA [35-38], or even than that of intramuscular α/β-arteether formulated with peanut oil [39-43] in India. It is clear that the efficacy of artemisinins *in vivo* (animal species and humans) is different compared to that of artemisinin drugs *in vitro*.

Table 3. In *vivo* sensitivity profiles with 50% curative total dose (CD_{50}, mg/kg) in mice (mg/kg) of artemisinin and its derivatives against *P. berghei* by an isotopic microdilution drug sensitivity test using tritium-labeled hypoxanthine [17-20]

Compounds	Intragastric (b.i.d x 5D)	Subcutaneous (Single)	Subcutaneous (Daily x 3D)
Artemisinin	469 (365-641)	778 (348-1737)	161 (102-259)
Dihydroartemisinin	85 (66-109)	-	
Artemether		52-71	
Arteether		30-72	
Artesunate	170 (132-217)	-	421 (273-875)
Artelinic acid	170 (132-217)	-	211 (129-376)

Values are given as median (95% confidence limits).

2.2. Basic Pharmacokinetic Parameters of Five Artemisinin Derivatives

The pharmacokinetics of artemisinin and its five derivatives are not yet known in very much detail in humans, but it has been clearly defined in animal species [44-49]. The five-artemisinin analogues have been compared under the same conditions in rats following intravenous, intramuscular, and intragastric administration. The intravenous results showed the basic parameters of PK for the five compounds in table 5, and the intravenous results of DHA, AM and AE were first reported with cremophore formulation [44]. All five artemisinin derivatives exhibited a rapid elimination (0.4-1.4 hr) and biphasic decline in plasma concentration after intravenous administration.

The data shows that AL has the highest plasma level, the slowest elimination half-life, the lowest volume of distribution, and the slowest total clearance when compared with the other four artemisinins. Considering that the dose of AM or DHA is 140 or 147% the dose of artelinic acid in molecular weight, the equal-molecular weight is analyzed in deriving the results. When C_{max} and AUC are recalculated on a μM basis, AL C_{max} and AUC are still higher than other four-artemisinin analogues (table 5). AL was not only stable in vitro in aqueous solution and biological fluid, but also stable in vivo for biotransformation [18, 45, 50, 51]. The data also shows that AE and AS, which was converted almost immediately into DHA and other metabolites, had very low C_{max} and AUC when compared with the other three drugs, suggesting that these two compounds had been rapidly and extensively metabolized in rats.

Table 4. Summary of 54 clinical trials of artemisinin derivatives monotherapy in treatment of patients with uncomplicated, complicated, and severe malarias. Values are given mean ± SD. [21-43]

Drug and Regimen	PCT (hr)	FCT (hr)	% of Recru descence	Clinical Trials No.
AE with sesame oil (Artemotil) [21,22]				
(IM 3.2 mg/kg-1.6 mg/kg x 4)	70.2	81.0	40.0	1
(IM 4.8 mg/kg-1.6 mg/kg x 5)	59.2	61.5	22.2	1
AM [23-32]				
(IM 3.2 mg/kg-1.6 mg/kg x 4)	28.3 ± 13.0	38.8 ± 4.4	8.6 ± 6.2	8
(oral 200 mg-100 mg/kg x 5)	39.7 ± 2.2	34.8 ± 6.9	5.2 ± 2.2	9
AS [33, 34]				
(IV and oral in various regimens)	30.3 ± 10.7	35.9 ± 11.1	7.5 ± 3.1	23
DHA [35-38]				
(oral in various regimens)	49.1 ± 7.5	33.8 ± 7.7	6.0 ± 1.8	7
AE with peanut oil [39-43]				
(IM 150 mg daily for 3 days)	37.8 ± 12.2	49.9 ± 16.2	9.4 ± 4.1	5

IM = intramuscular, IV = intravenous, PCT = parasite clearance time, FCT = Fever clearance time.

Table 5. Comparison of main pharmacokinetic parameters of artemisinin derivatives (DHA, AM, AE, AS and AL) at 10 mg/kg in rats following single intravenous injection. Values are mean ± SD (n = 4) [44]

Parameters	DHA	AM	AE	AS	AL
MW =	284.9	298.4	312.4	384.4	418.5
Dose (mg/kg)	10	10	10	10	10
Dose (μM/kg)	35.1	33.5	32.0	26.0	23.9
IV Vehicles	CMP	1:3 CMP/saline		0.9% saline (pH 8.5)*	
C_{max}					
(ng/ml)	6683 ± 2405	6231 ± 1837	3724 ± 430	2106 ± 399	12706 ±1010
(μM)	23.5 ± 13.0	20.9 ± 6.2	11.9 ± 1.4	5.5 ± 1.0	30.4 ± 2.2
AUC					
(ng•h/ml)	3184 ± 659	1857 ± 432	842 ± 154	738 ± 114	5481 ± 1754
(μM•h)	11.2 ± 2.3	6.2 ± 1.4	2.7 ± 0.5	1.9 ± 0.3	13.1 ± 3.8
Vss					
(liter)	0.50 ± 0.19	0.67 ± 0.11	0.72 ± 0.09	0.87 ± 0.35	0.39 ± 0.12
CL					
(ml/min/kg)	55.4 ± 9.7	91.8 ± 21.0	200.0 ± 31.0	190.9 ± 30.3	32.1 ± 8.0
t1/2					
(distribution, h)	0.22 ± 0.04	0.10 ± 0.01	0.10 ± 0.02	0.15 ± 0.02	0.19 ± 0.08
t1/2					
(elimination, h)	0.95 ± 0.21	0.53 ± 0.14	0.45 ± 0.03	0.35 ± 0.08	1.35 ± 0.45

CMP = Cremophore EL, DHA = Dihydroartemisinin, AM = Artemether, AE = Arteether, AS = Artesunic acid , AL = Artelinic acid, MW = Molecular weight, IV = intravenous; *pH adjusted to 8.5 with 1N $NaHCO_3$.

2.3. Neurotoxicity of Artemisinins in Animal Species

CNS neurotoxicity has been demonstrated in mice, rats, dogs, and rhesus monkeys that have been repeatedly administered with oil-soluble analogues of AM or AE at multiple doses of 5-24 mg/kg /day [52-55]. Studies show that AM and AE are toxic to the central nervous system and induce neuropathologic changes in these animals. The neurotoxic findings produced by artemisinins in animal species are summarized in table 6. Neuropathology has been detected in dogs given an AE dose of 5.0 – 6.75 mg/kg daily for 28 days [56-58]. The same neuropathology was found in rats at a dose of 12.5 mg/kg of AE given daily for 7 days [59] and in monkeys at 8 mg/kg of AE for 14 days [55]. However, clinical signs (ataxia and shaking) of neurotoxicity appeared at significantly higher doses in dogs (20 mg/kg, 7 days), in rats (50 mg/kg, 7 days), and in monkeys (24 mg/kg, 14 days) [54-56, 60]. This suggests that by the time neurological signs are observed in those animals, the drug concentrations are already three or four times higher than the doses known to cause neuropathologic changes.

Table 6. Neurotoxicity findings in pathological and behavioral evaluation in animal species treated with dihydroartemisinin (DHA), artemether (AM), arteether (AE), artesunate (AS) and artelinate (AL) following multiple intramuscular (IM) and intragastric or oral administrations (n = 4-20) [53-65]

Drug	Species	Pathological Neurotoxicity				Behavioral Neurotoxicity			
		Dose mg/kg	Route	Regimen	Refs	Dose mg/kg	Route	Regimen	Refs
AE	Rats	12.5	IM	7 daily	[53, 59]	50	IM	7 daily	[60]
	Dogs	5-7	IM	28 daily	[56-58]	20	IM	7 daily	[56]
	Monkeys	8	IM	14 daily	[55]	24	IM	14 daily	[55]
AM	Dog	20	IM	8 daily	[66]				
	Mice					150	IM	28 daily	[62, 64]
	Mice					300	oral	28 daily	
	Mice	300	oral	28 twice daily	[63]				
AS	Mice					250	IM	28 daily	[62, 64]
	Mice					200	oral	28 daily	[62, 64]
	Mice	300	oral	28 twice daily	[63]				
AL	Rats	160	oral	9 daily	[61]				
DHA	Mice	200	oral	28 daily	[63]	200	oral	28 daily	[63]

DHA = dihydroartemisinin, AM = artemether, AE = arteether, AS = artesunic acid, AL = artelinic acid; IM = intramuscular, Refs = References.

Despite extensive studies with AM and AE neurotoxicity, there is limited evidence of neurotoxicity in animals related to the water soluble artemisinin derivatives, for example AS, the most widely used artemisinin in humans. AL, another water-soluble artemisinin derivative, has also been reported to have some pathological neurotoxicity in rats following intragastric dose at 160 mg/kg daily for 9 days [61]. These studies help us see that the neurotoxicity of oil-soluble artemisinins is more potent than that of water-soluble analogues (table 6). The neurotoxicity of AL has been investigated in beagle dogs following daily oral administration at 25, 100, and 300 mg/kg dose levels for 14 days. No behavioral neurotoxicity has been observed in these beagle dogs at these doses. The considerable lack of toxicity detected in these dogs very well may be caused by very low oral bioavailability at these doses. Actually, in the highest dose level (300 mg/kg), the animals only received one-fifth of total dose due to the very low bioavailability (22%, our unpublished data). A recent study looked at AM, AS, and DHA orally administered daily for 28 days has helped us compare the two groups. There were little clinical or neuropathologic evidence of the neurotoxicity found at high dose levels of over 200 mg/kg/day in mice for the 3 drugs [62-64]. At the highest doses of intramuscular AM and AS, there was neurotoxicity and behavioral deficits of potentially irreversible abnormalities in balance and equilibrium. AM was determined to have much greater neurotoxicity than intramuscular AS though [64, 65].

The water-soluble artemisinin derivatives, AS and AL, were designed for intravenous injection. To date, no neurotoxicity (pathologic or behavioural) has been observed in animal species following intravenous administration at any repeated doses up to maximum tolerated doses (MTD). The MTDs of AS and AL are 240 and 80 mg/kg, respectively, following intravenous injection daily in rats for 3 days, but no neurotoxicity was detected in these animals [66]. In another study, intravenous AS had no effect on the neurotoxic scores at 120 mg/kg in sodium carbonate daily for 7 days (our unpublished data). After one intramuscular injection, a high dose of 420 mg/kg of AS and AL did not produce any neuronal necrosis in the rats. Also, up to 200 mg/kg of AS used orally daily for 5-7 days did not exhibit neuronal changes or any specific clinical signs [56].

Although artemisinin agents, mainly oil-soluble drugs, induced fatal neurotoxicity in animal models, a striking fact in treating patients with the artemisinins is the lack of any serious adverse events, despite careful monitoring in several clinical studies. Severe malarial infection itself, particularly cerebral malaria in multi-drug resistant strains in the developing world, often leaves patients with decreases in neural function. This development has made characterization of potential neurotoxic effects of the artemisinin derivatives very difficult to ascertain, even though these drugs are clinically utilized in ever growing numbers [67-69]. In a study of 3500 patients in Thailand, evidence of serious toxicity was not noticed [70]. From other reports, rare neurological side effects have been noted in humans receiving artemisinin drugs [71-76], and these findings were difficult to dissect from effects due to the concomitant malarial infection.

2.4. Neurotoxicity of Artemisinins in Humans?

A number of studies indicate that no neuralgic side effects are noted in humans from QHS, AM, AS, and DHA treatments. Even AE was safely used from phase I to III clinical trial studies [77-79]. However, a 36-year-old American geologist had neurological symptoms two days after completing AS treatment with worsening ataxia and slurred speech nine days after completing AS treatment [80]. Two months later, the patient still had slurred speech; a wide-based, ataxic gait; and impaired heel-to-shin and rapid alternating movement. He was re-treated with oral quinine and doxycycline after testing positive again for *Plasmodium* species (too scant to speciate) in a smear. Four months later, his ataxia was moderately improved, and his speech was nearly normal. In another case report, a 39-year-old man who returned from Sierra Leone with probable extrapyramidal syndrome that was self-limiting. He had an undetermined febrile illness for which he had received inappropriately long and repeated courses of both AS and chloroquine [81, 82]. Franco-Paredes et al. concluded that the patient's condition "suggests neurotoxicity due to multiple courses of AS therapy, perhaps compounded by chloroquine therapy [83]. However, Newton et al. pointed out that the patient was most likely suffering from the adverse effects of excessive chloroquine [84].

Certainly, these two reports do not constitute proof of any causal association, but the possibility that repeated administration of artemisinin drugs in malaria endemic areas will result in cumulative damage cannot be ruled out [85], especially since these drugs are often freely available for use in tropical countries [86]. However, another four patients experienced neuropsychiatric adverse events. One patient with history of epilepsy, seizure-free for 10 years, had an episode of tonic-clonic seizures; one patient suffered from anxiety, palpitations and sleep disturbance; one developed frank psychosis and another, depression. These patients were also receiving mefloquine though, a known cause of neuropsychiatric disturbances [87].

In the Gambian children with cerebral malaria described by van Hensbrock [23], intramuscular AM was associated with more convulsions (39 vs. 28%, P = 0.01) and more prolonged coma than was intramuscular quinine (26 vs. 20 hr, P = 0.05). Similar results were found in Vietnamese adults [24]. Survival analysis indicated a significant divergence in the times to recovery from coma among patients who remained unconscious for more than two days. In these patients, treatment with AM was associated with slower recovery than that of quinine dosing (66 vs. 48 hr, P = 0.003). Although in the current reports there was no increase in neurological sequelae in patients after multiple treatments with AM, significantly prolonged coma in both studies and increased incidence of convulsions in the AM group of Gamnian children indicates the need for further attentiveness and active investigation of the neurological side effects of artemisinin drugs. A recent report from Mozambique describes a small but significant and irreversible hearing loss in patients exposed to AM-lumefantrine [88, 89]. The results of this trial are controversial though as the treatment group had both malaria and treatment with AM-lumefantrine and the control group had neither. In another case control study, there were no differences in the test results between cases and controls. There was no neurophysiologic evidence of auditory trainstem toxicity that could be attributed to AM-lumefantrine in this study population [90].

Either intravenous followed by oral AS, or oral followed by intravenous AS were given at a dose of 2 mg/kg for 2 days to patients with uncomplicated acute *P. falciparum* malaria [91]. At the time of presentation the patients had been ill for a median of 3 days (range, 1 to 10 days) with fever, headache, anorexia, nausea, and vomiting. No adverse effects of the study drug were observed. In another trial, quinine plus tretracycline versus oral AS given at a total dose of 700 mg over 5 days was studied in patients with acute uncomplicated falciparum malaria [92]. The occurrence of adverse effects, such as tinnitus, was significantly higher in the quinine-tetracycline group. Nausea and dizziness were rather commonly associated with the AS group in this study. Toxicity has also been observed after 5 days of multiple intramuscular doses with AE. One person out of 14 subjects developed shiverers, clammy hands and feet, dizziness, headache, nausea and a 'metallic taste' 1 hr after the injection; the symptoms lasted about one hour and then were resolved spontaneously [93]. In view of their potential for neurological adverse effects, artemisinin analogues after multiple treatments should be borne in mind. Karbwang [92], Kager [93], Hoffeman [94], and Park [95] expressed concern about the potential neurotoxicity of all artemisinin derivatives, which are the drugs of choice for treating severe malaria caused by parasites with suspected resistance to chloroquine and quinine.

2.5. Reproductive Toxicity of Artemisinins in Animals

The artemisinin derivatives (mainly AM and AS) have been extensively studied in animals and in humans, and the experience in human pregnancy are encouraging. However, artemisinins have been shown to be very toxic to animal embryos in repeated preclinical studies. This preclinical data included in vivo embryo–fetal developmental toxicity studies carried out on mice, rats, hamsters, guinea pig, and rabbits, by different laboratories using for the most part ICH-compliant protocols [96-103].

Early study of QHS and AM were conducted in mice, rats and rabbits that were intramuscularly from gestation day (GD) 6 to 15 to observe for reproductive toxicity. The no observed adverse effect level (NOAEL) was 5.4 mg/kg in mice, 2.7 mg/kg in rats and 0.7 mg/kg/day in rabbits; above these doses, there were increased resorptions of fetuses: 100% resorption at 21.4 mg/kg/day in mice, > 90% resorption at 10.7 mg/kg/day in rats and >90% resorption at 2.7 mg/kg/day in rabbits [96, 97]. By subcutaneous administration, the study of AS was dosed in rats from GD 6 to 15, and the developmental retardation of sterna and ribs was noted in surviving fetuses in groups treated with 0.54 mg/kg of AS respectively. The dose that induced 50% fetuses resorbed (ED_{50}) was 0.58 mg/kg [98]. When rats were given a dose of 26 mg/kg/day at GD 1–6, 82.3% of fetuses survived. When the same dose was given in early organogenesis, GD 6–8, only 17.1% of fetuses survived, and treatment occurring after GD 8 resulted in 100% fetal resorption [98]. Recently, our study of AS was also performed in rats following intravenous and intramuscular injection from GD 5 to 15. The ED_{50} of AS after intravenous dosing was 0.61 mg/kg [99].

In experiments carried out in mice, hamsters, guinea pigs and rabbits both DHA and AS intragastrically, intramuscularly, or subcutaneously showed from mild to severe embryolethality effect. In mice and rabbits they caused embryo absorption whereas in hamsters and guinea pigs they induced abortion [100]. In rats, oral AS was administered from GD 6–19. The primary reported effect was embryo–fetal loss manifested as abortion in rabbits and resorption in both rats and rabbits. The no or low adverse effect levels were in the range of 5 to 7 mg/kg/day AS [101]. All preclinical studies of the reproductive toxicity in animal species are summarized in table 7. AS has the greatest toxicity to animal embryos by routes of subcutaneous, intramuscular and intravenous injections with less than 1 mg/kg of the ED_{50}, which is lower than therapeutic dose of 2-4 mg/kg in humans. [103]

Table 7. Embryotoxic effects (NOAEL and ED_{50}) of artemisinin (QHS), dihydroartemisinin (DHA), artemether (AM), artesunate (AS) given intragastrically, intramuscularly, subcutaneously, and intravenously on pregnant animal species (female mice, rats, hamster, guinea pig, and rabbits) [97-102]

Animals (Drugs)	Dose Duration (daily)	Dose Regimens	Dosing Routes	No-observed-adverse-effect-level (NOAEL)				ED_{50} (95% CL) (mg/kg)
				Oral	IM	SC	IV	
Mice (AM) [97]	GD6-15	Multiple x 10	IM		5.4			11.3 (10.6-12.0)
(DHA) [100]	GD7	Single	SC			10		32.8 (27.7-38.9)
Rats (QHS) [96]	GD1-6	Multiple x 6	Oral	5.6				11.5 (10.5-12.2)
(DHA) [102]	GD9.5, 10.5	Single	Oral	7.5				NA
(AM) [97]	GD6-15	Multiple x 10	IM		2.7			6.13 (4.52-8.26)
(AM) [97]	GD6	Multiple x 10	Oral	2.5				14.4 (10.4-17.8)
(AS) [98]	GD6	Multiple x 10	SC			0.2		0.58 (0.55-0.61)*
(AS) [99]	GD6-18	Multiple x 11	IM		0.5		0.4	0.61 (0.59-0.62)*
(AS) [101]	GD6-17	Multiple x 12	Oral	5-7				7.74 (6.92-8.57)
Hamster (DHA) [100]	GD7	Singl	SC			4.2		6.06 (5.90-6.21)
(DHA) [100]	GD7	Singl	Oral	20				51.0 (37.9-68.7)
(AS) [100]	GD5	Singl	SC			0.35		1.0 (0.9-1.2)*
Guinea Pig (DHA) [100]	GD18	Single	IM		2.5			18.3 (13.9-24.2)
Rabbits (AM) [97]	GD7-18	Multiple x 12	IM		0.7			NA
(AS) [101]	GD7-19	Multiple x 13	Oral	5-7				NA
(DHA) [100]	GD9	Single	IM		5			7.57 (7.48-7.67)

DHA = Dihydroartemisinin; AM = Artemether; AS = Artesunate; IM = intramuscular; SC = subcutaneous; IV = intravenous; ED_{50} = drug concentration induces 50% fetus resorbed; GD = gestation day (The day of mating was defined as day 0 of gestation.); * The severe toxic effects were detected in the animals treated with AS after single or multiple intramuscular, intravenous or subcutaneous injections. Values of ED_{50} are given as median (95% confidence limits). NA = not available.

Some recent studies found that tissue damage in embryos exposed to DHA affect primarily red blood cells during yolk sac hematopoiesis and higher concentrations and/or longer exposure inhibited angiogenesis [102, 104, 105]. Another study in rats showed that AS subcutaneous injection at a dose of 40 mg/kg/d during days 6-10 of gestation significantly decreased the concentration of serum progesterone in early pregnant rats and discontinued the degeneration of decidual cells and fetuses [106]. In cell culture, AS significantly decreased rat embryonic and placental glutathione peroxidase (GSH-Px) and increased malondialdehyde (MDA) level in these tissues [107].

The WHO expert panel judged from their review of these and 28 other experimental laboratory reports that in animals "all the artemisinin analogues have been associated with embryolethality over a narrow dose range and that there are instances of effects on development of the cardiovascular system, the axial skeleton and the limbs", but that "these do not suggest the nature of the toxic action." They considered that "because the safety data are limited, artemisinin compounds should only be used in the second and third trimester when other treatments are considered unsuited" [108].

Thus, an important population at high risk for malaria will continue to be excluded from treatment with artemisinin based combination therapy unless these treatments are shown to be effective and safe in pregnancy. Two early reports in China on pregnant women described that the effects of QHS, AM or AS were not found evident of drug toxicity [109, 110]. There were 94 cases of first trimester exposure to AS identified in the published literature [111, 112] and no unexpected adverse effects were reported. In areas of multi-drug resistance, only treatments based on artemisinin compounds were effective, and pregnant women have been treated for malaria with these drugs throughout pregnancy. Data from limited series of pregnant women (2,045 cases) exposed to artemisinin compounds, including a small number (108 cases) in the first trimester, did not show an increase in the rates of abortion or stillbirth or evidence of abnormalities. There were no clinically significant adverse effect of the drugs, on the outcomes of the pregnancies, or the development (neurological and physical) of the infants, including 44 infants exposed during the first trimester [112-120]. Treatment with AS during pregnancy is associated with higher birthweight, which may have resulted from clearance of malaria parasites, as placental malaria is associated with reduced birthweight [121]. However, the influence of confounding factors should not be excluded.

2.6. Current Use of Artemisinins Alone and Combination Regimens

In view of the fact that certain artemisinin drugs have produced fatal neurotoxicity and reproductive toxicities (in animals only), high recrudescent rate, poor oral bioavailability, and short half-lives, especially, intramuscular AE and AM were not successful in the clinical trials by monotherapy [21-24]. Artemisinin-based combination therapies (ACTs) are most preferred for their enhancement of efficacy [122-124], lower malaria incidence and their potential to lower the rate at which resistance emerges and spreads [125, 126]. Four ACTs recommended by a WHO Expert Consultative Group in 2001 are AM-lumefantrine (Coartem), AS-mefloquine (Artequin), AS-amodiaquine, and AS-sulfadoxine/pyrimethamine

[127]. Recently, WHO has endorsed ACTs as the "policy standard" for all malaria infections in areas where *P. falciparum* is the predominant infecting species [128].

The rapid parasite clearance of artemisinin drugs in the treatment of early cases of uncomplicated malaria with ACTs may prevent its progression to severe disease with consequent reduction in severe cases and mortality rate. AM-Lumefantrine was the first registered, fixed, ACT treatment, and constitutes about 70% of all current clinically-used ACTs [129]. It is highly effective when given twice a day for three days (6-dose) and with a small amount of fat [130, 131]. This is because lumefantrine has to be given with food (preferably containing fat) to ensure adequate absorption and thus efficacy. In an initial study with a 4-dose AM-lumefantrine regimen, there was a relatively high rate of late treatment failure (E1) [132]. In the study in an area with high-grade mefloquine resistance, the 6-dose AM-lumefantrine regimen was associated with a 28% treatment failure at 14 days (E3) [133]. Another ACT treatment, AS-mefloquine, has been used in South-East Asian countries such as Thailand and Cambodia, widely since 1994 and remains highly effective for uncomplicated falciparum malaria. Under the WHO system of efficacy assessment, more than 95% of patients will remain free of malaria 28 days after such treatment (E2) [134, 135]. However, the failure rate of AS-mefloquine combination has been reported to be up to 13% in Thailand and Cambodia [136], and the neuropsychiatric effects of mefloquine as well as its relative expense are problematic [137].

Monotherapy with the artemisinins was significantly decreased after 2001 to prevent the experiencing resistance. For complicated and severe malaria, however, intravenous AS, as monotherapy, is still in first line treatment for both adults and children in Asian countries [138], and some areas in Africa [139]. Trying to replace quinine (which has been the principal drug used to treat severe malaria for nearly 400 years) with a more effective, less expensive, and better tolerated drug [140], an initial trial using intramuscular AM demonstrated less toxicity but no clear mortality benefit over quinine [141, 142]. More recent trials have used intravenous AS with a more favorable pharmacokinetic profile [143, 144]. The SEAQUAMAT trial, a multicentre randomized trial conducted in Bangladesh, Thailand, Myanmar, Indonesia, India and Vietnam, recently reported a 34.7% reduction in all cause mortality associated with intravenous AS compared with intravenous quinine [138, 145, 146]. This is the largest trial ever performed in severe malaria and the first to demonstrate conclusively a mortality benefit over standard quinine therapy. There is convincing evidence that for those who do develop severe malaria, intravenous AS will reduce the risk of death by one-third when compared to quinine therapy. For the 202 children included in the trial, artesunate injection was equally safe and effective [145].

Almost immediately intravenous AS was recommended for patients with severe malaria by The European Network on Imported Infections Disease Surveillance (TropNetEurop) [147]. The most recent advance in antimalarial chemotherapy has been the use of artemisinin derivatives, especially intravenous AS, which may well revolutionize the management of complicated and severe malaria [148]. Therefore, we still need AS monotherapy [149]. However, there is currently no product available that is produced under good manufacturing practice (GMP) conditions. Walter Reed Army Institute of Research (WRAIR) has being developed a novel cGMP injection of AS since 2003, which is in the process of US FDA approval [66, 150].

2.7. The Objectives of the Chapter

Several perplexities continue to vex us with the artemisinins [151]. Why does this neurotoxicity mostly occur in animals treated with oil-soluble artemisinins (with sesame oil vehicle), but not or less with water-soluble agents? Why does the neurotoxicity induced by artemisinins depending on drug exposure time but not on drug exposure level? Why does the neurotoxicity and reproductive toxicity so easily observed in animal models not occur in humans getting equal or even higher doses of the drug? Why does the efficacy of artemisinins depend upon drug peak concentration (C_{max}) but not drug exposure level or time? In this review based on WRAIR and other research data from recent two decades, the pharmacokinetic characteristics will be evaluated and discussed that may shed light on some of these questions. Principally, the discussion will be: 1) neurotoxicity concerning drug pharmacokinetics; 2) pharmacokinetic role in reproductive toxicity; 3) relationship between drug efficacy and pharmacokinetics; and 4) how to maintain rapid efficacy and avoid lethal toxicities.

3. Neurotoxicity Concerning Drug Pharmacokinetics

3.1. The Role of DHA in Neurotoxicity

DHA is obtained by sodium borohydride reduction of artemisinin, an endoperoxide containing sesquiterpene lactone; this was isolated by Chinese researchers and characterized as the antimalarial principle of the plant *Artemisia annua*. Through *in-vitro* bioassay tests, DHA has been shown to be 1.4-5.2 folds more active than other artemisinins [1-3, 18-20] but has also been shown to be 2-4 folds more toxic than other artemisinins in vitro and in vivo [152-156]. Due to its poor solubility in water or oils, DHA has only been formulated as an oral preparation and has been used primarily as a semisynthetic compound for derivatization to other oil soluble and water-soluble artemisinins [33]. The effectiveness of AS has been attributed to its rapid and extensive hydrolysis to DHA [16, 44, 143, 157, 158). The efficacy of AM and AE has also been credited to the conversion to DHA, but their conversion rates were significantly lower and less complete than in AS [16, 44]. AL is a very stable artemisinin agent *in vitro* and *in vivo*, and has almost no biotransformation to DHA in animal species [18, 45].

Thus, evaluating the conversion rates of various artemisinin drugs is very important for assessing the risk of neurotoxicity for the four compounds that are the focus of this article. A conversion evaluation of AM, AE, AS, or AL to DHA is summarized in table 8 [27, 29, 65, 159-176]. The summary shown illustrates that the conversion of artemisinin drugs to DHA in humans, which seem to be much more efficient than that in other animal species. Compared to the data from animal species and humans treated with AM or AS, the ratios of AUC_{DHA} to $AUC_{AM\ or\ AS}$ are significantly higher in humans (0.4-9.7) than in animal species (0.04-2.7), suggesting that the human hydrolysis system is more active and complete.

Table 8. Mean ratios of AUC_{DHA} (an active metabolite) /$AUC_{AM\ or\ AE,\ AS,\ and\ AL}$, and the concentration values of $AUC_{DHA}/AUC_{AM\ or\ AE,\ AS,\ and\ AL}$ in ng·h/ml as the conversion evaluation of artemisinin derivatives (AM, AE, AS, and AL) to DHA in animal species and humans. [27, 157-163]

Drugs	Animal Species		Humans	
	Rats [44]	Dogs	Volunteers	Patients
Artemether (AM)				
Intravenous	0.04 (65/1857)			
Intramuscular	0.07 (71/1007)		0.41–1.62 a	1.06 b
Oral	0.10 (38/366)		1.12-7.69 c	1.42–8.55 d
Arteether (AE)				
Intravenous	0.04 (29/842)			
Intramuscular	0.15 (43/286)	0.23 (181/804) [159]		
Oral	0.17 (50/298			
Artesunate (AS)				
Intravenous	0.64 (474/738)	0.50 (778/1533)[160]		2.81–8.12 e
Intramuscular	0.31 (236/773)	0.73 (1109/1521)[160]		
Oral	2.74 (595/217)	0.45 (299/660) [160]	4.29–5.36f	6.35–9.7[illegible] g
Rectal			2.31[170]	
Artelinic acid (AL)				
Intravenous	0.01 (63/12706)	0.001 (7/11262) [45]		
Intramuscular	0.01 (44/5023)	0.003 (23/10195) 45]		
Oral	0.03 (62/1650)	0.002 (14/8849) [45]		

References: [a] = [27, 161], [b] = [162], [c] = [161-171], [d] = [161-172], e = [158, 173], f = [174-176], g = [91, 157, 158, 161, 176]; DHA = dihydroartemisinin.

In the animal species, the conversion rates are different with the four artemisinin agents. The highest hydrolysis found for AS are in rats and dogs with the DHA/AS ratio in the range of 0.31-2.74, whereas less than 0.23 of the ratio of DHA to their parent drugs have been measured for AM and AE. Moreover, the ratio in the range of 0.001-0.03 for AL conversion to DHA calculated in rats and dogs, suggests that DHA should not contribute as much toxicity for the 3 drugs (AM, AE, and AL) as that for AS (table 6). The concentration with AUC data has demonstrated that DHA hydrolyzed from AS is in the range of 236–596 ng·h/ml compared to that from AM and AE in the range of 29-71 ng·h/ml at same dose level in rats [44]. However, while AM and AE induce neurotoxicity in the animals, AS does not [177]. Similar results are observed in dogs, 1109 ng·h/ml of DHA is produced from AS at a dose of 10 mg/kg without neurotoxicity symptoms [160], whereas 181 ng·h/ml of DHA from AM at a dose of 20 mg/kg has resulted in fatal neurotoxicity following intramuscular injection for the drugs [65].

Data from our recent work found the maximum tolerant dose (MTD) for AS to be 240 mg/kg daily for 3 days after intravenous injection [66]. The animals were sacrificed at 24 hrs (1 day) and 192 hrs (8 days) after last dose. Histopathological evaluation demonstrated mild and moderate tubular necrosis in uninfected rats treated with AS 240 mg/kg; interestingly, fewer pathological lesions (minimal tubular necrosis) were observed in malaria infected rats. Renal injury was reversible in all cases by day 8 after cessation of dosing and no neurotoxicity was found in any case with all intravenous regimens [66]. In this case, the AUC of 6984–15768 ng·h/ml of DHA, which is converted from AS, can be simulated daily in this regimen of rats according to our previous study [44]. Although DHA is 2-4 folds more active and more toxic than other artemisinin derivatives [152-156], the high level of DHA generated from AS does not seem to have a role in neurotoxic induction in animal species.

In other comparative studies of toxicokinetics and hydrolysis, AL and AS were administered to malaria-infected rats using 3 daily equimolar doses (96 μmoles/kg) via intravenous administration. Plasma concentration of AS with a daily dose of 36.7 mg/kg was one-third less on day 3 than on day 1, resembling that of its active metabolite, DHA. The results were similar for other artemisinin drugs, but not for AL. Toxicokinetic parameters of AL were very comparable from day 1 to day 3 at the same molecular doses of AS at 40.6 mg/kg. AS was the pro-drug of DHA with a DHA/AS ratio of 5.26 compared to the ratio of 0.01 for DHA/AL. Other toxicokinetic parameters revealed that the total $AUC_{1\text{-}3\ days}$ (84.4 μg·h ml^{-1}) of AL was 5-fold higher than that of AS (15.7 μg·h/ml of AS plus DHA). In this study, the two drugs did not produce any CNS toxicity [178], but the general toxicity of AL was 3-fold greater than that of AS in malaria-infected rats [179]. The minimum doses of AS and AL producing parasitemia suppression were 2.3 and 2.5 mg/kg, respectively. The suppressive doses for decreasing the parasitemia by half (SD_{50}) were 7.4 and 8.6 mg/kg, respectively. The MTD for artesunate was 240 mg/kg with a therapeutic index of 32.6, whereas the MTD for AL was 80 mg/kg with a therapeutic index of 9.3 [179]. It is barely comprehensible that AS with 4893 ng·h/ml of DHA was not only significantly safer than AL with only 160 ng·h/ml of DHA, but it also did not produce neurotoxicity [178].

Therefore, we believe that DHA is not an important factor in neurotoxicity induction in animal species even though DHA is 2-4 times more toxic than other artemisinin derivatives in direct in vitro and in vivo studies [152-156].

3.2. The Role of Drug Distribution in the CNS

Data on the distribution of artemisinin analogues in the brain have few available studies, and of the published data, their methods all differ significantly. So to date, there are no comparative published results for quantitative analysis of the artemisinin drugs in brain tissue.

Using the thin-layer chromatography densitometry method, artemisinin (QHS), AM, and AS are found to cross the blood-brain and blood-placenta barriers with intravenous injection in rats [180]. QHS seems easier to detect in the brain after oral administration than after intravenous injection [181]. By radioimmunoassay, the highest level of AS was found in the rat intestine 10 minutes after intravenous administration, followed by the brain, liver, kidney, and other organs, in decreasing order. After one hour, the drug levels dropped significantly but not uniformly in all tissues, with high levels still remaining in the brain, fat, intestine and serum [182]. The highest levels were found in rat brains 5 minutes after intravenous injection. Moderate levels of AM were also found in the heart, lung and skeletal muscles, while liver and kidney levels were low [183].

At 24 h after intramuscular injection of ^{14}C-arteether, the tissue homogenate method was used to identify that the highest levels of radioactivity were present in the intestinal tracts, liver, kidneys, and spleen. Lower amounts of radioactivity were found in brown fat and brain.

The lowest levels of radioactivity were present in the heart, testes, muscle and residual carcass. High-performance liquid chromatographic data from this work indicated that three metabolites of arteether, but not arteether itself, could cross the blood-brain barrier (BBB). The calculated apparent concentration in the whole brain was 0.89% of the total radioactivity after intramuscular injection of 25mg/kg arteether [our unpublished data].

Autoradiographs of rats sacrificed 1 h following administration of ^{14}C-AL showed widespread distribution of the radiolabel. The relative activity of tissues (as density per unit area) were intestinal tract > liver > kidney > bone marrow > spleen > brown fat and salivary glands > heart and testes > brain. At 48 h, the relative activities were as follows: intestinal content > spleen > kidney > liver > salivary glands > brown fat and bone marrow > testes > brain. The low residual activity found in the brain appeared uniformly distributed. Autoradiographic evidence confirmed the presence of ^{14}C-AL in the brain from 1 to 192 h. However, the presence of ^{14}C-AL in the brain was at a lower level than the presence of ^{14}C-AL in most other tissues. There was no evidence of a label concentration in any area of the brain that was visible in the whole body sections. It was found that ^{14}C-labelled AL could not easily penetrate through the blood-brain barrier. An apparent concentration of 0.1% of total radioactivity/brain was calculated from an intravenous and oral administration of 10 mg/kg AL [178].

More recently, a neurotoxic dose range study showed that neuronal damage occurred in all beagle dogs at 40 and 80 mg/kg of AM following multiple intramuscular daily treatments. At 20 mg/kg, minimal neuronal effects occurred in 5 out of 8 dogs. Two hours after the 8th administration (on day 8), only low levels of AM were found in cerebrospinal fluid (CSF) with 25, 60, and 71 ng/ml for 20, 40, and 80 mg/kg dosing, respectively [65]. AM levels in the CSF were < 10% of plasma concentration.

These limited and incomparable data indicates that the oil-soluble derivatives, AE (0.89% of total dose in brain) and AM (10% of plasma level in CSF) seem to have the ability to cross the BBB more readily than water-soluble artemisinin compounds, like AL (0.1% of total dose). If this is true, then the differential neurotoxicity of AE and AM with the water soluble forms is easily understood. However, this deduction is not supported by the observation that AS, a water-soluble drug, has the ability to easily cross the BBB. The largest fraction of AS has been found in rat brain after intravenous administration by radioimmunoassay [182]. Recently it was found that the levels of ^{14}C-AS in rat brain were higher (>2-fold) than that in plasma; the AUCs of radioactivity in brain and plasma were 70.7 and 29.4 μg·h/g, respectively. During a 192 hour period, 1.27% of total radioactivity dose was detected in the rat brain. The half-life of ^{14}C-AS in brain tissue was 94.2 hours, significantly longer than that in plasma with only a 63.7 hour half-life [184]. These results indicated that the resident time of ^{14}C-AS was longer in the brain than in plasma. This may reflect a "sink effect" of DHA uptake transfer by lipid-rich brain structures [185].

If the absence of AS in CSF is consistent with its low lipid solubility and a decrease of concentration in plasma after intravenous injection [143], then the types of metabolites present in the brain tissue are unknown [184]. Whether these metabolites in the brain are associated with neurotoxicity is also unknown. Artesunate is converted stoichiometrically to DHA, concentrations of which peak at 5-10 min [143, 173] in plasma. DHA is highly lipid soluble and has a low molecular mass (284 Da) - both factors favoring penetration of CSF

[185]. Since DHA has relatively low solubility in water, it should be able to cross cell membranes and the BBB. After treatment with AS in patients, the parent drug (AS) can not be detected in the CSF. However, DHA levels in the CSF increase with time while DHA levels in plasma decrease. These finding suggest a continuing influx but a slower efflux of DHA in which DHA might accumulate in CSF during frequent AS dosing [185].

Although (i) radiolabeled AS has been shown to easily cross the BBB and have more accumulation in brain tissue when compared to other artemisinins, as described above [180-185], and (ii) other investigators has found increasing DHA levels in CSF (1100-1450 ng/ml) than in plasma (104-120 ng/ml) after intravenous injection of 120 mg AS in malaria patients [186], but no neurotoxicity has been observed. Therefore, while the artemisinin agents distribute in brain tissue and CSF, they do not appear to be a major factor in neurotoxicity.

3.3. The Role of Drug Exposure Levels in Neurotoxicity

Pharmacokinetic (PK) data demonstrate that AE and AM accumulation is observed in the plasma of rats [187], beagle dogs [65], rhesus monkeys (our unpublished data), and humans [188] following multiple intramuscular injections. Data collected from rat studies have demonstrated that the accumulation of AE in plasma is due to a slow and prolonged absorption from the injection sites [187]. The drug formulation, administration route, and plasma accumulation all appear to be associated with both general toxicity and neurotoxicity [62, 64, 177, 187, 189]

3.3.1. Drug Exposure Level in Rats

An accumulation and prolonged exposure of AE in plasma was first reported in rats with severe neurotoxicity due to slow and prolonged absorption in the muscle injection site following daily intramuscular injections of 25 mg/kg for 7 days [187]. The absorption of AE from muscle (at the injection site) was incomplete in the first 48 hours after a single injection. At 24 and 48 hours after dosing, 38% and 22% of the total dose of AE still remained in the injection site, respectively. The amount of AE in muscle rapidly decreased for 1-2 hours and then exhibited a much slower rate of decrease. Half-lives for the fast and slow absorption phases in the muscle were 1.0 hour and 26.3 hours, respectively. It is expected that the remaining dose amount would be absorbed later because an intramuscular total dose of AE with sesame oil should be 100% absorbed in the absence of decomposition or metabolism at the injection site.

The analysis of TK parameters on day 1 was similar to that of the single intramuscular dose. However, after day 1, the kinetic data estimates from days 2-7 showed a notable change in the PK parameter estimated for day 1 (figure 2, top). The elimination $t_{½}$ of AE after 7 daily doses was prolonged from 13.7 hours on day 1 to 31.2 hours on day 7, suggesting that the exposure time of AE had been greatly extended. C_{max} of AE (410 ng/ml) on day 7 was found to be three times higher than that on day 1 (130 ng/ml). AUC intramuscular dose was found to be 4.5-fold higher on day 7 at steady state (4367 ng·h/ml) than on day 1 (905 ng·h/ml). This indicates that the exposure concentration of AE has been greatly increased and the system of excretion and biotransformation in the rats may not have been normal [190].

Only a pathophysiological factor could change the slopes of the distribution and elimination due to biotransformation, excretion, and protein or tissue binding [191, 192].

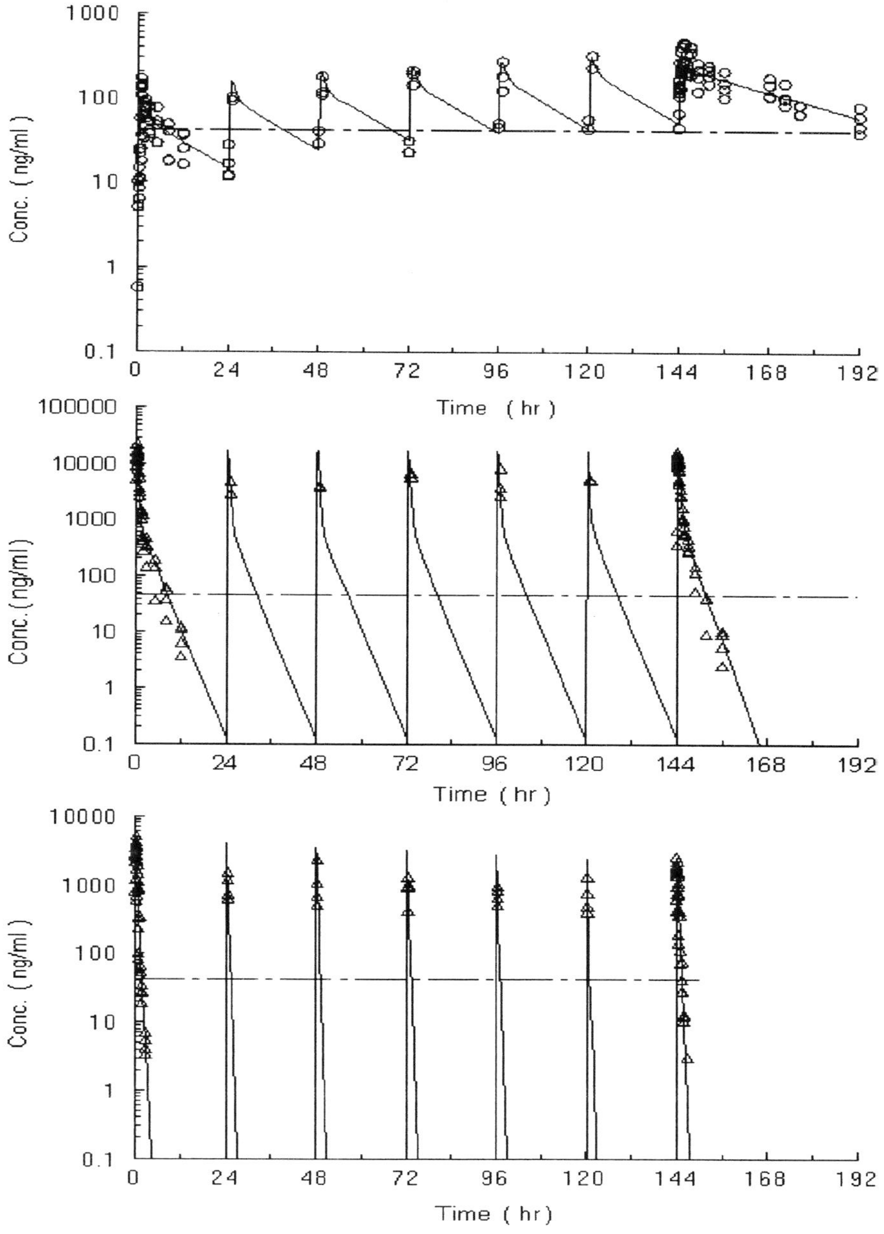

Figure 2. Pharmacokinetic profiles measured by HPLC-ECD (markers) and computer fitted curves (solid line) of 25 mg/kg of arteether with sesame oil (top, n = 4, Reference 187). Artelinate (middle) and artesunate (bottom) with 5% $NaHCO_3$/0.9% saline following daily intramuscular injection 25 mg/kg daily for 7 days in male rats. (n = 3, Reference 202). The minimal detected pathological effect level (MDPEL) from arteether measurement was estimated with 41.32 ng/ml (dashed line) in rats as described in Section 3.4.1.

Table 9. Neurotoxicity effects with exposure concentration (total AUC) and neurotoxic exposure time of artemisinin derivatives at an over 41.32 and 40.92 ng/ml of the minimal detected pathological effect level (MDPEL) of arteether, respectively, after intramuscular or oral administrations in rats (7 days dosing) and dogs (14 days dosing). [65, 152, 159, 187, 193, 194]

Rats	Arteether [187] Intramuscular (Sesame oil)	Arteether [152] Intramuscular (1:2 CRM/saline)	Artelinic acid [193] Intramuscular (5%NaHCO3)	Artesunate [193] Intramuscular (5%NaHCO3)
Dose	25 mg/kg x 7	25 mg/kg x 7	25 mg/kg x 7	25 mg/kg x 7
Neurotoxicity	Severe and death	Moderate	No	No
AUC total 7D, μg·h/ml	16.92 ± 4.04	46.29 ± 2.06	86.84 ± 5.59	8.57 ± 3.34
AUC total 7D (DHA)	3.43 ± 0.76	5.35 ± 0.83	0.56 ± 0.18	5.06 ± 1.21
AUC Day 1 (μg·h/ml)	1.31 ± 0.34	4.17 ± 0.68	12.46 ± 1.85	1.89 ± 0.80
AUC Day 7 (μg·h/ml)	11.37 ± 2.05	7.31 ± 0.59	10.56 ± 0.76	0.99 ± 0.34
Cmax Day 1 (ng/ml)	130.4 ± 39.0	1227 ± 171	20044 ± 3459	3981 ± 992
Cmax Day 7 (ng/ml)	410.0 ± 90.9	1826 ± 118	15585 ± 1476	2078 ± 416
Exposure time (hr)	164.28 ± 7.91	102.96 ± 5.26	42.48 ± 6.80	22.26 ± 4.87
Dogs	Artemether [65] Intramuscular (Peanut oil)	Arteether [159] Intramuscular (Sesame oil)	Artelinic acid a Oral (Suspension)	Artelinic acid [194] Oral (Capsules)
Dose	20 mg/kg x 7	15 mg/kg x 14*	20 mg/kg x 14	25 mg/kg x 14
Neurotoxicity	Moderate	Severe and death	No	No
AUC 7 or 14D (μg·h/ml)	32.13	24.39 ± 18.04	231.58 ± 115.81	191.14 ± 90.80
AUC Day 1 (μg·h/ml)	2.39	0.81 ± 0.32	13.97 ± 3.11	10.46 ± 4.89
AUC Day 7 or 14 (μg·h.ml)	5.11	7.09 ± 3.74	12.78 ± 3.37	11.35 ± 5.78
Cmax Day 1 (ng/ml)	190	90.11 ± 14.74	12360 ± 2706	6279 ± 2995
Cmax	346	352.7 ± 202.6	9780 ± 2885	7177 ± 6248
Exposure time (hr)	174	277.59 ± 10.67	57.98 ± 14.55	47.41 ± 11.78

[a] = Report from our contract company (Southern Research Institute); DHA = Dihydroartemisinin, CRM = cremophore, AUC = area under the curve.

Drug exposure levels of 25 mg/kg AE after a 7 day treatment was 16.92 ± 4.04 μg·h/ml for the AUC (a total of 7 days of AUC data), which induced severe neurotoxicity and animal death [187]. However, this exposure concentration level of AE was just one-fifth of the total AUC of AL (86.84 ± 5.59) with the same regimen of AE following intramuscular injection [202] (table 9). The clinical observation did not show any neurotoxicity effect in those animals treated with AL (figure 2, middle), even at high AL doses of 100 mg/kg after multiple intramuscular doses in rats [our unpublished data]. Computer simulation indicated that the total AUC for the high dose treatments (100 mg/kg) throughout the 7 days was 341.88 μg·h/ml and was 21 times higher than that of AE treated rats. This result suggests that the 5-21 times higher exposure concentrations of AL did not seem to be a principal independent factor in causing neurotoxicity.

In order to demonstrate that the neurotoxicity of AE is related to drug accumulation in blood and is due to the slow and prolonged absorption from the intramuscular injection sites, a study was designed to decrease the accumulation and toxicity of AE through the replacement of traditional sesame oil with a cremophore vehicle [152]. When administered at a daily dose of 25 mg/kg for 7 days, AE blood accumulation with sesame oil (AESO) had a 7.5-fold higher AUC (on last versus first day dosing), while AE with cremophore (AECM) had only a 1.8-fold higher AUC. Although the accumulation of AECM was greatly reduced, its total exposure level (46.29 μg·h/ml) was still 2.7-fold higher than AESO (16.92 μg·h/ml) due to a higher bioavailability of AECM (74.5%) compared with AESO (20.3%) (table 9, figure 3). While histopathological examinations of the brain demonstrated neurotoxic changes in both groups, the AESO group was significantly more severe than the AECM group. Brain injury scores with AECM were mild to moderate (2.3 to 3.0), but with AESO they were moderate to severe (3.0 to 4.7) on day 7 and day 10, respectively (table 10). This study further demonstrated that the toxicity of AE was not dependent on its exposure level in rats.

Table 10. Average effects in rat brain areas of repeated arteether (AE) injection with vehicle sesame oil (AESO) and cremophore (AECM) by daily intramuscular dosing of 25 mg/kg for 7 days (n = 3) [152]

	Finding	Vehicle Control	AESO	AECM	Student Test
Day 7	Neuronal chromatolysis	0	3.00 ± 1.00	2.33 ± 1.15	P = 0.092
Day 10	Neuronal chromatolysis	0	4.67 ± 0.58	3.00 ± 1.00	P = 0.019

*Finding were grading as 0 = no significant lesions, 1 = minimal, 2 = mild, 3 = moderate, 4 = marked, and 5 = severe.

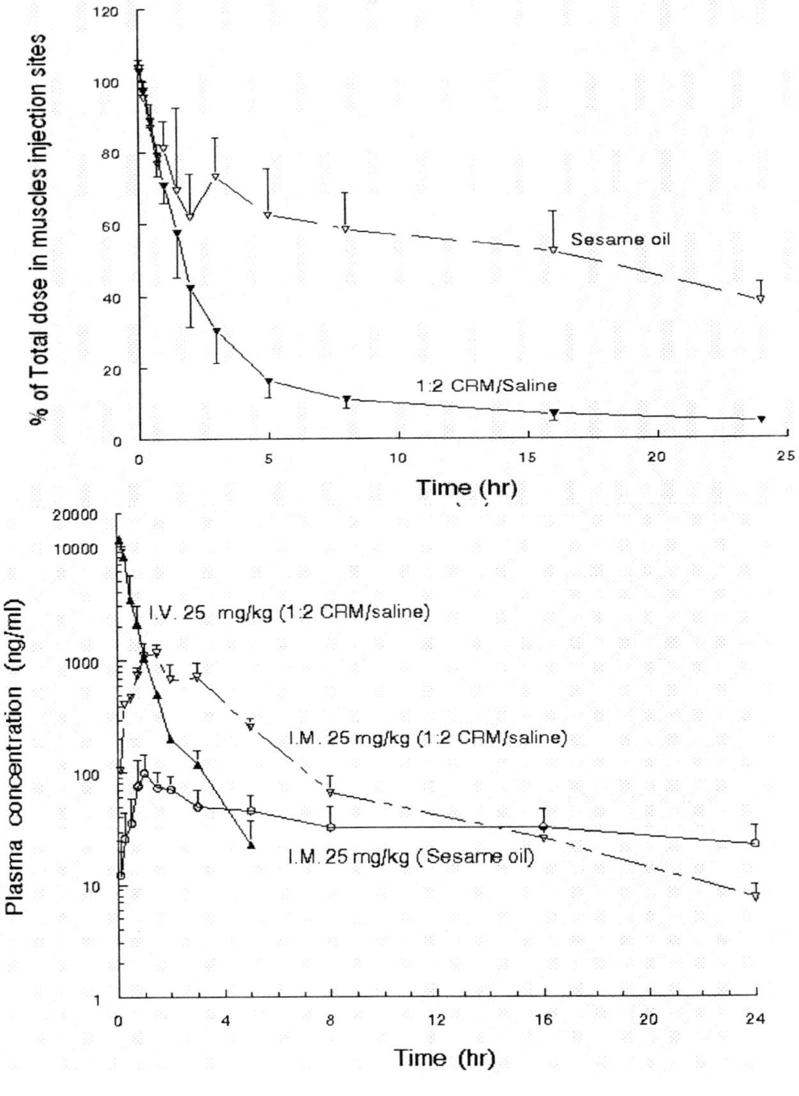

Figure 3. Mean amounts of arteether (AE) in muscle (injection site) measured by HPLC-ECD (top chart, n = 3) and mean plasma concentration-time profiles (bottom chart, n = 3) and by using 25 mg/kg of AE with sesame oil (dashed-line) and with 1:2 cremophore/0.9% saline (sold-line) after 7 days intramuscular injection in male rats [152, 187].

3.3.2. Drug Exposure Level in Dogs

AE accumulation was also observed in beagle dogs' plasma with severe neurotoxicity and death after daily intramuscular administration of 15 mg/kg for 14 days [159]. C_{max} of AE (352 ng/ml) was found to be four times higher on the last day (day 14) compared to the C_{max} on day 1 (90 ng/ml). AUC (7.09 μg·h/ml) on the last day was 8.7-fold higher than AUC of the intramuscular dose on the first day (0.81 μg·h/ml) indicating that the exposure concentration of AE had been greatly increased (figure 4, top). The total AUC during the 14 days at 15 mg/kg AE daily intramuscular repeated injection was 24.39 μg·h/ml (table 9),

Similar accumulation results for AM were reported in dog plasma after daily intramuscular administration of 20, 40, and 80 mg/kg for 7 days [65]. The concentration-time profile of 20 mg/kg AM in the beagle dog is shown in table 9. The analysis of the toxicokinetic (TK) parameters on day 2-7 was changed, with the parameter estimated on day 1. The elimination t½ of AM after 7 daily dosing was prolonged from 9 hours on day 1 to 37 hours on day 7, suggesting that the exposure time of AM had been significantly increased (figure 5, top). C_{max} of AM (340 ng/ml) doubled on day 7 from that on day 1 (190 ng/ml). AUC (6.79 μg·h/ml) on day 7 was 2.8-fold higher than AUC of the IM dose on day 1 (2.39 μg·h/ml), also indicating that the exposure concentration of AM had been increased.

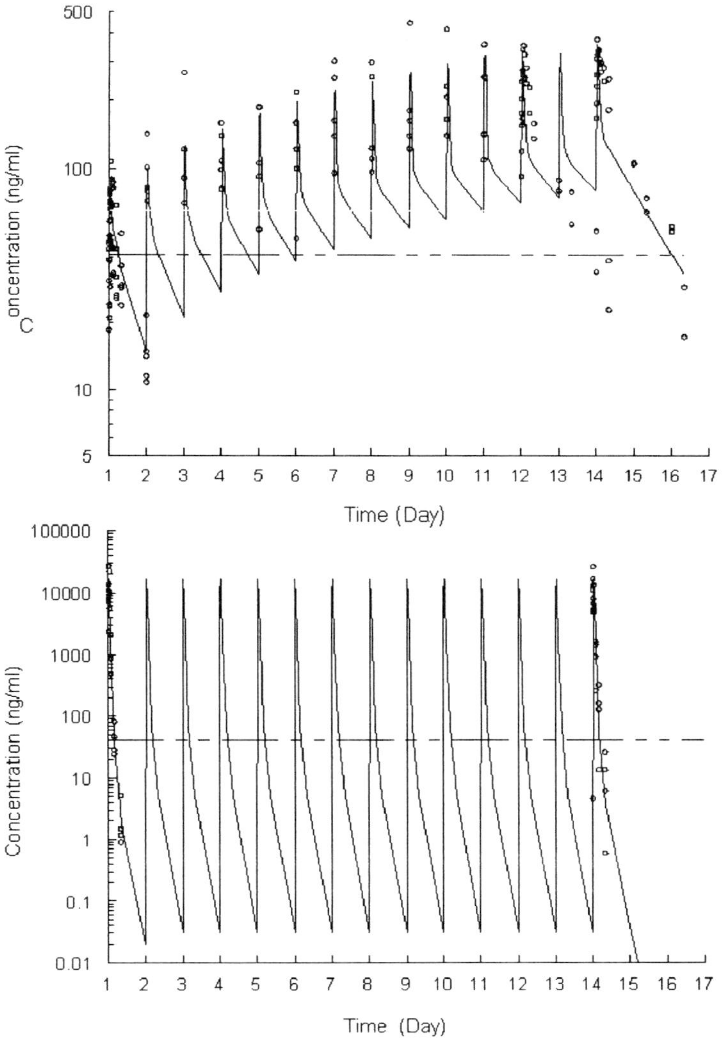

Figure 4. Pharmacokinetic profiles measured by HPLC-ECD (open circle) and computer fitted curves (solid line) of 15 mg/kg of arteether [159] with sesame oil after intramuscular injection (top, n = 5); 20 mg/kg suspension of artelinic acid with carboxymethyl cellulose (CMC) and water (bottom, n = 4) following intragastric administration daily for 14 days in beagle dogs [194]. The minimal detected pathological effect level (MDPEL) of AE was estimated as 40.92 ng/ml (dashed line) in male dogs as described in Section 3.4.2.

Compared to drug exposure levels, much higher plasma concentrations were found in dogs treated with AL following oral administration. An AUC value produced by AL at 20 mg/kg in a suspension formulation was 231.6 ± 115.8 μg·h/ml following daily oral doses for 14 days (figure 4, bottom). However, the value dropped to 191.14 ± 90.80 μg·h/ml for oral AL in a daily 25 mg/kg capsule formulation for 14 days (table 9). The animals in both groups did not show any clinical toxicity [193]. The two dose regimens in dogs treated with AL showed at least 7 times higher exposure concentrations than those in dogs treated with AE. Neurotoxicity was neither detected in those animals with 20 or 25 mg/kg oral dose levels for 14 days [193, 194], nor in animals treated at even very high AL doses of 320 and 300 mg/kg after multiple oral doses [194, 195]. The drug exposure levels of these treatments suggest that a much higher exposure concentration of AL in the dogs does not produce neurotoxicity compared to AE and AM, which induce neurotoxicity with much lower exposure concentrations (table 9) in dogs.'

3.3.3. Drug Exposure Level in Monkeys

Similarly, great plasma accumulation of AE was shown in rhesus monkeys' plasma after daily intramuscular administration of 16 mg/kg for 14 days (figure 6, top). The concentration-time profile of 16 mg/kg AE in the monkeys showed that the C_{max} of AE (1230 ± 577 ng/ml) on day 14 was 19-fold higher than that on day 1 (63.36 ± 9.08 ng/ml). AUC (53101 ng·h/ml) on the last dosing day was 60-fold higher than the AUC of the intramuscular dose on the first dosing day (877 ng·h/ml), indicating that the exposure concentration of AE was greatly increased [our unpublished data].

3.3.4. Drug Exposure Level in Humans

Except for AE and AM intramuscular injections with oils, no plasma accumulation is found for all artemisinin drugs by other administration routes in human. On the contrary, four artemisinin drugs (QHS, AS, AM, even DHA) have reported a declining concentration in plasma during multiple oral treatments in malaria patients and health subjects. The C_{max} and AUC values are markedly reduced from one-third to one-seventh on last dose day compared with first day. The decrease in drug exposure during treatment is not disease-related, since the artemisinin drug PK on day 1 is similar to that reported in healthy subjects [95, 196-199]. Similar time-dependent declining of oral AM was also found in animals (figure 5, bottom) [65]. One possible explanation for the decrease in plasma concentration-time during treatment is an increase in metabolic capacity due to auto-induction of hepatic drug-metabolizing enzymes. However, the drug decrease did not occur for AE in sesame oil after intramuscular administration in humans.

Kager reported on the first use of AE in humans on the studies of safety, tolerance and preliminary pharmacokinetics [93]. An initial AE intramuscular dose of 3.2 mg/kg was used in 27 healthy subjects on day 1. The dosage was then decreased to 1.6 mg/kg for four additional days. The PK data showed a long elimination half-life of 25-72 hr, explaining the marked accumulation in plasma observed in the multiple dose injection (figure 6, bottom). Recently, another study reported administering AE by intramuscular injection to human subjects in multiple doses in a clinical treatment trial. Two dose regimens of AE (AE with 3.2 mg/kg intramuscular start and then 1.6 mg/kg for 4 days as low dose regimen, and high dose of AE regimen with 4.8 mg/kg at 0 hr and 1.6 mg/kg at 6, 24, 48, 72, and 96 hr) were administered for the patients with uncomplicated falciparum malaria [21, 200]. Although these dose regimens have been designed as loading (high) and maintaining (low) doses, AE accumulation was still observed in the human plasma for both of those two dose regimens (table 11).

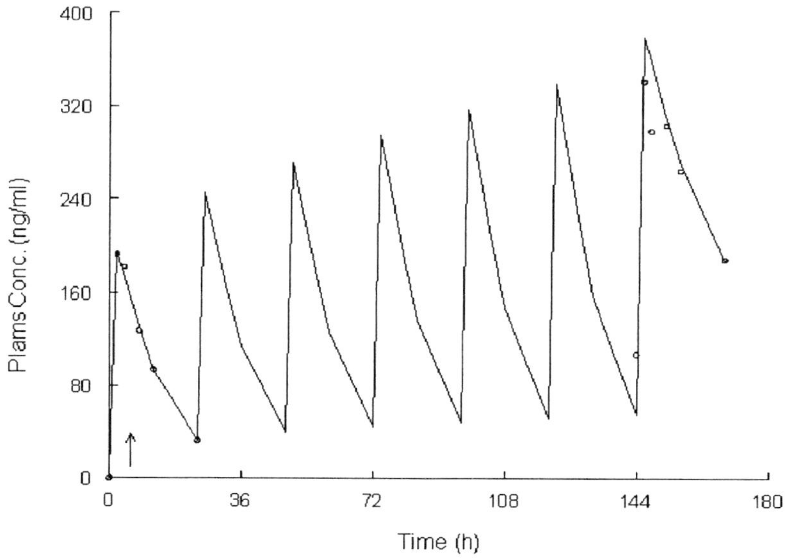

Figure 5. Pharmacokinetic profiles measured by HPLC-ECD (open circle) and computer fitted curves (solid line) of 20 mg/kg of artemether with sesame oil (top, showing drug accumulation) after intramuscular injection and 600 mg/kg of artemether in capsule (bottom, showing drug decline) following oral administration daily for 7 days in beagle dogs. [65].

In the low dose regimen, the elimination t½ of the low dose of AE regimen in human after 5 daily dosing was prolonged from 12.5 hr (day 1) to 40.7 hr (day 5), suggesting that the exposure time of AE had been greatly extended. The C_{max} of AE was two times higher on day 5 (140.8 ng/ml) than that on day 1 (63.6mg/ml). $AUC_{96\text{-}120h}$ (8409 ng·h/ml) on day 5 was 3.5-fold higher than $AUC_{0\text{-}24h}$ of the intramuscular dose on day 1 (2521 ng·h/ml), indicating that the exposure concentration of AE had been greatly accumulated. Similar profiles of the prolonged half-lives and increased C_{max} and AUC were also confirmed in the high dose regimen of AE in humans (table 11). These dose regimens proved to be safe and had potent antimalarial efficacy in reducing parasitemias from the peripheral blood.

3.3.5. Prolonged Absorption Effect on the Accumulation of AE and AM

Many scientists believed that the intramuscular administration of AM and AE was associated with the slowest elimination because the drugs were dissolved in oil (sesame or peanut oil) and, when injected, formed a depot from which drug was slowly released [44, 62, 74, 93]. The inference of slow elimination was recently demonstrated in a rat study, which also found a great deal of accumulation in plasma at injection sites [187]. Following 25 mg/kg of AE in sesame oil daily intramuscular injections for 7 days, the study confirmed and extended the results of earlier studies [44] by demonstrating that the absorption of AE from muscle (injection site) was incomplete. This study also indicated that up to 38% of the total single dose of AE remained in the injection site 24 hr after dosing and 22% of the total single dose still remained in the muscle after 48 hr. The dose amounts of AE remaining in the injection site vs. time are shown in figure 3 (top). The amount of AE rapidly decreased for 2-3 hours and then exhibited a slower decrease. The half-lives for the fast and slow absorption phases were 0.97 ± 0.48 hr and 26.3 ± 1.2 hr, respectively. Following 7 days of multiple dosing of AE (25 mg/kg), 91.4% of a single dose (25 mg/kg) was still left in the muscles from the 7 injection sites 24 hrs after last dose [187].

Table 11. Main pharmacokinetic parameters of ß-arteether with sesame oil (Artemotil) following multiple intramuscular administration of low dosage regimen (3.2 mg/kg on day 0 and 1.6 mg/kg on day 1-4, n = 11) and high dosage regimen (4.8 mg/kg on day 0 and 1.6 mg/kg on time 6, 24, 48, 72, and 96 hr, n = 44) in Thai patients with severe *P. falciparum* malaria* [200]

Parameters	Day 1	Day 5	Day 1-5	Ratio of Day 5/Day 1
Low dosage regimen (n =11)				
Dose (mg/kg)	3.2	1.6		
Cmax (ng/ml)	63.6 ± 39.9	140.8 ± 74.2		2.9 ± 2.4
$AUC_{inf. Artemotil}$ (ng·h/ml)	2521 ± 1950	8409 ± 4730	16242 ± 9113	4.5 ± 2.9
$AUC_{inf. DHA}$ (ng·h/ml)			2842 ± 1119	
$t_{1/2}$ absorption (h)	3.20 ± 0.64	2.13 ± 1.44		
$t_{1/2}$ elimination (h)	12.53 ± 3.91	40.66 ± 14.82		3.4 ± 1.1
High dosage regimen (n = 44)				
Dose (mg/kg)	6.4	1.6		
Cmax (ng/ml)	110.1 ± 56.9	241.1 ± 121.4		2.7 ± 1.5
$AUC_{inf. Artemotil}$ (ng·h/ml)	4702 ± 2964	9484 ± 4365	19782 ± 7725	2.9 ± 1.9
$AUC_{inf. DHA}$ (ng·h/ml)			3209 ± 1058	
$t_{1/2}$ absorption (h)	3.18 ± 2.90	3.46 ± 1.96		
$t_{1/2}$ elimination (h)	22.36 ± 9.24	31.62 ± 12.73		2.0 ± 1.3
Patient 151 (who likely got first dosing intravenously, n =1)				
Dose (mg/kg)	6.4	1.6		
Cmax (ng/ml)	2407.5	317.3		0.1
$AUC_{inf. Artemotil}$ (ng·h/ml)	12259	7403	24529	0.6
$AUC_{inf. DHA}$ (ng·h/ml)			2432	
$t_{1/2}$ elimination (h)	9.4	28.9		3.1

*Values were indicated are the mean ± SD. Min = minutes; AUC = area under the curve; Vss = volume of distribution at steady state; F = fraction of drug absorbed into blood; CL = clearance rate; MRT = mean residence time; DHA = dihydroartemisinin.

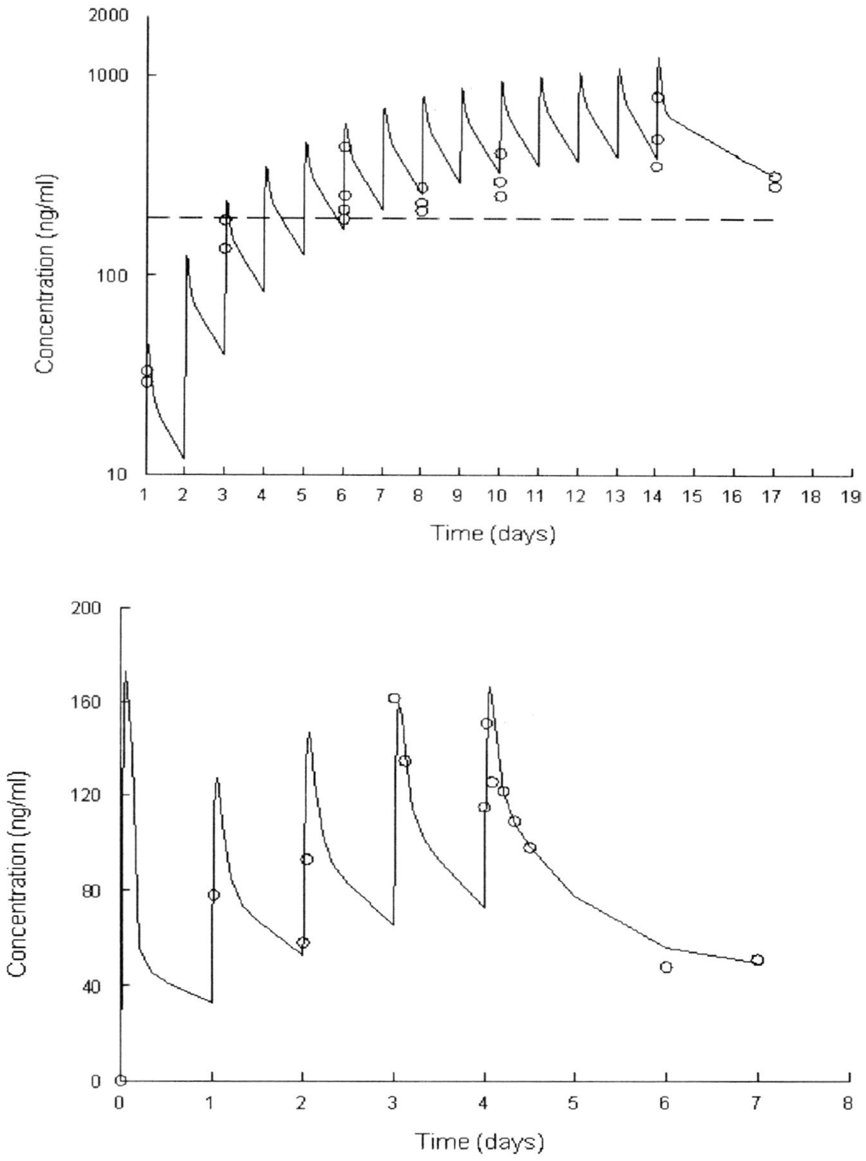

Figure 6. Pharmacokinetic profiles measured by HPLC-ECD (empty diamonds) and computer fitted curves (solid-line) of 16 mg/kg daily for 14 days in rhesus monkeys (top, n = 2) [our unpublished data], and the minimal detected pathological effect level (MDPEL) of AE was estimated as 193.8 ng/ml (dashed line) in male dogs as described in Section 3.4.3. In humans, 3.2 mg/kg in first day and then 1.6 mg/kg for another 4 days of arteether with sesame oil from health subjects (bottom, n = 27) [93]. Both data showed the drug accumulation in monkeys and humans after the 5 days treatments.

After intramuscular multiple dosing, accumulation of AE levels in plasma and muscle were evaluated. Plasma concentration after 7 days of dosing increased 3-4 fold, from an increase in C_{max} of 130.4 ng/ml to 410.0 ng/ml to an increase in AUC from 905 ng·h/ml to

4367 ng·h/ml. When compared with single dosing, AE accumulations in the muscle at injection sites increased 2.4-fold after multiple injections from 38% (day 1) to 91.4%, (day 7) of the total single doses following the 7 daily doses. When muscle absorption data from the single dose study was used to simulate the amount of dose remaining in the muscle after 7 days of dosing, 89% of a single dose was calculated to be present, which is similar to the actual measured amount [187]. This suggested that the change in TK observed during day 1 was not due to a change in absorption, but rather a change in body distribution or/and elimination. Therefore, the volume of distribution at a steady state on day 7 (41.8 L) was 40% of the volume on day 1 (104.3 L). Clearance value was increased by 89% from day 1 to day 7, 0.98 L/h to 1.85 L, respectively. The elimination t½ of AE after 7 daily dosing was also prolonged from 13.7 hr (day 1) to 31.2 hr (day 7).

Furthermore, the histopathological study demonstrates that the slow and prolonged absorption of AE in rat muscle is due to a slow release of AE from the sesame oil phase and therefore associates the cytotoxicity of the drug on the muscle cell at the injection site [our unpublished data].

3.4. The Role of Drug Exposure Time in Neurotoxicity

3.4.1. Drug Exposure Time in Rats

Genovese et al. [59] found that a minimal daily dose of AE at 6.25 mg/kg for 7 days is the no detectable pathological effect dose (NDPED), which does not produce clinical neurotoxicity in rats. Statistically significant neuropathology in brain stem nuclei was observed in the group of rats (6/6 affected) treated with 12.5 mg/kg. These results demonstrate that AE-induced brainstem neuropathology in rats could occur at the relatively high dose of 12.5 mg/kg (double the NDPED dose) for 7 days. The pharmacokinetic parameters and the minimal plasma AE concentration of 41.32 ng/ml at 12.5 mg/kg dose has been determined by our previous studies [152], as the minimal detected pathological effect level (MDPEL) in plasma that should result in clinical neurotoxicity and neuropathology [56, 201].

When calculating the exposure time of AE with sesame oil spent over the MDPEL (41.32 ng/ml) period in rats, neurotoxic exposure time was 164.28 ± 7.91 hours in the 7 day treatment after daily 25 mg/kg intramuscular injections (figure 7, top; table 9). This exposure time affected neurotoxicity is seen at 85.6% of the total dose treatment period (192 hours) with AE [152]. The total exposure time of AE with cremophore was 102.96 hours during the treatment period (192 hours, figure 7, bottom), which was about a third (37%) less than the exposure time of AE with sesame oil (164.28 hours). Neurotoxicity effects in those rats were reduced from severe to moderate, and the drug exposure time seems to be related to the effects of neurotoxicity (table 10) [152].

Compared with AL treatment, drug accumulation and neurotoxicity were not found in animals treated at the same dose (25 mg/kg), same period (7 days) and same conditions as the AE study [187, 202]. The drug exposure period of AL spent over the MDPEL was 42.48 ± 6.80 hours (figure 2, middle, table 9) in rats, which was significantly shorter (4-fold) than the AE study (164.28 hours). Therefore, the animals treated with AL would have avoided the risk and the neurotoxic outcome. An even wider safety margin is seen in animals treated with AS. With the same conditions, 25 mg/kg of AS daily for 7 days generated 22.26 ± 4.87 hours of exposure time in rats (figure 2, bottom; table 9), is 7-fold shorter than that in animals treated with AE (figure 2, top; table 9). This result suggests that the 4-7 time shorter exposure times of AL and AS over the MDPEL compared to the exposure times of AE seem to play a major role in avoiding clinical neurotoxicity.

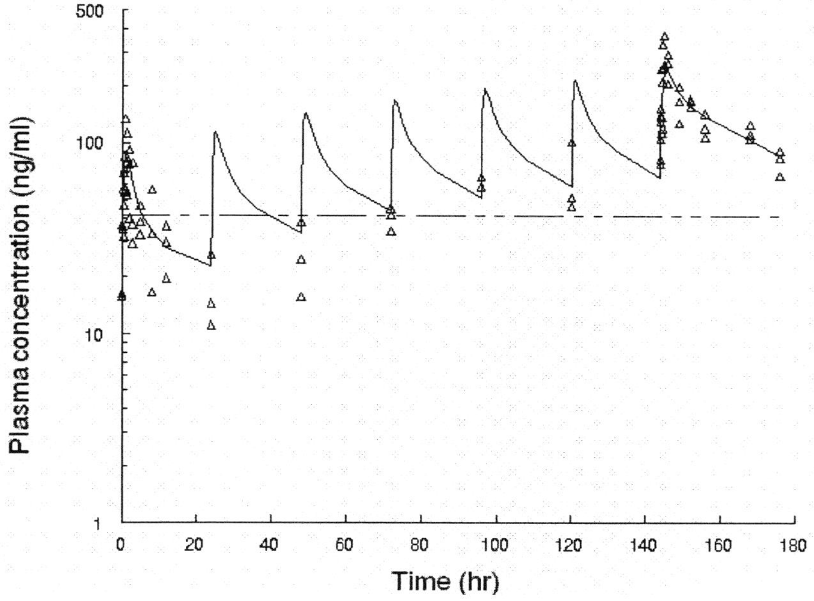

Figure 7. Toxicokinetic profiles in plasma measured by HPLC-ECD (open circle) and computer fitted curves (solid-line) of 25 mg/kg of arteether with sesame oil (AESO, top, n = 3) and arteether with cremophore (AECM, bottom, n = 3) following daily intramuscular injection for 7 days in male rats [152]. The minimal detected pathological effect level (MDPEL) was estimated as 41.32 ng/ml (dashed line) [section 3.4.1].

Changing administration route from intramuscular to intragastric, AL showed severe neurotoxicity in rats treated with 160 mg/kg daily in 9 multiple doses for 9 days but not in animals with 288 mg/kg every other day in 5 multiple doses for 9 days [61]. When calculating the neurotoxic exposure time with AE's MDPEL (41.32 ng/ml), 234.76 hours was measured as the exposure period threshold to affect neurotoxicity (figure 8, top). These results indicate a correlation between neuropathology of rats and a prolonged AL exposure. The AL exposure was related to drug accumulation in the blood resulting from a delayed gastric emptying-induced prolonged absorption of the drugs from the stomach [61]. When rats were treated intermittently with AL at 288 mg/kg every other day in 5 multiple for 9 days, the neuronal degeneration was not identified (not significantly different from that of vehicle control group) until day 7 after the last treatment. The neurotoxic exposure time was calculated as 55.21 hours in the animals (figure 8, bottom). The data further indicated that by shortening the drug exposure time at MDPEL level, it was possible to reduce the neurotoxic risk in the animal treated with the artemisinins.

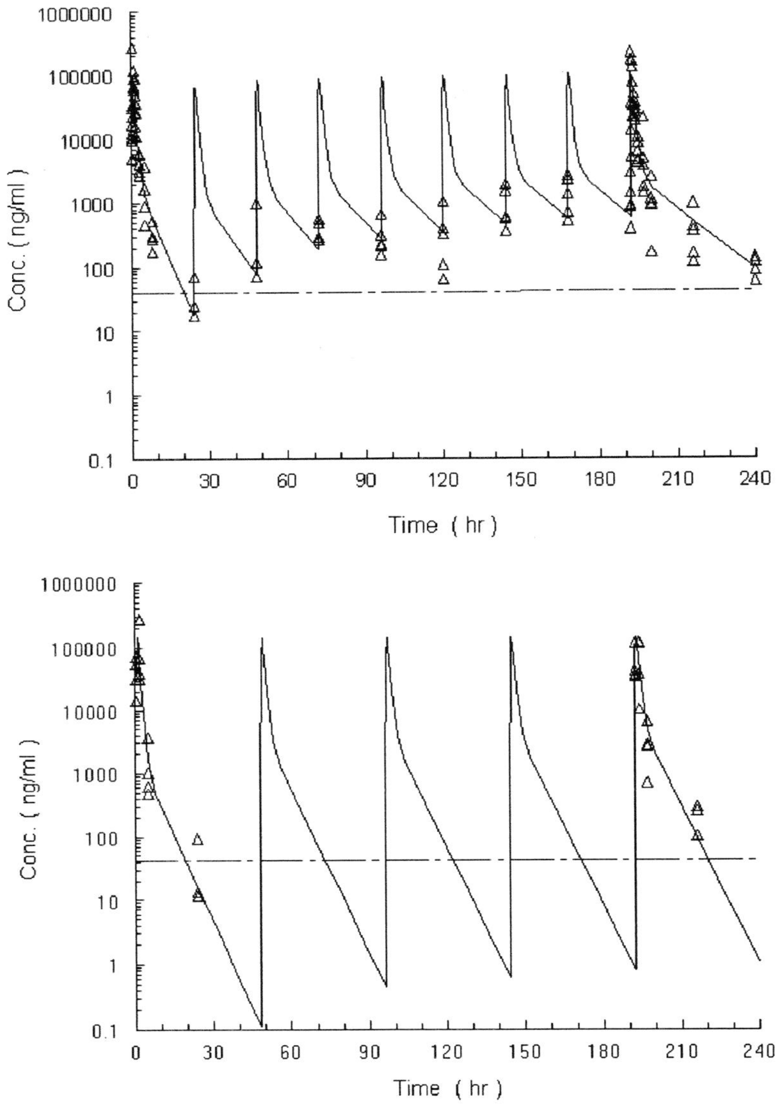

Figure 8. Pharmacokinetic profiles measured by HPLC-ECD (markers) and computer fitted curves (solid line) of artelinic acid (AL) in suspension at 160 mg/kg daily for 9 dosages (top, n = 5), and artelinic acid in suspension at 288 mg/kg every other daily for 5 dosages in rats (bottom, n = 4). The two regimens have same total dose with 1440 mg/kg and same treatment period for 9 days [61]. The minimal detected pathological effect level (MDPEL) from arteether (AE) measurement was estimated as 41.32 ng/ml (dashed line) for rats.

3.4.2. Drug Exposure Time in Dogs

Davidson [58] showed that a minimal daily dose of AE at 3 mg/kg for 28 days is a no detectable pathological effect dose (NDPED) that does not cause neurotoxicity in beagle dogs; this was confirmed by histopathological examinations. AE-induced brainstem neuropathology has been detected though in some dogs with a dose as low as 5 mg/kg/day from Brewer [52, 57], 6.25 mg/kg from Dayan [56], and 6.75 mg/kg from Davidson [58], based on a daily dose for 28 days. Thus, the average of the minimal dose to produce neurotoxicity in dogs should be 6 mg/kg (calculated from the three findings.) The minimal plasma concentration of AE with this low dose (6.0 mg/kg) has been simulated by previous publications in figure 4 (top) [159]. The concentration level of 40.92 ng/ml could be calculated as the MDPEL in plasma that should be the first risk for causing neurotoxicity in dogs.

AE accumulation was also observed in plasma of the beagle dogs after daily intramuscular administration of 15 mg/kg for 14 days [159]. The mean concentration-time profile of AE in the beagle dog is shown in figure 4 (top). The kinetic data from toxicokinetic parameters indicated notable changes on the last dosing day from the pharmacokinetic parameters estimated on day 1. The important change was the elimination t½ of AE during the two weeks of daily dosing. The elimination was prolonged from 11.9 hours on the first dosing day to 22.5 hours on the last dosing day, suggesting that the exposure time of AE had been doubly extended. Also, a MDPEL (40.92 ng/ml) of AE in beagle dogs first appeared in that study on day 6-7. Therefore, day 6-7 would be the earliest time that neurotoxicity occurred in the beagle dogs, based on the toxicities and the toxicokinetic data analysis.

When estimating the exposure time of AE over the concentration level of 40.92 ng/ml (MDPEL) in dogs with severe neurotoxicity and death, the exposure period was 277.59 ± 10.67 hours in a 14-day study after daily intramuscular injections of 15 mg/kg (table 9). The neurotoxic exposure time of AE was 82.6% of the total dosing treatment period (336 hours). Compared with AL dosing by suspension or capsules orally, the neurotoxic exposure times were calculated to be 57.98 ± 14.55 hours for AL suspension (figure 4, bottom), and 47.41 ± 11.78 hours for AL capsules (table 9). All animals treated with AL were not observed to have any neurotoxicity [194].

The evaluations from above strongly support the findings that neurotoxicity is exposure time dependent in the animal species regardless of formulation and administration route. As a result, the artemisinins exposure time in animal species has an imperative role in the induction of neurotoxicity. Other factors of the pharmacokinetic parameters, such as drug distribution in the brain, toxicity of active metabolite (DHA), or drug exposure level, tend to be of minor importance.

3.4.3. Drug Exposure Time in Monkeys

AE was present in rhesus monkeys plasma after daily intramuscular administrations of 16 mg/kg for 14 days [our unpublished data]. The concentration-time profile of 16 mg/kg AE in the monkeys showed that the C_{max} of AE (1230 ± 577 ng/ml) on day 14 was 19 fold higher than that on day 1 (63.36 ± 9.08 ng/ml). AUC (53101 ng·h/ml) on the last dosing day was 60-fold higher than the AUC of the intramuscular dose on the first dosing day (877 ng·h/ml), indicating that the exposure concentration of AE had been increased (figure 6, top). Since AE-induced brainstem neuropathology in monkeys occurred at a minimal dose of 8 mg/kg daily doses for 14 days [55], the minimal plasma concentration of AE 193.8 ng/ml with this low dose (8.0 mg/kg) had been simulated by our unpublished data, as the minimal detectable pathological effect level (MDPEL) in plasma that should be at first to risk causing neurotoxicity in monkeys. The MDPEL value (193.8 ng/ml) of monkeys is 4-fold greater than that of rats (41.32 ng/ml) and dogs (40.92 ng/ml), indicating that the rat and dog seems to be more sensitive than monkey species to suffer neurotoxicity.

3.5. Drug Exposure Time Resulting in Neurotoxicity

To date, there have been no neurological side effects noted in humans due to DHA, QHS, AM, AE and AS treatments. After intramuscular administration, AE and AM provide a longer exposure time in humans the same way they did in animal species (rats, dogs and monkeys) [21, 188, 200]. The conversion of AM and AS to DHA in human is much higher than that in animal species [156-171], but why humans are able to avert the fatal neurotoxicity described in animal species is unknown. This review finds that the drug exposure time is the principle factor in the induction of neurotoxicity in rats, dogs and monkeys. The minimal detected pathological effect level (MDPEL) has been used to measure the exposure period at neurotoxic effect levels in the animals in the present discussion. When using the rats (41.32 ng/ml) or monkeys (193.8 ng/ml) MDPEL to calculate human samples treated with AE with regimen of 4.8 mg/kg at 0 hr and 1.6 mg/kg at 6 hr and then daily in 2-5 day following intramuscular injection, the 162.4 or 33.2 hours (figure 9, top), respectively, of drug exposure time is estimated during the 5 days treatment in the subjects [200]. However, in the 42 patients treated with this regimen there was a failure to detect any neurotoxicity even under the very carefully monitored design in those clinical trials. With regard to acute toxicity, monkeys have fewer responsive than rats, whereas humans appear to be less sensitive than animals [203, 204] and humans have much better repair capabilities than do animals [205].

Other possible explanations for the neurotoxicity discrepancy observed between animal and human can be:

i) The therapeutic dose (2-4 mg/kg) in humans is never higher than the minimal dose that exhibited neuropathologic findings in rats (12.5 mg/kg for 7 days), dogs (6 mg/kg for 28 days), or monkeys (8 mg/kg for 14 days). Also, it is never higher than the minimal doses that showed clinical signs in rats (50 mg/kg for 7 days), in dogs (20 mg/kg for 7 days), or in monkeys (24 mg/kg for 14 days), all of which are 3-4 times higher than the doses resulting in neuropathologic findings;
ii) The treatment period (3-7 days) in humans is never longer than the minimal time for the development of neurotoxicity in rats (7 days), dogs (28 days), or monkeys (14 days);
iii) Many of the patients followed had been seriously ill with cerebral malaria due to severe *falciparum* infection. The resulting evidence may lead to future studies on whether the pattern of neurotoxicity occurred from the illness or from the drug(s);
iv) A number of early reports did not pay sufficient attention to the feasibility of associating brain damage and neurological disorders in patients with such treatments of malaria; and

v) Post-marketing surveillance is limited in developing countries and the potential neurological side-effects of the drug are not recorded.

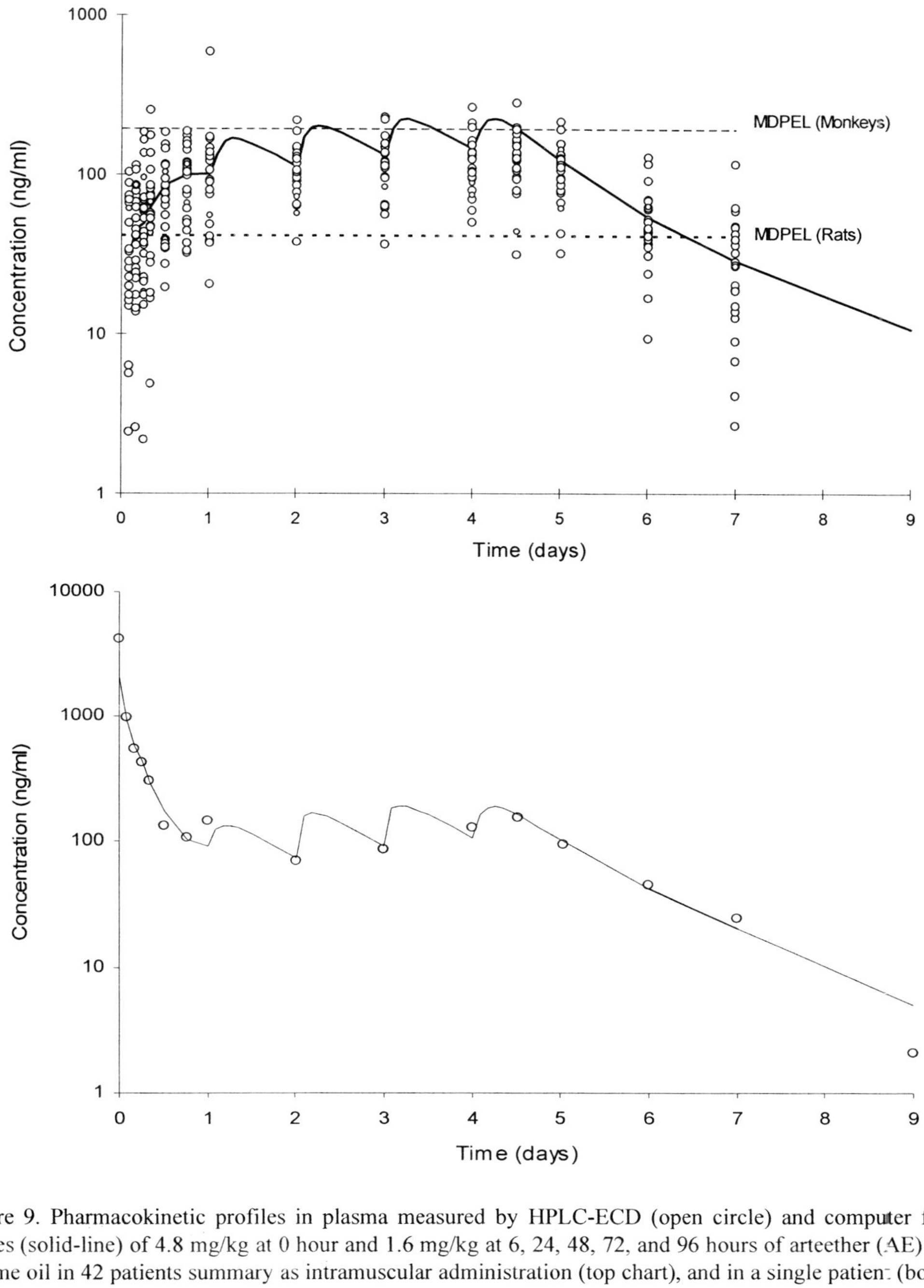

Figure 9. Pharmacokinetic profiles in plasma measured by HPLC-ECD (open circle) and computer fitted curves (solid-line) of 4.8 mg/kg at 0 hour and 1.6 mg/kg at 6, 24, 48, 72, and 96 hours of arteether (AE) with sesame oil in 42 patients summary as intramuscular administration (top chart), and in a single patient (bottom chart), who seemed to be injected into vessel as intravenous injection at first dosing and appeared a great efficacy [200].

In conclusion, the drug exposure time of artemisinins is the principle factor responsible for the induction of neurotoxicity in animal species. Therefore, the active metabolites (DHA), the drug distributed in CNS, and/or the drug exposure levels do not play important roles in inducing neurotoxicity. The oil-soluble artemisinins, AM and AE, possess the ability to induce fatal neurotoxicity because their sesame oil vehicle delays and prolongs the absorption from the intramuscular injection sites leading to an enormous drug accumulation, notably extending the exposure time to the toxic effect level. This would indicate that relinquishment of sesame oil as a vehicle should be considered. The water-soluble artemisinins, AS and AL, have very short half-lives and produce limited exposure time in animal species and humans, indicating that once-daily oral or intravenous administrations of AS are relatively safe.

4. Drug Pharmacokinetic Role in Reproductive Toxicity

4.1. Pharmacokinetics of Artemisinins and other Antimalarials in Pregnancy

Physiological changes in pregnancy – beginning during the first trimester, and most marked during the third trimester – alter the absorption, distribution and clearance of drugs. In addition, most drugs gain access to the feto-placental unit. These changes are detailed below before considering specific effects for individual classes of drugs. The pharmacokinetics of antimalarials is altered in pregnancy. This is the consequence of multiple factors: expansion of the distribution volume, increase in clearance, change in the protein binding, lipid distribution and absorption of drugs, as well as influence of hormonal changes on the drug metabolism [206].

4.1.1. Drug Absorption

Gastric emptying and small intestine motility are reduced in pregnancy due to elevation of progesterone. The elevation may increase T_{max} and reduce C_{max}, although effects on total bioavailability may be relatively minor. An increase in gastric pH, due to a reduction in H^+ secretion and an increase in mucus production may increase the ionization of weak acids, reducing absorption of acid material more than that of weak bases. Such effects are unlikely to be important during repeated dosing. They may, however, reduce the efficacy of a single dose of an oral drug such as an analgesic or anti-emetic for which T_{max} and C_{max} are important. A more practical problem for drug absorption is the nausea and vomiting associated with pregnancy. If nausea is reduced in the evening its effects on absorption can be minimized by deferring dosing until the evening (in the case of once-daily dosing). For example, dose optimizations for antimalarial drugs, such as AS, are needed in pregnancy [207].

4.1.2. Drug Distribution

During pregnancy there is an expansion of intravascular (plasma volume) and extra-vascular (breasts, uterus, peripheral edema) water content. Thus, total body water increases, creating a larger space within which hydrophilic drugs may distribute, i.e. increasing V_d. As a result of this apparent dilution, C_{max} of many antimalarial drugs is reduced, although the clinical effect of the reduction is compensated by changes in protein-binding. Total plasma concentration of albumin-bound drugs decreases as a result of haemodilution and the subsequent fall in plasma albumin concentration. In addition, steroid and placental hormones displace drugs from their protein-binding sites. There is the possibility of a rise in free (active) drug concentration of agents that are normally albumin-bound. This would be expected to produce an increased drug effect. However, the unbound drug is distributed, metabolized and excreted; therefore, the free concentration of drug is little influenced. These changes in protein binding are of clinical importance when monitoring plasma concentrations of drugs. Although body fat increases, creating a larger volume of distribution for lipophilic drugs - this has little practical importance.

4.1.3. Drug Metabolism snd Elimination

Some enzymes of the hepatic cytochrome P-450 and G6PD systems are induced by estrogen/progesterone, resulting in a higher rate of metabolism (and hence elimination) of drugs. For example, primaquine (8 aminoquinoline) is not prescribed in pregnancy because of the intravascular hemolysis risk in the mother and the fetus. This risk is linked to the dose administered and the degree of G6PD deficiency [208]. Clearance of drugs (such as artemisinins) that are secreted via the biliary system may be attenuated due to the cholestatic property of estrogen [209]. Some extra-hepatic enzymes, such as cholinesterase, have diminished activity during pregnancy. Renal blood flow is increased by 60 ± 80% during pregnancy, and glomerular filtration rate rises by 50%, leading to enhanced elimination of drugs that are normally excreted unchanged - for example, mefloquine and halofantrine [209]. This leads to slightly lower steady-state drug concentrations; however this rarely necessitates increasing the dosage [210].

4.1.4. Feto-Placental Unit

Drug transfer occurs mainly via diffusion across the placenta, thus favouring the movement of lipophilic agents; the rate-limiting step is placental blood flow.

Protein-bound drugs do not cross the placenta. Both the immature fetal liver and the placenta can metabolize drugs. Immature phase I (hydrolysis, oxidation and reduction) and phase II (conjugation) metabolism can only occur in the fetus early gestation post-conception. Some antibiotics (tetracycline and doxycycline) are used in combination with quinine or artesunate in areas of multi-drug resistance [211]. Use of these antibiotics in human pregnancy is associated with disturbances of bone growth of the fetus [212] and with irreversible teeth coloration when given in the late gestation [213]. Congenital cataract has also been reported [214]. Furthermore, the hepatotoxicity of tetracycline is increased in pregnancy [215] and fatal fatty liver degeneration occurs when large doses are used [216]. Most antimalarial drugs are weak bases and are mainly non-ionized (lipophilic), diffuse across the placental barrier and become ionized in the more acidic fetal blood, leading to a net movement from the maternal to fetal system.

4.1.5. Pharmacokinetic Role of Artemisinins in Pregnancy

These physiological changes in pregnancy can cause a decrease in plasma concentrations and AUCs, resulting in reduced efficacy. Few studies in women have been published for artemisinins and other antimalarials. For example, chloroquine in oral treatment [217] by using prophylaxis [218], oral mefoloquine [219], oral progunil [220, 221], oral atovaquone [118], as well as oral DHA [207] all have altered kinetics in pregnancy, and plsama levels are significantly lower than in non-pregnant patients with malaria [118, 207, 217-221]. This is likely due to increased clearance, larger volume of distribution and perhaps altered absorption following the oral administration. A similar observation is also found in animal studies for oral administration of AS [101]. It is clear that oral dosages of these antimalarials need to be adapted to keep efficacy when given to pregnant patients and animals with malaria [210].

However, the pharmacokinetic parameters for the antimalarial agents show no significant difference between pregnant and non-pregnant women and animal species after intravenous or intramuscular injections [91, 222, 223]. The pharmacokinetics of chloroquine is determined in pregnant and non-pregnant rabbits following intravenous administration. Chloroquine rapidly crossed the placenta, resulting in equivalent fetal and maternal blood concentrations 15-30 min after dosing the mother. The subsequent 1 and 2 hr fetal blood concentrations are about two-fold higher than the corresponding maternal blood concentrations. The desethylchloroquine metabolite blood concentrations are low relative to the drug, although the metabolite is detected in all blood samples including the initial 5 min maternal blood samples and 15 min fetal blood samples. Comparing the pharmacokinetics of chloroquine in the pregnant and non-pregnant animals reveals no difference in total body clearance. However, there is an approximately two-fold decrease in the apparent volumes of distribution and terminal half life in the pregnant rabbits. Because of the relatively large inter-animal variability of these parameters, the differences are not statistically significant ($p > 0.05$), but do indicate a trend toward changes in chloroquine pharmacokinetics during pregnancy [223].

4.1.5.1. Pharmacokinetics of AS in Pregnant and Non-Pregnant Rats

Preclinical studies of the reproductive toxicity in animal species (table 7) suggested that AS contains the greatest toxicity to animal embryos by routes of subcutaneous and intramuscular injections (single or multiple doses) with less than 1 mg/kg of the ED_{50}, which is much lower than the therapeutic dose (2-4 mg/kg) in humans. The comparative pharmacokinetics of AS was determined in pregnant and non-pregnant rats following 3 daily multiple intramuscular administrations [224]. Since the bioequivalence of AS by intravenous regimen was fulfilled for AS by intramuscular injection in rats [224], the results after intramuscular regimen could refer to a study by intravenous administration. Comparing the pharmacokinetics of AS in the pregnant and non-pregnant animals revealed no difference in plasma concentrations, body volume distributions, and total body clearance only one day after injection. However, the pharmacokinetic parameters changed significantly on day 3 and on the conversion of AS to DHA during the 3 days of treatments. On day 3, the plasma concentration of AS decreased from C_{max} 8668 ng/ml on day 1 to 5037 ng/ml on day 3 and from AUC 3984 ng·h/ml on day 1 to 2239 ng·h/ml on day 3 in the non-pregnant rats, but no significant changes showed in pregnant animals (table 12). The body volume distribution (Vss) and total body clearance (CL) remarkably increased two-fold from Vss/F 2325 ml/kg on day 1 to 4624 ml/kg on day 3 and from CL/F 139.7 ml/min/kg on day 1 to 231.7 ml/min/kg on day 3 in non-pregnant rats, but there was no significant difference showed in pregnant animals [99, 224].

Similar no-change results of pharmacokinetics were exhibited for DHA, an active metabolite of AS, from day 1 to day 3 in the pregnant rats. The AUC value of DHA was even higher on day 3 (4820 ng·h/ml) than that on day 1 (3681 ng·h/ml). However, the significant decrease of plasma concentration in non-pregnant animals was on day 3 when compared to day 1 in values of C_{max} and AUC (table 12). In addition, the conversion rates of AS to DHA were much greater in pregnant rats than that in non-pregnant rats. The ratios of AUC_{DHA}/AUC_{AS} were 0.99-1.02 for pregnant rats and 0.42-0.48 for non-pregnant animals, indicating that the total AUC from day 1 to 3 (15049 ng·h/ml) in pregnant rats was more 3-fold higher than that (4015 ng·h/ml) in non-pregnant rats [224].

Table 12. Main pharmacokinetic parameters of artesunate (AS) and dihydroartemisinin (DHA), an active metabolite of AS, following multiple intramuscular administration of 30 mg/kg daily for 3 days (on GD11-13) in pregnant (n = 3) and non-pregnant rats (n = 4)* [99]

Parameters	Pregnant Rats		Non-pregnant Rats	
	GD 11	GD 13	Day 1	Day 3
Artesunate (AS)				
Cmax (ng/ml)	16545 ± 2873	14927 ± 7292	8668 ± 1068	5037 ± 805
Tmax (hr)	0.08	0.08	0.15 ± 0.04	0.23 ± 0 08
$AUC_{inf.}$ (ng·h/ml)	3749 ± 311	4758 ± 849	3984 ± 620	2239 ± 470
$t_{1/2}$ absorption (h)	0.08 ± 0.02	0.10 ± 0.02	0.13 ± 0.02	0.13 ± 0 04
$t_{1/2}$ elimination (h)	0.35 ± 0.02	0.49 ± 0.09	0.43 ± 0.02	0.41 ± 0 05
Vss/F (ml/kg)	2133 ± 589	2378 ± 769	2325 ± 511	4624 ± 827
CL/F (ml/min/kg)	133.3 ± 13.2	107.7 ± 25.1	139.7 ± 24.0	231.7 ± 58.8
$AUC_{D1\text{-}3\ total}$ (ng·h/ml)		13630 ±1952		8893 ± 1690
AUC_{Day3}/AUC_{Day1}		1.27 ± 0.23		0.61 ± 0 12
Dihydroartemisinin (DHA)				
Cmax (ng/ml)	10335 ± 1475	9087 ± 1437	3049 ± 1499	2409 ± 344
Tmax (hr)	0.08	0.14 ± 0.06	0.23 ± 0.08	0.25 ± 0 07
$AUC_{inf.}$ (ng·h/ml)	3681 ± 238	4820 ± 625	1636 ± 273	1049 ± 95
$t_{1/2}$ absorption (h)	0.08 ± 0.01	0.10 ± 0.01	0.13 ± 0.01	0.11 ± 0.02
$t_{1/2}$ elimination (h)	0.37 ± 0.04	0.53 ± 0.13	0.51 ± 0.09	0.53 ± 0.14
Vss/F (ml/kg)	3164 ± 305	3342 ± 395	10314 ± 4081	8450 ± 3734
CL/F (ml/min/kg)	135.8 ± 12.9	106.3 ±13.5	321.5 ± 63.1	393.6 ± 183.6
$AUC_{D1\text{-}3\ total}$ (ng·h/ml)		15049 ± 3092		4015 ± 326
AUC_{Day3}/AUC_{Day1}		1.48 ± 0.29		0.66 ± 0.16
Ratio AUC_{DHA}/AUC_{AS}	0.99 ± 0.09	1.02 ± 0.11	0.42 ± 0.10	0.48 ± 0.07

* Values were indicated are the mean ± SD. min = minutes; AUC = area under the curve; Vss = volume of distribution at steady state; F = fraction of drug absorbed into blood; CL = clearance rate; MRT = mean residence time; GD = gestation day.

As described previously, four artemisinin drugs (QHS, AS, AM, even DQHS) have reported a declining concentration in plasma during multiple oral treatments in malaria patients and health subjects. The C_{max} and AUC values are markedly reduced from one-third to one-seventh on last dose day compared to the first day. The decrease in drug exposure during treatment is not disease-related, since the artemisinin drug PK on day 1 is similar to that reported in healthy subjects [95, 196-199]. One possible explanation for the decrease in plasma concentration-time during treatment is an increase in metabolic capacity due to auto-induction of hepatic drug-metabolizing enzymes. The declining results are also demonstrated in rats following intramuscular and intravenous injections of AS [178, 202]. Why didn't the concentrations decrease after multiple doses of AS were given to pregnant rats?

4.1.5.2. Tissue Distribution of Radiolabeled as in Pregnant Rats

Tissue distribution and pharmacokinetics of [^{14}C] artesunate (^{14}C-AS) related material following single intravenous administration were reported recently in pregnant Sprague-Dawley rats using quantitative whole-body autoradiography [225]. After dosing, rats were deeply anesthetized with isofluorane, euthanized, and frozen by submersion in a bath of hexane cooled to approximately -70°C with solid carbon dioxide at 0.5, 3, 8, 24, 48, 72, 96, and 192. Carcasses were stored at approximately -20°C prior to preparation for whole-body autoradiography. Sagittal, whole body sections, which were approximately 40 µm thick, were obtained from each rat, and were supported using adhesive tape (Scotch Tape No. 8210, 3M Ltd., St. Paul, MN, USA). Sections were taken of various levels from each carcass until samples of the following tissues or biological matrices along with QC blood standards were obtained (where possible): Adipose (brown and white), adrenal gland, bile (in bile duct), blood (cardiac), brain (cerebrum, cerebellum), bone, bone marrow, epididymis, esophagus, uveal tract of the eye and lens, Harderian gland, heart, kidney cortex and medulla, large intestine (and contents), liver, lung, lymph node, nasal turbinates, pancreas, pituitary gland, prostate gland, salivary gland, seminal vesicles, skeletal muscle, skin, amnion, amniotic fluid, fetal body, mammary, ovary, placenta, uterus, vagina, stomach (and contents), small intestine (and contents), spleen, spinal cord, testis, thymus, thyroid, and urinary bladder (and contents).

Sections were allowed to dry by sublimation in the cryomicrotome at -20°C for approximately 2 days. Sections were then mounted on cardboard backing and exposed along with [^{14}C] spiked blood calibration standards to [^{14}C] sensitive imaging plates (Molecular Dynamics, Sunnyvale, CA, USA). The imaging plates and sections were enclosed in exposure cassettes and were allowed to be exposed in a lead safe at room temperature for four days. At the end of the exposure time, the sections were removed from the imaging plate. The plates were then scanned and the images stored onto a dedicated QPS computer server using the Typhoon 9410, phosphor image acquisition system (Molecular Dynamics, Sunnyvale, CA, USA).

Quantification, relative to the calibration standards, was performed by image densitometry using MCID image analysis software (Imaging Research, St. Catherine's, Ontario, Canada). Image optical density data was acquired as MDC/mm2. The autoradiographic standard image data (calibration and internal standards) were sampled using the MCID software to create a calibrated standard curve and to verify section thickness uniformity. The actual whole body sections were used as a reference to identify tissues.

Specified tissues, organs, and fluids regions of each image were analyzed, and the tissue concentrations were interpolated from each standard curve as microcuries per gram. Tissue concentration data were determined for the tissues and/or contents listed previously. Tissue concentrations were converted to microgram equivalents per gram of tissue based on the specific activity of the test material [226-228].

Upper and lower limits of quantitation were determined and employed for these data. The results and conclusions described in this report are based on digital images that were selected from a complete set of autoradiographs. The clarity observed in the digital images may not be apparent in reproductions obtained by photocopying.

Similar to our previous publication in male rats [209], the mean terminal half-lives of radioactivity in blood (97.73 h) and other tissues (131.69 hr on average) in the present study were greatly prolonged compared with that of unchanged AS (0.43 h) and unchanged DHA (0.75 h), an active metabolite of AS. The drug was widely distributed after 0.5 hr in select tissues and the total amount of radioactivity in all measured tissues per gram was 217.19 μg equivalents (table 13). The highest concentration of radiolabel was found in small intestine contents (81.21 μg equivalents), followed by the bile (13.22 μg equivalents), small intestine (8.85 μg equivalents), liver (8.12 μg equivalents) and the rest. At the same time point, the total radioactivity was 17.41 μg equivalents detected in feto-placental unit (amnion, amniotic fluid, fetal body, mammary, ovary, placenta, uterus and vagina), indicating that ^{14}C-AS could rapidly cross the placenta and are deposited in fetal pigmented tissues [225].

Three hours after the injection, the radioactivity level in all tissues had increased up to 271.0 μg equivalents; the remarkable increase of radioactivity level in other tissues at 3 hours may relate to the re-distribution from tissues or enterohepatic circulation [209]. However, the drug distribution slightly decreased in productive tissues from 17.41 μg equivalents (0.5 hr) to 14.20 μg equivalents (3 hr). From 8 to 192 hours, measured radioactivity level rapidly declined in all tissues except for the spleen and bone marrow (table 13). At 192 hours after dosing, residual activity (close to 3.58% of total amount collected) was still detected in some tissues and the highest levels of radioactivity were measured in the spleen, bone marrow, kidney, bile (in duct), and adrenal gland; trace amounts were also found in other tissues. The total $AUC_{0\text{-}192h}$ of the radioactivity in all measured tissues of pregnant rats was 22879 μg equivalents·h/g, and only 6.54% (1480 μg equivalents·h/g) of the total radioactivity was present in the feto-placental tissues. During the treatment period, measured levels of radioactivity were more than 2-4 fold higher in the ovary, placenta, and uterus, respectively, than in blood; the AUC of radioactivity from 0 to 192 hours was 555, 367 and 216 μg equivalents·h/g in the ovary, placenta, and uterus, respectively, but 134 μg equivalents·h/ml in the plasma. The half-life of radioactivity was measured in the blood at 97.73 hr, whereas that in the ovary, placenta, and uterus were 159.90, 200.55, and 152.60 hr, respectively, suggesting that ^{14}C-AS remained in those reproductive tissues longer than in blood [225].

Table 13. Mean concentrations and main pharmacokinetic parameters of ^{14}C-AS following single intravenous injections at 5 mg/131.4 μCi/kg in the tissue or organs of the pregnant rats by quantitative whole body autoradiograph (QWBA) [225]

Tissue Type	Tissue	0.5 hr	3 hr	8hr	24 hr	48 hr	96 hr	192 hr	Cmax	$t_{1/2}$	AUC	% total
Adipose	Adipose (brown and white)	8.30	4.91	3.86	2.76	2.17	4.47	1.26	6.49	118.72	807.67	3.53
Alimentary Canal	Large Intestine	1.56	1.40	1.82	1.48	0.62	0.65	0.25	1.82	99.08	173.41	0.76
	Large Intestine (contents)	0.12	0.14	3.35	7.34	1.28	5.30	0.06	7.34	49.00	617.83	2.70
	Stomach and Contents	4.30	1.64	4.15	1.25	1.11	2.15	0.40	3.44	141.53	361.46	1.58
	Small Intestine	8.85	5.35	4.35	1.48	0.47	0.74	0.17	9.47	68.61	204.78	0.90
	Small Intestine (contents)	81.21	97.04	47.50	9.67	1.58	26.84	0.06	120.3 5	27.55	3172.53	13.8 7
Central Nervous System	Brain	2.11	0.85	0.68	0.28	0.20	0.20	0.18	2.11	155.21	88.84	0.39
	Spinal Cord	2.72	1.20	0.81	0.31	0.27	0.30	0.25	2.72	168.31	127.65	0.56
Endocrine	Adrenal Gland	6.38	6.76	3.82	2.99	2.17	2.30	2.19	7.59	207.79	1145.58	5.01
	Pituitary Gland	2.93	1.84	1.32	0.74	0.57	0.58	0.37	2.93	172.50	213.82	0.93
	Thyroid Gland	1.96	2.52	1.76	0.89	0.95	1.23	1.05	2.58	139.81	323.57	1.41
Excretory/ Metabolic	Bile (in duct)	13.22	14.71	7.54	8.02	2.06	2.65	2.89	16.84	153.87	1387.64	6.07
	Renal Cortex	5.78	5.49	4.53	2.85	4.30	4.42	3.38	6.71	179.10	1490.90	6.52
	Renal Medulla	5.44	5.45	2.66	1.11	1.20	1.02	0.56	6.19	117.97	326.73	1.43
	Liver	8.12	7.52	4.77	2.48	2.78	2.43	1.75	9.06	160.42	903.65	3.95
	Urinary Bladder	4.66	19.13	23.66	6.44	1.81	0.91	0.51	23.66	74.39	674.17	2.95
	Urinary Bladder (contents)	3.62	44.27	23.74	3.17	0.66	1.01	0.06	44.27	41.79	592.24	2.59
Ocular	Eye Uveal Tract	1.08	0.23	0.78	0.16	0.15	0.22	0.06	1.08	71.83	45.09	0.20
	Eye Lens	0.15	0.23	0.20	0.07	0.03	0.11	0.02	0.29	70.75	17.22	0.08
Reproductive	Amnion and Amniotic Fluid	1.34	1.19	1.25	0.29	0.17	0.29	0.13	1.56	76.91	64.32	0.28
	Fetal Body	2.12	1.64	1.31	1.15	0.19	0.16	0.08	2.26	83.63	80.91	0.35
	Mammary	3.00	1.25	1.06	0.50	0.35	0.23	0.16	2.99	120.76	100.03	0.44

Table 13. (Continued).

Tissue Type	Tissue	0.5 hr	3 hr	8hr	24 hr	48 hr	96 hr	192 hr	Cmax	$t_{1/2}$	AUC	% total
	Ovary	4.80	5.12	4.86	2.15	1.94	1.40	0.98	5.84	159.90	555.13	2.43
	Placenta	3.00	2.85	2.05	0.86	0.85	0.61	0.71	3.21	200.55	366.77	1.60
	Uterus	2.19	1.41	1.58	0.66	0.38	0.43	0.46	2.19	152.60	215.58	0.94
	Vagina	0.99	0.74	1.37	0.51	0.31	0.39	0.14	1.46	88.96	96.98	0.42
Respiratory Tract	Lung	1.97	1.83	1.52	0.73	0.55	0.57	0.19	2.13	93.92	135.31	0.59
	Nasal Turbinates	3.66	1.90	2.89	1.61	0.85	0.71	0.57	4.27	155.33	311.18	1.36
Secretary	Harderian Gland	4.34	2.22	1.65	1.14	0.55	0.70	0.20	4.34	78.01	157.18	0.69
	Pancreas	2.96	1.83	1.43	0.67	0.57	0.92	0.42	2.96	142.56	235.57	1.03
	Salivary Gland	2.34	1.58	1.31	0.74	0.76	0.77	0.57	2.34	206.18	313.67	1.37
Skeletal/ Muscular	Bone	0.26	0.15	0.07	0.03	0.05	0.09	0.06	0.32	171.66	25.79	0.11
	Heart	2.79	2.56	1.79	1.21	1.12	1.05	0.81	2.96	166.21	405.69	1.77
	Skeletal Muscle	1.91	0.91	0.84	0.39	0.35	0.51	0.22	1.91	158.88	135.96	0.59
Dermal	Skin	1.71	0.87	0.87	0.47	0.34	0.45	0.22	1.71	100.77	111.97	0.49
Vascular/ Lymphatic	Blood (cardiac)	1.57	1.50	1.33	0.80	0.53	0.52	0.20	1.57	97.73	133.50	0.58
	Bone Marrow	6.21	9.76	7.01	3.86	3.98	4.51	3.80	9.76	359.31	2822.62	12.34
	Lymph Nodes	1.55	2.20	1.01	0.43	0.82	1.09	0.63	2.27	200.63	357.48	1.56
	Spleen	4.27	7.44	6.29	6.49	6.58	6.55	5.95	8.68	246.06	3359.66	14.68
	Thymus	1.70	1.36	1.13	0.53	0.43	2.05	0.68	1.75	175.93	219.16	0.96
	Total	217.19	271.00	183.89	78.70	46.09	81.52	32.66		Mean	Total AUC	
	%	23.84	29.75	20.18	8.64	5.06	8.95	3.58		131.69	22879.22	100

*The procedures described in this paper were performed in accordance with Quest Pharmaceutical Services, L.L.C. (QPS, Newark, DE). This study was not conducted in compliance with the Food and Drug Administration Good Laboratory Practice Regulations and was not inspected by the quality Assurance department of QPS.

4.2. Damage to the Angiogenesis of Embryos Induced by Artemisinins

Artemisinin derivatives are not currently recommended for use during the first trimester of pregnancy in women because the derivatives cause embryo death and some abnormalities in early pregnancy in animals [96-103]. In order to better understand the mechanism of the developmental toxicity in animals, the main animal experiments have been listed here for the discussion.

With big doses (40 mg/kg subcutaneously on day 6-10 of gestation), Lou and Zhou observed that AS significantly decreased the concentration of serum progesterone in early pregnant rats; decidual cells and fetuses of treated groups were found to be degenerated at day 11. Drug was shown to directly damage the decidual cells. Similar results were found in human decidual cell cultures with AS for 48 h. The damage of AS on the decidua and placenta may be the mechanism of its contragestational action [106]. These results also suggested that in order to examine the effect and mechanism of AS on embryo development, rat embryo and placental glutathione peroxidase (GSH-Px) and malondialdehyde (MDA) must be identified by using dithionitrobenzene (DTNB) direct method and thiobarbituric acid (TBA). They found that AS induced developmental toxicity in rat embryos and placenta by neutralizing the antioxidant defense mechanism [107].

Chen et al. reported that AS [105] and DHA [229] were found to inhibit angiogenesis in vivo and in vitro. The anti-angiogenic effect in vivo was evaluated in nude mice by means of human ovarian cancer HO-8910 implantation and immunohistochemical staining, vascular endothelial growth factor (VEGF) and VEGF receptor KDR/flk-1. The in vitro effect of AS was tested on models of angiogenesis, namely, proliferation, migration and tube formation of human umbilical vein endothelial cells (HUVEC). The results showed that AS and DHA significantly inhibit angiogenesis in a dose-dependent form. Additionally, the inhibitory effect of AS and DHA on HVUEC proliferation was stronger than that on Hela, JAR, HO-8910 cancer cells, NIH-3T3 fibroblast cells and human endometrial cells, indicating that AS and DHA were selectively against HUVEC. These findings and the known low toxicity of AS and DHA are clues that artemisinins may be a promising angiogenesis inhibitor [105, 229].

The effects of DHA in rat's whole embryo cultures (WEC) were recently conducted by Longo et al. [104]. DHA was added to the culture medium for the entire 48-hour culture, 1.5 hours after the beginning or 1.5 hours before the end of the culture dose of 0.01–2 μg/ml. DHA affected primarily red blood cells during yolk sac hematopoiesis. Higher concentrations and longer exposure inhibited angiogenesis. More studies the inhibition of angiogenesis by artemisinins were conducted by various investigators [230-235]. AS strongly reduced angiogenesis in vivo in terms of vascularization of Matrigel plugs injected subcutaneously into syngenic mice. Based on these studies, AS represents a promising candidate drug for the treatment of the highly angiogenic Kaposi's sarcoma. As a low-cost drug, it might be of particular interest to areas of Kaposi's sarcoma endemics. These results and the known low toxicity are clues that AS and DHA may be promising novel candidates for cancer chemotherapy [232, 235].

It is clear that the embryotoxicity and contragestational effect of artemisinins (AS and DHA) in pregnant animal species is mainly due to the angiogenesis and the expressions of vascular endothelial growth factor on embryos and fetuses. Further research has demonstrated that the embryotoxicity of artemisinins is drug exposure level dependent [104, 229].

4.3. Artemisinins Exposure Level and Time on Inhibition of Angiogenesis

To study the effects of DHA on embryonic development, a rat whole embryo culture (WEC) study was conducted by Longo et al. [104]. This model allowed the investigation of early embryonic developmental stages, which reportedly were highly susceptible to artemisinin compounds in vivo, in the absence of maternal interaction. Ultimately, the WEC study was conducted in order to understand better the mechanism of the developmental toxicity and to identify the initial target of action of DHA.

On gestation day 9, pregnant female rats were euthanized to extract embryos (9.5 days of age, 1–3 somites). The extracted embryos were randomly distributed to experimental groups and cultured in a 25-ml glass bottle (5 embryos/bottle) containing 5 ml of heat-inactivated sterile rat serum. DHA was dissolved in DMSO and added to the culture medium (5 μl/bottle) in order to obtain a range of final concentrations of 10 – 2000 ng/ml. Group 1: control, DMSO 0.1% from GD 9.5 to 11.5; Group 2: DHA 10, 50, 100, 500, 1000 and 2000 ng/ml from GD 9.5 to 11.5; Group 3: DHA 50, 100, 500, 1000 and 2000 ng/ml at GD 9.5 for 1.5 h, thereafter the medium was changed and embryos were cultured in normal serum until GD 11.5; Group 4: DHA 1000 and 2000 ng/ml at GD 11, 1.5 hr before the end of the culture. At the end of the culture period, the embryos (11.5 days old) were transferred into Tyrode's salt solution (Sigma) and examined under the stereomicroscope.

All embryos exposed to DHA for 48 hr at all concentrations were alive at the end of the culture period. At DHA concentrations ≥ 50 ng/ml, the visceral yolk sac was well vascularized but pale; yolk sac vessel formation and circulation appeared normal but blood was visibly paler than in controls. This effect increased in proportion to increasing DHA concentrations. At concentrations ≥ 500 ng/ml, the vasculature was also affected. Vessel diameter was reduced, small anastomotic vessels were not visible, and the number of circulating cells was further reduced. At 1 μg/ml, yolk sac vasculature and circulating cells were markedly reduced and at 2000 ng/ml only a few poorly organized yolk sac vessels were present.

The allantois, although well developed up to the DHA concentration of 500 ng/ml, showed pale umbilical vessels starting from 50 ng/ml. At 1 μg/ml, the allantois was present but attached ectopically to the yolk sac (fusion with the chorion did not occur near the ectoplacental cone but in other regions of the yolk sac). At 2000 ng/ml, the allantois was lying free in the exocelom. At DHA ≥ 1000 ng/ml, the heart-rate was reduced and irregular. Analysis of cytospin blood preparations showed a reduction in the number of RBCs starting at concentrations ≥ 100 ng/ml, and deformed or damaged RBCs at concentrations ≥ 500 ng/ml. At 2000 ng/ml, DHA induced complete embryonic disruption with multiple non-specific abnormalities. Histological examination showed areas of cell death in the branchial arches, in the mesenchyme of the caudal region and near the dorsal aorta at 100, 500 and 1000 ng/ml. Complete tissue disorganization was detected at 2000 ng/ml. Histological examination confirmed the reduced presence of RBCs in the heart and aorta of embryos exposed to DHA at 100 ng/ml concentrations. For embryos exposed to DHA for 48 hr, the no observed adverse effect level (NOAEL) was 10 ng/ml.

Similar observation of the embryotoxicity was also found at 1.5 hr after culture with DHA. The embryos exposed to DHA at all concentrations tested were alive at the end of the culture period and had normal heart rate. At DHA concentrations ≥ 100 ng/ml, the visceral yolk sac, although well vascularized, was pale; yolk sac vessel formation and circulation appeared normal, but blood was visibly paler than in control embryos. This effect was more obvious with increasing concentrations. Starting from 1µg/ml, the circulation was also affected, and small anastomotic vessels were not visible. The allantois, although well developed at all concentrations tested, showed pale umbilical vessels starting from 100 ng/ml and cases of ectopy from 1000 ng/ml. At DHA concentrations ≥ 2000 ng/ml, the heart rate was reduced and irregular in the majority of embryos. The analysis of cytospin blood preparations showed a clear reduction in the number of RBCs starting from 500 ng/ml and deformed or damaged RBCs from 1000 ng/ml. For embryos exposed to DHA for 1.5 h at the start of the culture, the NOAEL was 50 ng/ml.

The results evidently indicated that the drug exposure level is more important to induce the embryotoxicity than drug exposure time; this was evident because the AS and DHA have very short half lives [44] in clinical therapy. When concentrations of DHA were increased to100 ng/ml for 1.5 hr, the initial damage could be seen on the embryos. At 500 ng/ml, the analysis of cytospin blood preparations showed a clear reduction in the number of RBCs. At 1000 ng/ml level, the significant ectopy, irregular heart rate, and deformed or damaged RBCs were observed and detected. Those indicators would be great references for the clinical monitoring on the embryotoxicity induced by artemisinins. The literature on human trials and animal experiments concluded that a range of 1000-2000 ng/ml was an acceptable estimation of median AS or DHA maximum concentration [162-176].

4.4. Drug Sensitivity Period in Pregnant Animals and in Pregnant Women

Although the drug exposure level is a major factor in the development of embryotoxicity in animals, the sensitive duration period of the embryos during the gestation is another important factor for the toxic investigation. In most studies in the rat, treatment usually started around implantation on day 6 and continued thereafter. A common effect seen was a dose-related increase in post-implantation loss with total resorptions at higher dose levels. Some studies show instances of morphological abnormalities at doses that cause fetal resorption, without maternal toxicity. All studies using AS, AM or AE show a steep dose–response curve and some have demonstrated marked sensitivity to the day of dosing between Days 9–14 of gestation in the rat. In particular, in Chinese studies on rats, with AS, a dose of 0.4 mg/kg produced no increase in resorptions (5.8%), but 0.8 mg/kg caused 98% resorption [98]. Total resorption was also induced by AS at 25 mg/kg SC, when administered during GD 9–11 or 12–14, while no effect was seen when treatment was given prior to GD 8 or after GD 14. Further comparative in vivo experiments with AS, DHA, AM and AE indicate that the critical period for induction of resorption is GD 9–14; GD 10 is identified as the most sensitive day [104].

From day 9.5 of gestation in rats (day 7.5 in mice) and day 15 in humans, simple diffusion is no longer sufficient to meet the increasing demand for oxygen supply of the growing embryo. At that point, undifferentiated mesenchyme on the yolk sac condenses to form angiogenetic cell clusters, the blood islands that give rise to hematopoietic stem cells (the precursors of the blood cells) and angioblasts (the precursors of blood vessels). As soon as a capillary network is created, mature erythroid cells formed within the yolk sac enter the embryos and reach the vitelline vessels. Hematopoiesis within the yolk sac occurs in rats during GD 9–14 (GD 7–12 in mice) and in humans between GD 15 and 6 weeks of gestation, when it is replaced by late embryonic, fetal and subsequently definitive adult sites of hematopoiesis (the liver, spleen and bone marrow) [236]. The effects of exposure to artemisinins during this special period of organogenesis can be noticed especially on the embryotoxicity.

During the development period embraced by this experiment, it becomes more apparent that a transition occurs from predominantly anaerobic to aerobic glycolysis, with active Krebs cycle and oxidative phosphorylation; this requires significantly higher oxygen concentrations as well as an adequate circulation. Accordingly, culture conditions are changed from 5 to 20% O_2. Under the latter conditions, the probability of reactive oxygen species (ROS) formation is increased. The visceral yolk sac has a protective role for the embryo proper by removing ROS and antioxidant defenses increase several times in the yolk sac from GD 9 to 13 [237].

Longo's results are compatible with the hypothesis that DHA also affects RBC precursors (hemoangioblasts) and the Wolffian blood islands, thus explaining why hematopoiesis as well as vasculogenesis and angiogenesis are affected, although with different sensitivities. Some of the features observed in embryos seem to point to similar mechanisms as those described above for the malaria parasite. Embryonic RBCs derived from the yolk sac have transferrin receptors as they react with anti-rat CD71 monoclonal antibody. Moreover, some of the in vivo studies reported fetal growth retardation, delayed skeletal development and cardiovascular malformations in the animals [97-107]. The damage to the hematopoietic system and angiogenetic process may all be induced by exposure to those artemisinins. Finally, the days of marked sensitivity correspond to the period of yolk sac hematopoiesis, which occurs during GD 9–14 in rats and, correspondingly, GD 15 to week 6 in humans.

4.5. Drug Exposure Duration and Peak Level Concerning the Reprotoxicity

The adverse impact of malaria in pregnant women is largely caused by *P. falciparum*; approximately 90% of clinical cases globally occur in sub-Saharan Africa. Every year there are approximately 50 million pregnancies in women living in malarious areas [222]. Artemisinins have been used to treat pregnant women since 1987 [110]. Data from limited clinical trials in pregnant women (2101 cases) exposed to artemisinin compounds, including a small number (108 cases) in the first trimester, do not show an increase in the rates of abortion or stillbirth or evidence of abnormalities. There were no clinically significant adverse effects of the drug, neither in the outcomes of the pregnancies, nor in the development (neurological and physical) of the infants, including 44 infants exposed during the first trimester [109-120, 238, 239]. Are artemisinins really not toxic to either the women, the fetuses during pregnancy, or to the infants during lactation? Without other relevant human pharmacokinetic data, it is difficult to quantify the risk of possible embryonic death or teratogenicity with exposure to artemisinin compounds in the first trimester in women. However, the two factors of the pharmacokinetic characteristics (including tissue distribution) and the drug sensitive period of the embryos during the gestation (summarized above) may assist us in avoiding the low birth weight, abortion, and even potentially fetal death for pregnant women requiring malaria therapy.

In the summary of embryotoxicity in animals (table 7), the severe toxic effects were detected in the animals treated with AS after single or multiple intravenous, intramuscular or subcutaneous injections. The three ED_{50} doses (0.58-1.0 mg/kg) are all below human therapeutic dose (2-4 mg/kg). Other dosage regimens of AS, AM and DHA produced the high ED_{50} doses with values of 6.1-32.8 mg/kg in those animal species, which seems to be safe in clinical usage because those dosages are higher than the human therapeutic doses with wide safety margin. Why is the situation so severe such that there is AS only following the single or multiple injections intravenously, intramuscularly and subcutaneously? The possible explanations could be:

1 The administration is during the days of marked sensitivity corresponding to the period of yolk sac hematopoiesis, which occurs during GD 9–14 in rats;
2 The bioequivalences of AS by intramuscular and subcutaneous administration are fulfilled for AS by intravenous injection in rats [224], and the 3 administrations of AS can produce a significantly higher peak concentration than AS, AM, and DHA after oral administration or AM with oil vehicle after intramuscular injection in rats [44]. Again, the data revealed that the peak concentration is a major issue that causes the toxicity;
3 As with multiple administrations, a single subcutaneous injection of AS also induced severe embryotoxicity in hamsters, demonstrating that the drug exposure level (even with just one exposure) is the principal role for persuading the toxicity when compared to longer drug exposure time with multiple doses;
4 When the peak concentrations are high in the blood, the concentration could be even higher in the location of the feto-placental unit because the drug distribution of AS in feto-placental tissues was always higher (2-4 folds) than that in the blood of the pregnant rats [225].

To treat women with artemisinins, a recent WHO consultation has recommended that: i) because of the limited experience with artemisinins in pregnancy they should only be used when other treatments are considered unsuitable; ii) presently, they cannot be recommended for treatment of malaria in the first trimester. They should not, however, be withheld if they are considered lifesaving for the mother; iii) to further document the safety of artemisinin compounds in pregnancy, careful follow-up is required, with documentation of pregnancy outcome and the subsequent development of the child whenever possible; and iv) to guide further development of policies on the use of artemisinin derivatives during pregnancy, alone or in combination, there is an urgent need for further research/documentation of their efficacy and safety for use as therapy for malaria [108].

In accordance with WHO recommendations and the new research described above, the two major issues for considering artemisinin drug use in a program for prevention or management of malaria in pregnant women are safety and effectiveness. First, the exposure to artemisinins should be avoided during the early sensitive days (GD 15 to week 6 in humans), which is the critical period for induction of embryo damage and resorption, to protect pregnant women from malaria with treatment of artemisinin derivatives. This is essentially the same recommendation as WHO consult above that the artemisinin drugs should not be used in the first trimester of pregnancy in women. Secondly, WHO recommends that artemisinin compounds should only be used in the second and third trimester when other treatments are considered unsuited. However, we feel that oral doses or oral doses in combination regimens could be used to treat pregnant women at in the first trimester when other treatments are considered unsuited, because the oral regiments provides a lower peak concentrations, and that can make the agents safer than intravenous or intramuscular injection of AS. In fact, reprotoxicity was not found in humans treated with artemisinins during the past twenty years; this conclusion resulted from the more than 90% of pregnant women treated orally or intramuscularly with AM in sesame oil over that period whose tests resulted in a much low plasma concentration and prolonged absorption from muscle [65, 109-120].

In addition, further studies to define the precise mechanism of damage in animal models are warranted. Reliable pharmacovigilance on the use of these drugs in pregnancy and the careful monitoring of safety after exposure in the first trimester of pregnancy, when treatment may occur inadvertently or be necessary to save life even with injection AS, are needed.

To date, there have been no convincingly documented cases of embryotoxicity or other reprotoxicity side effects noted in humans due to QHS, DHA, AM and AS treatments [109-120, 238, 239]. After the four oral drugs and one intramuscular drug (AM) administration, the conversion of AM and AS to DHA in humans was been much higher than that in animal species although they produced lower peak concentrations in plasma [156-171]. It remains unknown how humans have been able to avert the death embryotoxicity described in animal species. Data from limited clinical trials in pregnant women (2,101 cases) exposed to artemisinin compounds, including a small number (108 cases) in the first trimester, have not shown an increase in the rates of abortion or stillbirth; they have also not shown evidence of abnormalities. With regard to acute toxicity, humans appear to be less sensitive than animals [203, 204] and humans have much better repair capabilities than do animals [205]. Other possible considerations for the reprotoxicity discrepancy observed between animal and human:

I. The animal data revealed that only intramuscular or subcutaneous (including intravenous) AS causes reprotoxicity at lower dose than the therapeutic dose (2-4 mg/kg) in humans. Other doses in different regimens (oral or intramuscular AM) are safe at higher levels than the therapeutic doses. Since more than 90% of pregnant patients have been treated with oral or intramuscular AM in our counted trials (2101 cases), it may be the reason for the lack of toxicity observed;

II. Many of the pregnant patients followed have been seriously ill with malaria, which is responsible for 5-12% low birth weight (LBW), 35% of LBW that is preventable during pregnancy [240], and contributes to 70,000-200,000 infant deaths each year [241]. The resulting evidence may lead to future studies on whether the pattern of reprotoxicity has occurred from the illness or from the drug(s) [238, 242];

III. A number of early reports have not paid much attention to the feasibility of associating low birth weight, abortion, and/or infant disorders in patients with such treatment of malaria with artemisinins; and

IV. Post-marketing surveillance has been limited in developing countries, and the potential reproductive side-effects of the drug have not been well recorded.

5. Relationship between Drug Efficacy and Pharmacokinetics

Artemisinin derivatives have been found to kill not only asexual blood stages, but also early stages of gametocytes of *P. falciparum* [243-246]. DHA is highly effective against all parasitical blood stages [5] and gametocytes of *P. falciparum* [247]. Other artemisinin drugs (AM, AE, AS and AL) are most active against rings and schizonts stages but are not as active against trophozoites stage of *P. falciparum, P. cynomolgi, P. vinckei petteri and P. berghei* [5-15]. The results of clinical trials to date indicate that artemisinins are relatively non-toxic and rapidly effective against multi-drug resistant strains of *P. falciparum* [248, 249]. However, patients treated with artemisinin drugs alone have been found to exhibit high recrudescence rates [250]. The pharmacodynamic properties of these drugs have been relatively addressed with pharmacokinetic findings [161, 164, 166, 250].

5.1. Drug Exposure Level and Time Affect on Efficacy *In Vitro*

At dose range 10^{-7}-10^{-5} M (30 –3000 ng/ml), synchronous culture study showed that artemisinin was extremely effective against both of ring and schizonts stages, demonstrating 100% growth inhibition of these stages within 4-6 h. The inhibitory effects of AM were more gradual, requiring 8-10 hr of exposure time to achieve 70% growth inhibition of the ring stage and 40-50% inhibition of schizonts stage. DHA is found to be highly effective against all stages of the parasite, in most cases achieving 100% growth inhibition by 2-4 hr [5].

Classically, *in vitro* studies have addressed the effect of drug exposure against *P. Falciparum* for 48 hr (one life cycle). Recently, more life cycles of *P. falciparum* study on drug exposure time and concentration had been investigated [9, 251]. The parasite viability after exposure to artemisinin was assessed to explore any killing or suppressive effect of the compound in relation to its concentrations and exposure time. Concentration of 10^{-6}-10^{-5} M (280-2800 ng/ml) artemisinin showed a parasitical effect after only 3 hr of drug exposure, whereas 10^{-7} M (28 ng/ml) artemisinin required 24 hr of exposure for a cidal effect. At concentration of 10^{-8} M (2.8 ng/ml), artemisinin had no appreciable effect on the parasites. If the concentration was increased to 3×10^{-8} M (8.4 ng/ml), (with drug exposure time extending to 72-96 hr and the parasitemia reducing below the starting level of 0.5%), then the long exposure time to the lower concentration could be as effective as the high concentration [251].

It is clear that the low dose will increase the exposure time, and the high dose will shorten the treatment period. At a 10^{-8} or 10^{-7} dose level (3-30 ng/ml), artemisinin drugs require 24-96 hr of constant exposure to kill all parasites (IC_{99}). Therefore, the low dose range cannot be selected for artemisinin drugs in human treatments in malaria because 1) the artemisinins have very short half-life and 2) longer exposure time of artemisinins is a principle factor leading to fatal neurotoxicity because the exposure time is more likely responsible than other PK parameters resulting in fatal neurotoxicity.

Survival of the patient is obviously key in treating patients with severe and complicated malaria. Using a low effective dose would delay the treatment time period and should not be allowed. A high loading dose would best achieve switching off all the parasite's vital functions as soon as possible [252]. There is currently no evidence that rapid parasite killing with high doses is harmful. Similarly, there is no evidence of a Jarisch-Herxheimer reaction in malaria and therapeutic blood drug concentrations can be readily achieved without risking toxicity [247].

Because of these factors, the plasma concentration of the artemisinin derivatives in human against *P. falciparum* should be at least 10^{-6}-10^{-5} (300-3000 ng/ml) or higher for AS or DHA, the more potent of the artemisinin compounds. The concentration should be even higher for AE or AM, and ideally should be higher for AL due to its the lowest antimalarial potency among the five agents [1]. The relative antimalarial potency of artemisinin compounds against W-2 parasites is 0.72 (AL) < 1.0 (QHS) < 1.84 (AM) < 2.41 (AE) < 3.01 (AS) < 3.59 (DHA), and the potency against D-6 parasites is 0.32 (AL) < 1.0 (QHS) < 1.22 (AM) < 1.87 (AE) < 2.48 (AS) < 2.99 (DHA). In fact, higher plasma concentration of AS at 21098 ng/ml in humans [our unpublished data] and AL at 20044 ng/ml in animals did not result in the any toxicity, as discussed in section 3.3 (table 9).

5.2. Drug Exposure Level and Time Affect on Efficacy *In Vivo*

Human and animal species studies have shown unambiguously that artemisinin derivatives are very potent drugs against *falciparum* and *vivax* malaria. These drugs initiate immediate decreases in parasitemia and, in most studies; clinical recovery of the patient is faster than with other antimalarials. However, a high recrudescence (about 30-50% for 3 days, 6-15% fro 5 days, and 2-6% for 7 days regimens) is still a major disadvantage for all of these compounds after monotherapy [12, 33]. Although the clinical significance of the rapid killing advantage, in terms of mortality, has yet to be determined by using other artemisinins drugs [23, 24, 74], at least one published study has shown the potential in decreasing mortality. The SEAQUAMAT trial, a multicentre randomized trial conducted in Bangladesh, Thailand, Myanmar, Indonesia, India and Vietnam, recently reported a 34.7% reduction in mortality associated with intravenous AS compared with intravenous quinine [138, 145, 146].

Efficacy in Malaria (Animal Models)

Injectable AS is being developed as a potential agent for the treatment of severe and complicated malaria. A risk assessment of the therapeutic index and related hematological changes of AS and AL following daily intravenous injection for 3 days has been conducted in *P. berghei* infected and uninfected rats. The minimum doses of AS and AL for parasitemia suppression were 2.3 and 2.5 mg/kg, respectively, and the suppressive doses for decreasing parasitemia by half (SD_{50}) were 7.4 and 8.6 mg/kg, respectively. There seemed to be no significant difference between these two water-soluble compounds at suppressive dose levels [179].

However, with regards to parasite clearance time (PCT), equimolar doses of 96 μmoles/kg, AS (36.7 mg/kg) cleared parasitemia in 7 out of 18 rats with a 39% clearance rate. At this dose, the PCT of AS was 52.8 hrs and clearance time lasted only 2.7 days with recrudescence back in the 7 animals. Accordingly, AS did not clear 0.339% (Emax) of parasitemia in rats treated at this dose level. The EC_{50} was 8.86 hrs, and the area under the effect curve (AUEC) was 536 % of parasitemia·hr for this dosage of AS/$NaHCO_3$ in the 7 rats. Using the same equimolar dose of 96 μmoles/kg, AL (40.6 mg/kg) cleared the parasitemia in all of 19 rats with 100% clearance rate. At this dose level, the PCT of AL was 57.2 hrs with clearance lasting for 3.2 days before recrudescence. Computer fitting revealed that E_0 was 6.2 ± 2.3%, whereas Emax was measured at 0.008 ± 0.01% of parasitemia. The EC_{50} was 10.9 hrs, and the area under the effect curve (AUEC) was 313 % of parasitemia·hr for this dosage of AL [179].

It is comprehensible from this data that at the equimolar dose of AL (with 100% clearance) has much great efficacy than that of AS (with 39% clearance) in the malaria infected rat. However, the *in vitro* data indicate that, AS has a 5-8 fold greater antimalarial activity than AL (Section 5.1.). Why do the results contrast between *in vitro* and *in vivo* data? A pharmacokinetic analysis may provide the answer to the question. The comparative pharmacokinetics and hydrolysis studies of intravenously administered AL and AS were performed in malaria-infected rats using 3 daily equimolar doses (96 μmoles/kg). The drug concentration of AS with daily doses of 36.7 mg/kg was one-third less on day 3 than on day 1, and the mean Cmax of AS on day 1 was 16,492 ng/ml and 1,377 ng/ml on day 3. Similar to its active metabolite, DHA, it had peak plasma drug concentrations of 10,842 and 6,485 ng/ml on days 1 and 3, respectively, suggesting an auto-induction of hepatic drug-metabolizing enzymes for AS [95, 196-199].

The auto-induction of the enzymes were similar for other artemisinin drugs (QHS, DHA, AE and AM) [95, 196-199], but not for AL. Pharmacokinetic parameters of AL were very comparable from day 1 to day 3 with same AS molecular dose at 40.6 mg/kg. The mean Cmax of AL on day 1 was 48,453 ng/ml and 44,101ng/ml on day 3. AS is the pro-drug of DHA with a DHA/AS ratio of 5.26 compared to a ratio of 0.01 for DHA/AL. Although total $AUC_{1\text{-}3D}$ of 13,051 ng·h/ml DHA was produced by AS compared to 524 ng·h/ml DHA by AL, the peak level of AL was still 2-fold and 6-fold higher than that of AS plus DHA concentrations on day 1 and day 3, respectively. The increase in AL's peak concentration can explain why AL has a much great efficacy than AS *in vivo* (figure 10). Other pharmacokinetic parameters revealed that the total $AUC_{1\text{-}3}$ days (84.4 μg·h/ml) of AL was 5-fold higher than that of AS (15.7 μg·h/ml of AS plus DHA). The elimination half-life of AL

(7.1 h) was much longer than that of AS (0.36 h) or DHA (0.72 h) (table 14). The remarkable alteration of the pharmacokinetic shape of AL may be caused by poor conversion rates to DHA and an enterohepatic circulation, which has been confirmed by pharmacokinetics and tissue distribution studies [178, 209]. Compared to AS, higher drug peak and AUC values of AL in the rat blood may be the cause of its increased efficacy in vivo.

To evaluate the efficacy of AE and AM with two different intramuscular vehicles, sesame oil and cremophore, efficacy and pharmacokinetic investigation have been performed in rats [152]. AE and AM showed comparable efficacy against *P. berghei* when used cremophore vehicle to replace sesame oil following intramuscular treatment. The results of 50% cure dose (CD_{50}) were significantly different between the sesame oil and cremophore. AE and AM with sesame oil had the similar CD_{50} values of 34.1 (1.3-66.9) and 35.6 (7.6-63.6) mg/kg, respectively. However, the drugs with cremophore had 14.2 (6.8-21.5) and 21.0 (18.5-23.4) mg/kg for AE and AM, respectively, in malaria mice (table 15). The results showed that AE and AM formulated in cremophore had a significantly higher efficacy than the sesame oil formulation following the three daily multiple intramuscular injections in mice.

Table 14. Toxicokinetic parameters of artesunate (AS) and artelinate (AL) at 96 µmoles/kg following multiple intravenous injections daily for three days in *P. berghei* infected rats by using Culex automated blood sampler. [178]

TK Parameters	AS (36.7 mg/kg , n = 4)		AL (40.6 mg/kg, n = 6)	
	Parent drug (AS)	Metabolite (DHA)	Parent drug (AL)	Metabolite (DHA)
Day 1				
Cmax (ng/ml)	16492 ± 4205	10842 ± 1950	48453 ± 7177	124.2 ± 36.2
Tmax (h)	0	0.19 ± 0.03	0	
$AUC_{inf.}$ (ng·h/ml)	1324 ± 242	4893 ± 779	25857 ± 2114	160.4 ± 86.2
$t_{1/2}$ distribution (h)	0.04 ± 0.01	0.20 ± 0.02	0.29 ± 0.06	
$t_{1/2}$ elimination (h)	0.36 ± 0.03	0.72 ± 0.05	7.05 ± 2.01	
Vss (liter/kg)	8.10 ± 1.70	-	4.57 ± 2.01	
CL (ml/min/kg)	474.2 ± 89.8	-	25.93 ± 2.10	
MRT (h)	0.62 ± 0.33	0.43 ± 0.04	2.89 ± 1.11	
Day 3				
Cmax (ng/ml)	1377 ± 898	6485 ± 1053	44101 ± 21452	116.6 ± 74.3
Tmax (h)	0	0.18 ± 0.06	0	0.26 ± 0.12
$AUC_{inf.}$ (ng·h/ml)	490.6 ± 314.0	3327 ± 743	24650 ± 8663	204.2 ± 134
$t_{1/2}$ distribution (h)	0.12 ± 0.07	0.21 ± 0.02	0.30 ± 0.08	
$t_{1/2}$ elimination (h)	0.46 ± 0.06	0.65 ± 0.06	6.06 ± 0.64	
Vss (liter)	76.87 ± 8.54	-	5.24 ± 3.50	
CL (ml/min/kg)	2172 ± 1274	-	29.40 ± 8.24	
MRT (h)	0.53 ± 0.01	0.60 ± 0.11	2.78 ± 1.34	
Total $AUC_{1\text{-}3D}$ (ng·h/ml)	2717 ± 809	13051 ± 1926	84406 ± 19703	524 ± 277
Ratio of DHA/AS or DHA/AL (1-3D)		5.26 ± 2.22		0.01 ± 0.00

TK = toxicokinetics, DHA = dihydroartemisinin, MRT = Mean residence time; D = days.

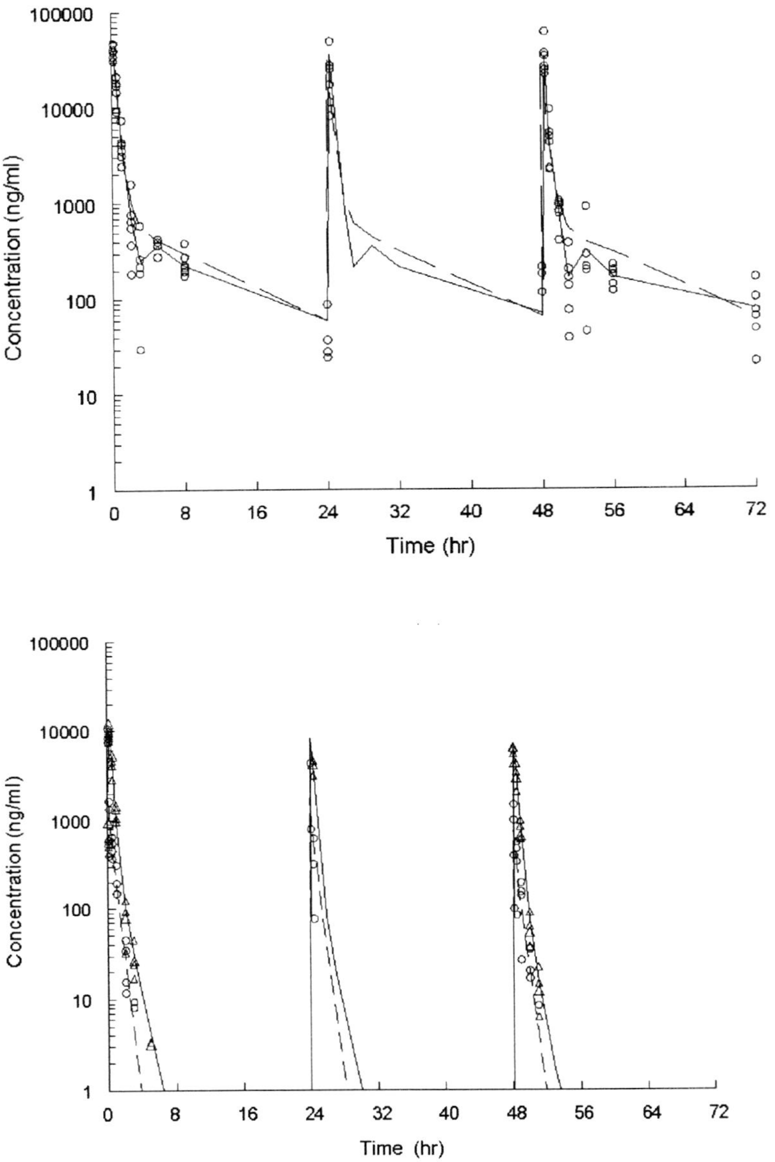

Figure 10. Individual plasma concentration-time profiles of artelinate (AL) measured by LC/MS/MS (markers) and mean concentration (solid line) as well as computer fitted curves (dashed line) by pharmacokinetic parameters at daily dosage of 40.6 mg/kg intravenously for three days in malaria-infected rats (top, n = 6). Individual plasma concentration-time profiles of artesunate (AS) measured by HPLC-ECD (markers) and computer fitted curves for parent drug, AS (dashed line), and its active metabolite, DHA (solid line), by pharmacokinetic parameters at dosage of 36.7 mg/kg once daily intravenously for 3 days in *P. berghei* infected male rats.(bottom, n = 4) [178].

Table 15. Antimalarial activity (50% cure dose, CD_{50})* and corresponding 95% confidence interval (95% CI) of arteether and artemether given intramuscularly in daily dose for 3 days against P. berghei in female mice (n = 8 for each dose level) [152]

Drug	Arteether (CD_{50})		Artemether (CD_{50})	
	mg/kg	95%CI	mg/kg	95%CI
Sesame oil formulation	34.1	1.3-66.9	35.6	7.6-63.6
Cremophore formulation	14.2	6.8-21.5	21.0	18.5-23.4

* When the mice have survived and showed negative smears at 60 days, they were considered cured.

The mean plasma concentration-time profile (n = 3) of AE formulated with sesame oil (AESO) and 1:2 cremophore/0.9% saline (AECM) after single intravenous and intramuscular doses is shown in figure 3 (bottom). AE with sesame oil and cremophore data showed a biphasic pattern of disposition and was fitted by a two-compartment open model after either intravenous or intramuscular injection. The concentration-time profiles of AE with the two vehicles are shown in figure 7 after daily intramuscular for 7 days with the multiple administrations. The trough plasma concentrations increased significantly up to the last dosing in AESO treated rats, but not in AECM rats. Obviously, the drug accumulated (7.5-fold) in the plasma of animals administered with AESO (comparing the 7th dosing day to the first dosing day). In the AECM rats, the AE level increased slightly (1.8-fold) on day 7 over that on day 1 following the multiple dosing.

Significant differences in pharmacokinetic parameters between AECM and AESO are summarized in table 16 after multiple intramuscular doses of 25 mg/kg. Plasma peak concentration on day 1 indicated that the Cmax of AECM (1227 ± 171 ng/ml) was more than 13-fold higher than that of AESO (92.2 ± 19.9 ng/ml). The area under the curve (AUC) of AECM (4165 ± 676 ng·h/ml) was about 4-fold greater than that of AESO (1135 ± 277 ng·h/ml) on day 1. Total AUC of AECM (46286 ± 2061 ng·h/ml) during the 7-day dosing period was about 2.7-fold higher than that of AESO (16922 ± 4038 ng·h/ml). The elimination half-life was 7.0 ± 0.9 hr for AECM and 17.7 ± 2.7 hr for AESO on day 1. Based on the AUC data, the bioavailability of AECM was 74.5 ± 12.1% and 20.3 ± 5.0% for AESO after a single intramuscular injection. The data suggested that AECM, a less oily formulation, was more easily absorbed by the muscle with a higher Cmax and AUC, which may be the explanation of its increased efficacy.

The *in vivo* efficacy model shows that AE and AM formulated with cremophore had a significantly higher efficacy than that with sesame oil. It is apparent that the higher plasma concentration of AE produced by cremophore formulation has principle role in the increased efficacy. Plasma concentration showed that the C_{max} and AUC of AECM were about 13-fold and 5-fold, respectively, higher than that of AESO on day 1. Even the total AUC of AECM (46286 ng·h/ml) during the 7-day period was 2.7-fold higher than with AESO (16922 ng·h/ml). The much higher level of AE exposure in the rats using a cremophore vehicle truly contributed to the antimalarial efficacy, and without a doubt, the antimalarial efficacy is drug concentration dependent [5, 9, 251, 252], especially with the 13-fold higher peak concentration.

Table 16. Pharmacokinetic parameters of arteether (AE) and dihydroartemisinin, a metabolite of AE, following single intravenous (25 mg/kg), and multiple intramuscular (25 mg/kg) administration with sesame oil and 1:2 cremophore (CRM)/0.9% saline daily for 7 days in male rats (n = 3-7) [152]

Dosing Parameters	IV single	Intramuscular Multiple			
	Vehicle:	Sesame oil (AESO)		1:2 Cremophore/saline (AECM)	
	CRM/Saline	Day 1	Day 7	Day 1	Day 7
Arteether					
Cmax (ng/ml)	14482 ±1023	92.2 ± 19.9	311.9 ± 54.6	1227 ± 171	1826 ± 118
Tmax (min)	0	1.42 ± 0.63	1.67 ± 0.58	1.33 ± 0.29	1.33 ± 0.58
AUC (ng·h/ml)	5593 ± 591	1135 ± 277	8527 ± 1006	4165 ± 676	7312 ± 588
AUC_{D1-8} (ng·h/ml)			16922 ± 4038		46286 ± 2061
Vss (liter)	0.98 ± 0.25	150.2 ± 33.7	54.1 ± 7.8	8.70 ± 1.21	5.06 ± 0.27
Cl (ml/min/kg)	71.3 ± 9.11	73.7 ± 2.8	147.9 ± 6.19	76.3 ± 2.9	76.0 ± 1.9
$t_{1/2}$ distribution (h)	0.22 ± 0.04	0.71 ± 0.47	1.08 ± 0.49	1.00 ± 0.04	1.18 ± 0.14
$t_{1/2}$ elimination (h)	0.82 ± 0.05	17.66 ± 2.68	29.57 ± 2.07	6.96 ± 0.93	9.06 ± 1.69
MAT (h)	-	0.76 ± 0.40	0.87 ± 0.39	1.04 ± 0.03	1.07 ± 0.10
MRT (h)	0.74 ± 0.18	23.56 ± 3.42	41.51 ± 2.84	6.21 ± 0.66	5.83 ± 0.09
Bioavailability (%)	100	20.3 ± 5.0	152.4 ± 17.9	74.5 ± 12.1	130.7 ± 10.5
% of single daily dose in muscle		37.6 ± 8.2	91.4 ± 11.6	4.7 ± 1.8	17.3 ± 3.3
Dihydroartemisinin (DQHS, a metabolite of AE)					
Cmax (ng/ml)	815.8 ±164.2	16.02 ± 4.05	123.8 ± 28.9	171.1 ± 79.4	188.4 ± 91.0
Tmax (min)	0	0.92 ± 0.14	0.86 ± 0.35	0.92 ± 0.14	1.33 ± 0.29
AUC (ng·h/ml)	350.0 ± 97.1	117.1 ± 33.0 790.3 ± 220.6	607.7 ± 101.5	708.2 ± 29.2	AUC (ng·h/ml)
AUC_{D1-8} (ng·h/ml)			3427 ± 759		5346 ± 831
$t_{1/2}$ elimination (h)	1.08 ± 0.16	9.17 ± 2.54	14.47 ± 2.17	4.71 ± 0.71	6.64 ± 1.25
Ratio of DQHS/AE	0.06 ± 0.02	0.09 ± 0.03	0.08 ± 0.03	0.14 ± 0.03	0.11 ± 0.01

* On day 1 the amount of dose in the muscle was measured at 24 h after first dosing, and on day 7 the amount of dose was measured at 24h after last dosing. IV = intravenous, CRM/saline = 1:2 cremophore/0.9% saline.

Efficacy in Malaria (Human Studies)

Karbwang reported on four patients, not cured of their malaria by the oral AM regimen used in his study, that had significantly lower plasma concentrations of DHA, an active metabolite of AM [25] than others in the study. Using the same AM dose amount, a much lower C_{max} (196 ng/ml at 6 h and 54 ng/ml at 12 h) of DHA was measured in the four patients than the Cmax (354 ng/ml at 6 h and 158 ng/ml at 12h) of DHA in 46 other subjects. Also, a lower AUC (834 ng·h/ml) of DHA was detected in these 4 patients but not in the remaining 46 patients (3684 ng·h/ml). Concentrations of the parent drug, AM, was not much different in these four patients (1044 ng·h/ml) when compared to the other subjects (1272 ng·h/ml). It is unknown how those patients resulted in such low DHA concentrations, but these low levels of DHA may be the cause for the treatment failure. The four patients, in whom most parasites may have been more mature, may have required higher concentrations of AM/DHA than patients with similar numbers of parasites.

More recently, Sharma reported on two patients who died with a very high degree of parasitemia (16% and 50%) and cerebral malaria. The dose regimen of AM at 80 mg was intramuscularly injected twice on first day and then once daily for another four days [253]. Intramuscular formulation of AM resulted in very low plasma concentration and low bioavailability [85] due to the prolonged absorption from the injection site [187]. This study showed that using a low dose regimen (total 480 mg) may not have enough drug concentration to cure the heavy parasitemia in these patients.

During a phase III clinical trial of intramuscular Artemotil (AE), a patient had inadvertently obtained a full or fractional intravenous injection with the intramuscular formulation on the first day of treatment. The difference in concentration profiles vs. time of AE and DHA for patient number 151 from the high dose group is shown in figure 9 (bottom). As first dosing, AE seemed to be accidentally injected in patient 151 through a vessel instead of the muscle. This resulted in an intravenous injection profile with very high C_{max} concentration right after injection and a rapid distribution phase. AE and DHA plasma concentrations decreased significantly after first dosing with an elimination $t_{1/2}$ of 1.1 hr in the first 6 hrs. After the second intramuscular injection at the 6th hour, the elimination $t_{1/2}$ of AE was immediately extended to 9.35 hr as a daily half-life. The Cmax (2407 ng/ml) was shown to be about 22-fold higher in patient 151 than the mean value (110 ng/ml) reported in other patients in high dose group. AUC value (12259 ng·h/ml) was 2 times higher than the mean value (7403 ng·h/ml) shown in other subjects. The same results were also reported for increasing DHA levels in patient 151. To be expected, this patient was successfully cure at 36 hr (PCT) and 4 hr (FCT) compared with other patients with 64.4 hr (PCT) and 70.1 hr (FCT) [200]. The clinical cure indicated that the intravenous formulation, like AS injection, is very important in the rapid treatment of malaria with high peak concentration (C_{max}), especially in the severe and complicated malaria. In the meantime, the C_{max} (22-fold) could have also been an important factor in the observed increase of drug efficacy.

Other cases of oral or intramuscular administration of AS and AM were compared in malaria patients [144, 254]. The first-dose pharmacokinetic properties of intramuscular AS at 2.4 mg/kg immediately followed by 1.2 mg/kg daily and AM at 3.2 mg/kg intramuscular start, followed by 1.6 mg/kg daily were compared in Vietnamese adults with severe falciparum malaria. A total of 19 patients were studied; 9 received AS, and 10 received AM. Intramuscular AS was rapidly absorbed. Concentrations of AS in plasma peaked between 523 and 3221 ng/ml (median, 2193 ng/ml) within 20 min of injection and then declined with a median (range) half-life of 30 (3 to 67) min. AS was hydrolyzed rapidly and completely to the biologically active metabolite DHA. Peak DHA concentrations in plasma ranged between 488 and 2011 ng/ml (median, 869 ng/ml) and declined with a t1/2 of 52 (26 to 69) min. The median times for fever and parasite clearance were 65 h and 38.2 h, respectively, in the AS group. All patients survived.

In contrast, AM was slowly and erratically absorbed. The absorption profile appeared biphasic. Maximum AM concentrations in plasma ranged between 20 ng/ml and 487 ng/ml (median, 171 ng/ml) and occurred at a median (range) of 10 (1.5 to 24) h. There was relatively little conversion to DHA. After intramuscular injection in cases of severe malaria, absorption of the water-soluble AS is rapid and extensive, whereas the absorption of the oil-based AM is slow and erratic with relatively little conversion to the more active DHA. The median times to fever and parasite clearance were 56 h and 48 h, respectively, in the AM group. Two out of ten patients died in the process (20% mortality). Based on this pharmacological study, parenteral AS seems preferable to AM as an initial antimalarial therapy, particularly in seriously ill patients. Also, with the peak concentration (2193 ng/ml) of AS being 13-fold higher than that (171 ng/ml) of AM, it indicates that a high peak concentration contributes greatly in improving efficacy and reducing mortality.

After oral dose, despite a 29% lower molar dose, oral AS administration result in a significantly larger drug concentration. It also resulted in higher antimalarial activity than after oral AM ($P \leq 0.02$). The mean (95% CI) oral antimalarial bioavailability of AM, relative to oral AS, corrected for molar dose was 58% (40–76). The mean (95% CI) relative antimalarial bioavailability of AM was lower on the first day of treatment, 31% (17–100), compared to the second day, 72% (44–118) ($P = 0.018$). In *vivo* parasite clearance and time above the *in vitro* IC_{90} were similar for the two drugs, despite considerable differences in C_{max} and AUC. The oral antimalarial potency following AM was significantly lower than that after AS. AM oral antimalarial bioavailability was reduced in acute malaria. Oral AS provided greater antimalarial activity than AM at the same molar dose [254].

All of the evidence shows that higher plasma concentration (C_{max} and AUC), especially the peak concentration (C_{max}), will greatly increase the efficacy and clinical therapeutic potentials of artemisinin drugs. As discussed above, from the severity of these complications, *P. falciparum* malaria constitutes a medical emergency, and appropriate treatment should be initiated as soon as infection is suspected. The appropriate treatment means that enough high dose regimens should be given as to provide a successful therapeutic efficacy for the malaria patients. It is known that 84% of all malaria related deaths occurs within 24 hr of hospital admission in African children [255]. Therefore, first exposure concentrations of artemisinin drugs are very clinically important.

5.3. Therapeutic Efficacy of Artemisinins in Monotherapy

The therapeutic potentials of all artemisinin drugs in monotherapy with 54 clinical trials have been summarized in the treatment for malaria with various dose regiments (table 4). Successful (or 100% cure) treatment is found neither in the 3-5 day treatments nor the high dose (4.8 mg/kg) regimens with monotherapy [21-45, 256]. The rates of recrudescence, fever, and parasite clearances are traditional evaluations for the efficacy of the antimalarial drugs in humans. These three parameters exhibit the therapeutic potential of intravenous, intramuscular and oral agents in various regimens. Results have shown that AE in sesame oil vehicle is not superior to that of the oral DHA, oral and intravenous AS, intramuscular AM, or even intramuscular α/β-arteether formulated with peanut oil.

With these data, and their known mode of rapid action, the artemisinin group of antimalarials is considered to be highly and independently effective compared with other traditional malaria drugs. Although there is no evidence that drug resistance has occurred *in vivo*, short treatment courses (3-5 days) are associated with high recrudescence rates. The data that emerges from all available artemisinin drugs is that given a dose sufficient to induce initial parasite clearance and clinical recovery, the duration of therapy is the ultimate determinant for recrudescence. The rates of recrudescence (30-50% for 3 day regimen, 6-15% for 5 day regimen, and 2-6% for 7 day regimen) continues to be a big problem for all these compounds described previously [12, 33]. It has been suggested that preventing recrudescence does not have the highest priority, but that a recrudescence should rather be treated with the same regimen again. Eventually, all patients would be radically cured with this strategy. The potential risk of development of resistance and recrudescence urges us to look for combination regimens that offer radical cure instead.

Reduction of parasitemia measured as the parasite clearance time (PCT), along with the fever clearance time (FCT) are primary measures of initial drug effect in *vivo.* Reviews of this therapeutic efficacy from multiple clinical studies demonstrate that when given alone (monotherapy) AM (oral and intramuscular administration), AS (oral and intravenous dosing), and DHA (oral) appear to have same effects for reducing PCT and FCT with various dose regimens (table 4). The finding that therapeutic potentials of AM and AS in oral formulation could be equal to DHA may be contributed to the great conversion rate of AM and AS to DHA in human and high peak concentrations as described above. AE after intramuscular injection appears to have fewer efficacies than the other 4 drugs, even with high dosage regimen or compared with AM intramuscular formulation (table 4), which may have much lower blood concentration due to slow and prolong absorption [144, 254, 257].

Parasitemia count and clearance time (PCT) do not always accurately reflect the total burden of parasitised red blood cells, but better parameters are not available. All artemisinin compounds induce a remarkably rapid reduction of parasitemia, starting almost immediately after administration [258, 259]. Fortunately the rapid parasite clearance induced by artemisinin drug treatment provides a simple pharmacodynamic measure that can be used in drug comparisons and assessment. Certainly, parasitological cure is the best end point measure of efficacy for patients with malaria. In this review, the available pharmacodynamic data of parasitemia reduction is evaluated with its associated PK result during the malaria treatment in human described as below.

5.4. Pharmacokinetic/Pharmacodynamic Evaluation of the Artemisinins

The pharmacokinetic/pharmacodynamic (PK/PD) results for artemisinin drugs in monotherapy may give us more comprehension in dosage regimen investigation. This section has analyzed the same subjects in one publication for the PK and PD analysis of artemisinin (QHS). However, for the other four drugs (AS, AE, AM, and DHA), the PK and PD with same drug, same administration route, and same dosage regimen are combined from two individual publications [37, 91, 200, 260-263].

Pharmacokinetics (PK), in general, shows an absorption phase of artemisinin drugs following oral or intramuscular administration. It then reaches peak concentration at 1-3 hours followed by a sharp decline in elimination phase. After multiple administrations, four drug concentrations (QHS, AS, AM, even DHA) has been reported to decline daily due to an auto-induction metabolism [95, 196-199]. Following oral administration, AS and DHA has short mean residence time (MRT) with 2.0 and 2.7 hr, respectively, and QHS has longer MRT with 7.4 hr. Due to prolonged absorption and accumulation in the injection sites, AE and AM have very long MRT at 13.9-42.9 hr in human treatment (table 17). For cases analysis, PK data of five artemisinin drugs (QHS, DHA, AE, AM and AS) associated with parasitological consequences in malaria patients are shown in table 17.

Table 17. Pharmacokinetics/pharmacodynamic (PK/PD) parameters of AS (oral, 100 mg and even 50 mg b.i.d x 4), DHA (oral, 200 mg and even 100 mg x 4), AM (IM, 3.2 mg/kg and 1.6 mg x 4), and QHS (oral, 500 mg and 250 b.i.d x 4 and then 500 mg on D6) in human treatment with uncomplicated and severe/complicated malaria [22, 37, 91, 200, 260-263]

PK/PD Paremeters	AS	DHA	AM	AE	QHS
	(tablets)	(tablets)	(sesame oil)	(sesame oil)	(capsules)
Route of administration	Oral	Oral	IM	IM	Oral
First loading dosage	100 mg	200 mg	3.2 mg/kg	4.8 mg/kh	500 mg
Maintaining dosage	50 mg x 4	100 mg x 4	1.6 mg x 4	1.6 mg x 5	250 mg x 5
Refs	[91, 260]	[37, 261]	[262, 263]	[22, 200]	[197, 260]
PK parameters (Day 1)					
Cmax (ng/ml)	1052 (DHA)	437.5	74.9	110.1	588.0
tmax (hr)	0.75	1.4	6.0	8.2	2.4
tlag (hr)		0.2			0.45
$AUC_{0\text{-}24\ hr}$ (ng·h/ml)	1334 (DHA)	1329	1230	4702	2601
$t_{1/2}$ (absorption, hr)	0.36	0.67	1.88	3.2	1.21
$t_{1/2}$ (elimination, hr)	0.70	0.85	7.83	22.7	2.3
MRT (hr)	1.95	2.71	13.94	42.9	7.41
PD parameters (Day 1)*					
Time of lag phase (hr)	2.81	4.03	7.26	8.89	5.76
AUEC (%·h/μl)	921.2	1167.9	1613.4	2463.5	1464.4
PC_{50} (hr)	8.48	10.05	15.63	19.68	13.95
Emax (%) or MPC	0.0016	0.2132	0.0030	0.5504	0.0100
Curative rate (%)	81.3	76.0	86.7	48.0	74.3-75.2

*The data was fitted with WinNonlin (V5.0) by author.

PK = pharmacokinetics; PD = pharmacodynamics; MRT = Mean residence time; PC_{50} = Mean time for parasitemia to fall by half; AUEC = area under effect-time curve; QHS = Artemisinin; DHA = Dihydroartemisinin; AM = Artemether; AE = Arteether; AS = Artesunic acid; MPC = minimum parasiticidal concentration; IM = intramuscular.

Pharmacodynamics (PD) is similar to PK profiles but measures efficacy parameters. The mean parasitemia-time curve following treatment with any antimalarial compounds presents a lag phase. The lag phase is then followed by a sharp decease in parasite counts (which presents a clearance phase), and is then slowly decreased to a very low parasitemia. This process is usually under the limitation of microscopic observation for both the dormant and terminal phases (figure 11, top). The artemisinin drugs affect these profiles in several ways. First, they appear to prevent the continuation of merogony at a later stage of parasite development than either quinine or mefloquine. This prevents or attenuates the occasional alarming sharp rise in parasitemia immediately following treatment described earlier (lag phase). Second, the decline in parasitemia is accelerated. This can be explained only by enhancement of clearance of erythrocytes infected with ring forms (clearance phase) [250, 264,]. After rapid termination, surviving and stage unaffected parasites have very low levels at a dormant status [265], which is a basis of the recrudescence (dormant and terminal phase). Different artemisinin drugs with different dosage regimens showed the different profiles of parasitemia-time (figure 11, bottom). Although the PK/PD publication is very limited, the possible PK and PD evaluations for individual drug with same regimens in monotherapy for human-malaria are described below.

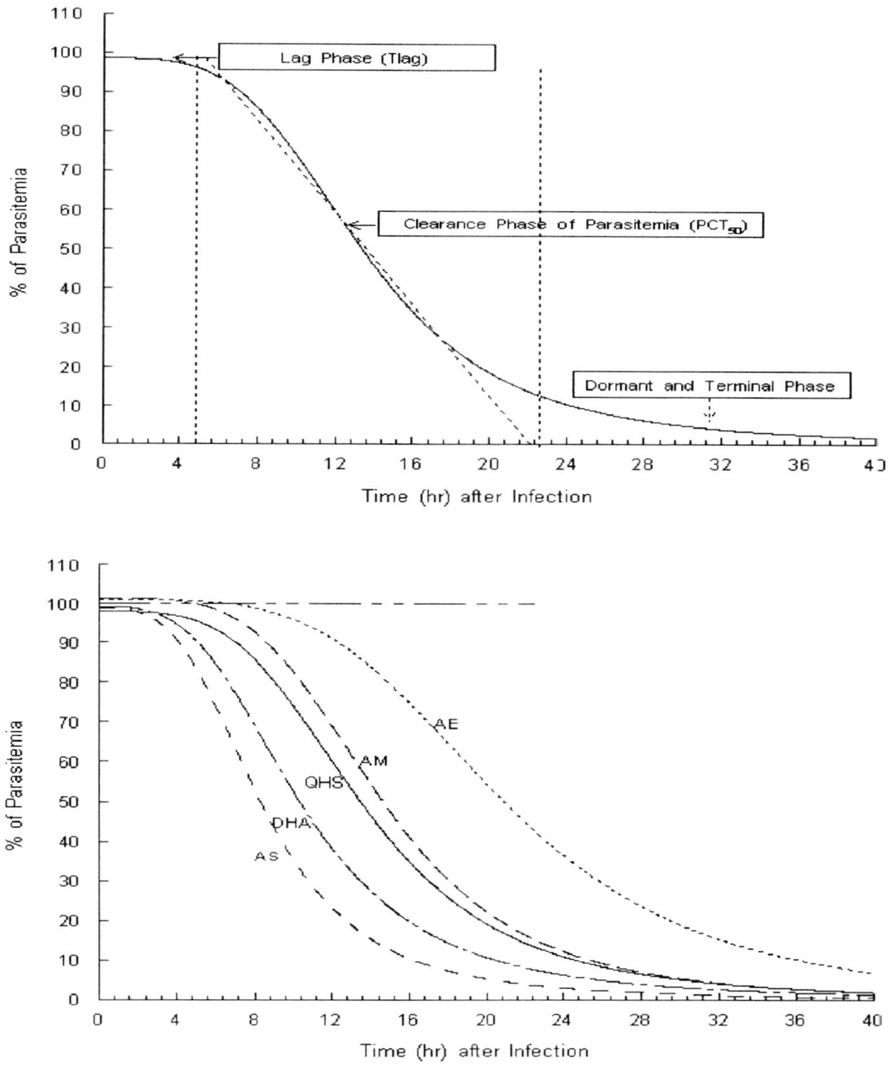

Figure 11. Standard parasite clearance curve in different stages (lag phase, clearance phase, dormant and terminal phase) and synchronicity of parasite development under antiparasitic drug received at 0 hour (top chart). The mean parasite clearance curves of AS (dashed line) at 100 mg first day and 50 mg b.i.d 2-6 days orally [91, 260]; DHA (dot and dashed line) at 200 mg first day and 100 mg 2-5 days orally [37, 160]; QHS (solid line) at 500 mg first day, 250 mg b.i.d 2-5 and 500 mg last day orally [197, 260]; AM (dashed line) at 3.2 mg/kg first day and 1.6 mg/kg 2-5 days intramuscularly [262, 263]; and AE (dot line) of 4.8 mg/kg at 0 hour and 1.6 mg/kg at 6 and then 2-5 days intramuscularly [22, 200] in malaria patients (bottom chart) (Table 17). The parasitemia at 0 hour was set as 100% of parasitemia.

5.4.1. Artesunate

Pharmacokinetic/pharmacodynamic profiles in plasma has been studied following AS oral administration in tablets of 100 mg/person dose on first day and then followed by 50 mg twice daily for 2-6 days (figure 12). The mean peak plasma concentration of DHA, a metabolite of AS, was reached at 1052 ng/ml and then declined with elimination half-life calculated at 0.75 hr (table 17). Also, the AS concentration declined daily during the 5 days of dosing [199]. Mean AUC of DHA was estimated at 1334 ng·h/ml, which was 6.4 times higher than that of its parent compound (AUC of 210 ng·h/ml), AS, in this clinical trial [91].At same dosage regimen, the time of lag phase in the parasitemia curve was 2.81 hr, which was the shortest lag time compared with other 4 drugs (figure 11, bottom), indicating that the effect of AS tablets was very fast and efficient with 0.36 hr absorption half-life and 1052 ng/ml of Cmax [260]. Similarly, very rapid parasite clearance produced a mean time of 8.48 hr for clearance of half the parasitemia (PC_{50}), the lowest PC_{50} and the lowest area under effect-time curve (AUEC) with 921.2%·h/µl (table 17).

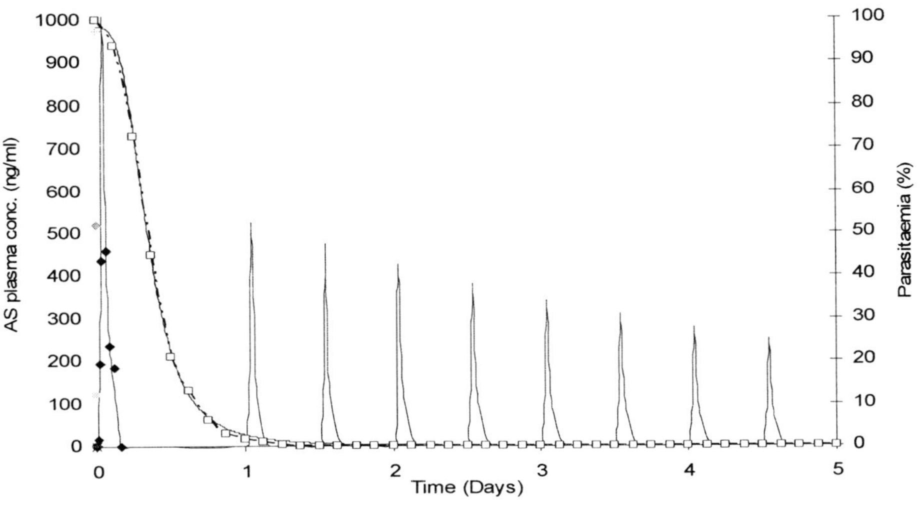

Figure 12. Pharmacokinetic/pharmacodynamic profiles are in plasma following artesunate (AS) oral administration of 100 mg/person dose on first day followed by 50 mg twice daily for 2-6 days by using tablets. DHA, a metabolite of AS, measured by HPLC-ECD (diamonds) and computer fitted curves (solid-line) [91], which was simulated by declining metabolism of AS in humans [199]. Mean parasite densities versus time measured by microscopy (empty squares) and computer fitting curve (dashed line) [260] are from malaria human trials. Relative PK/PD parameters are given in Table 17. The parasitemia was counted 100% at zero while the first dosing time.

After the computer fitting, the 0.0016% parasitemia of an E_{max} was estimated for the oral AS treatment in human (table 17) on the first day in (or for) computer modeling. The E_{max} was the principal pharmacodynamic parameter to determine the antimalarial response in maximum effect to the artemisinin derivatives, which had very steep concentration-effect relationships. The relationship may be caused by the time that blood concentrations exceed the minimum parasiticidal concentration (MPC), rather than the C_{max} or AUC [264]. For the data presented here, after 100 mg per patient of AS, the MPC was the lowest parasitemia remaining in blood when compared to other four artemisinin derivatives (figure 12).

5.4.2. Dihydroartemisinin

PK/PD profiles in plasma following DHA oral administration in tablets of 200 mg/person on day 1 and then 100 mg at day 2-5 are shown in figure 13. After 200 mg of DHA by oral dosing, the mean peak plasma concentration of DHA was reached at 437 ng/ml and then declined with elimination half-life calculated at 0.85 hr. Mean AUC of DHA was estimated at 1329 ng·h/ml. At 200 mg dosage regimen orally, the time of lag phase in the parasitemia curve was 4.03 hr. The lag time was longer than AS (2.81 hr) and still shorter than AM (7.26 hr), AE (8.89 hr) and QHS (5.76 hr) (table 17, figure 11, bottom), indicating that fast effect of DHA tablets was not as good as AS, but was more rapid than AM, AE and QHS regimens. In addition, the rapid parasite clearance resulted in a mean time of 10.05 hr of PC_{50} and the 1167.9 %·h/μl. of AUEC.

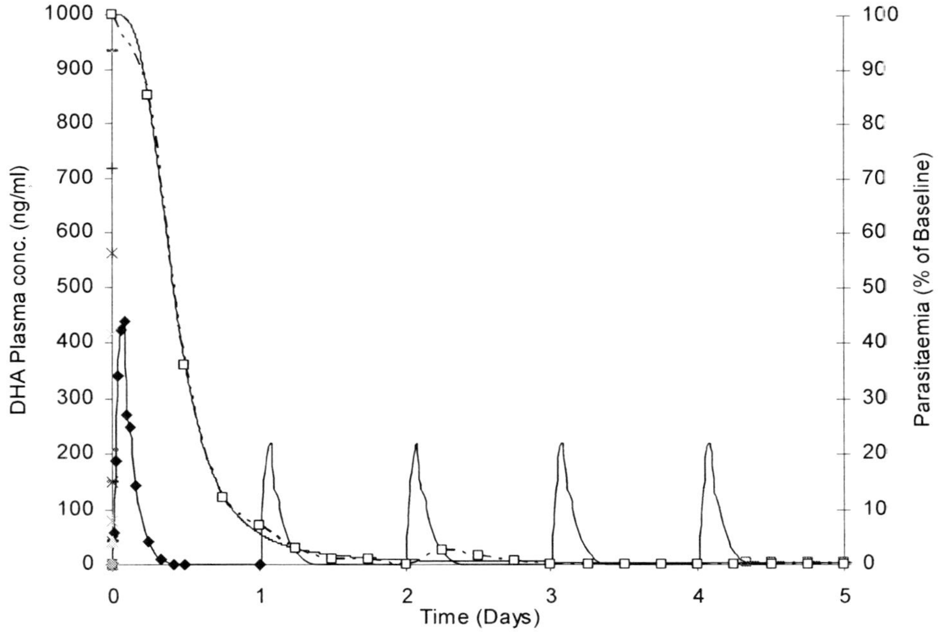

Figure 13. Pharmacokinetic/pharmacodynamic profiles are in plasma following dihydroartemisinin (DHA) oral administration of 200 mg/person on day 1 and then 100 mg daily at day 2-5 in tablets. DHA measured by HPLC-ECD (diamonds) and computer fitted curves (solid-line) [37, 261]. Mean parasite densities versus time measured by microscopy (empty squares) and computer fitting curve (dashed line) [261] are from malaria human trials. The parasitemia was counted 100% at zero while the first dosing time.

After first day computer modeling, the 0.213% parasitemia of an E_{max} was estimated for the oral DHA treatment in human. For the data presented here, after giving 200 mg per patient of DHA, more MPC remained in the blood when compared to the other three artemisinin derivatives (table 17). The absorption of DHA tablets with 0.67 hr half-life was 50% slower than the AS (0.36 hr) trial too, suggesting that the slow reduction of parasitemia may have resulted from the slow absorption. In addition, the AUCs of the two treatments (AS and DHA with double dose) were the same, only the C_{max} of AS dosing was two times higher than DHA treatment, indicating that the high peak concentration (C_{max}) may be another reason for the decrease of parasitemia in human [37, 261]. Compared with the AS study, DHA appeared to have very low bioavailability (< 50%). If calculated with an equal dose level, the C_{max} and AUC_{DHA} estimated from AS treatment was 4-fold and 2-fold, respectively, higher than the DHA dosage regimen. Our data demonstrated that the DHA tablet (Cotexin) in beagle dogs had only 24.4% obsolete bioavailability [160]. Rebound parasites (3%) on day 3 and one-fourth recrudescence rate (24%) were found in patients treated with DHA tablets in clinical work [37]. The 3% of rebound parasites was only found in DHA oral treatment in this comparison (figure 13).

5.4.3. Artemether

PK and PD profiles in plasma following AM intramuscular administration in sesame oil of 3.2 mg/kg on day 1 and then 1.6 mg/kg daily on day 2-5 can be seen in figure 14. The mean peak plasma concentration was reached at 74.9 ng/ml and then declined with elimination half-life calculated at 7.83 hr (table 17), indicating that this formulation had the lowest peak of drug concentration when compared to the other 4 artemisinin drugs. Mean AUC was estimated at 1230 ng·h/ml [262]. At the same dosage regimen the time of lag phase in the parasitemia curve was 7.26 hr, which was the second longest lag time compared with other 3 drugs except for AE, indicating that the effect of the AM intramuscular formulation had a very low and prolonged absorption from muscle injection sites [187]. Parasitemia counts in the beginning after dosing did not decrease due to the low peak concentration of AM, but increased markedly to 110% at 4 hours (parasitemia was counted 100% at zero while the first dosing time). That may be the reason why the lag time was longer at 7.26 hr with no parasites decrease after injection at hour 4. Similarly, there was very slow clearance to parasites produced at mean PC_{50} time of 15.6 hr, which was also the longest PC_{50} time compared to other 3 drugs (table 17). The highest AUEC of 1613.4 %·h/μl also revealed that the drug with the intramuscular regimen was not efficacious in reducing the parasitemia [263].

Although the intramuscular AM was not fast enough to kill parasites in patients, the long lasting exposure level of AM (7.83 hr elimination half-life) could reduce parasitemia at a good rate. The computer modeling estimated that the 0.003% parasitemia was the E_{max} in this clinical trial. The MPC (E_{max}) was only a little more than oral AS in the first day modeling, but much less than oral DHA, AE and QHS (table 17).

5.4.4. Arteether

PK and PD profiles in plasma following AE intramuscular administration in sesame oil of 4.8 mg/kg at 0 h and 1.6 mg/kg at 6 h on day 1 and then daily 1.6 mg from day 2-5 are illustrated in figure 15. The mean peak plasma concentration was reached at 110.1 ng/ml and then declined with elimination half-life calculated at 22.7 hr (table 17), indicating that this formulation has a low peak of drug concentration when compared to AS, DHA, and QHS. Mean AUC was estimated at 4702 ng·h/ml [200]. At the same dosage regimen the lag time in the parasitemia curve was 8.89 hr, which was the longest lag time compared with other 4 drugs, indicating that the effect of the AE intramuscular formulation had a very low and prolonged absorption from muscle injection sites [187]. Parasitemia counts in the beginning after dosing did not decrease due to the low peak concentration of AE, but increased markedly to 108% at 6 hours (100% parasitemia was counted at zero hour during the first dosing time). The increase may be the reason why the lag time is longer at 8.89 hr with no parasites killing after injection at 6 hours. Similarly, a very slow parasite clearance was produced at mean PC_{50} time of 19.68 hr, which was the longest PC_{50} time compared to other 4 drugs (table 17). The highest AUEC of 2463.5 %·h/μl revealed that the drug with the intramuscular regimen was not efficacious in reducing the parasitemia [263].

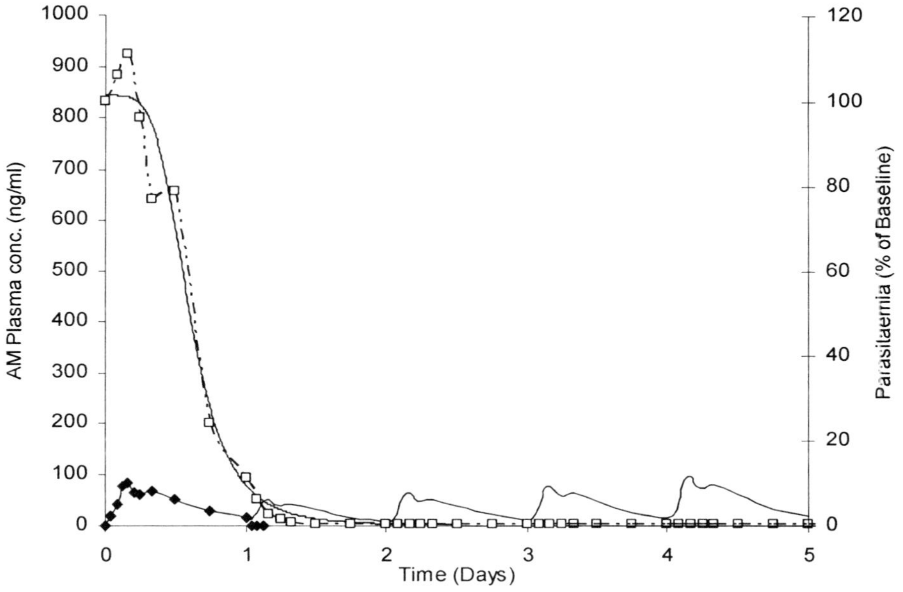

Figure 14. Pharmacokinetic/pharmacodynamic profiles are in plasma following artemether (AM) intramuscular administration of 3.2 mg/person on day 1 and then daily 1.6 mg at day 2-5 in sesame oil. AM measured by HPLC-ECD (diamonds) and computer fitted curves (solid-line) [262]. Mean parasite densities versus time measured by microscopy (empty squares) and computer fitting curve (dashed line) [263] are from malaria human trials. The parasitemia was counted 100% at zero while the first dosing time.

The intramuscular AE was neither able to exterminate parasites rapidly, nor to reduce parasitemia much in patients. The computer modeling estimated that the 0.550% parasitemia was the E_{max} in this clinical trial. In spite of two doses on day 1 (4.8 mg/kg at 0 hr and 1.6 mg/kg at 6 hr), the MPC was still the highest value compared to other four artemisinins (table 17).

5.4.5. Artemisinin

PK/PD evaluation in plasma following artemisinin (QHS) oral administration of 500 mg/person on first day followed by 250 mg twice daily for 4 days and then another 500 mg on 6th day is seen in figure 16. After 500 mg of QHS by oral dosing, the mean peak plasma concentration of QHS was reached at 588 ng/ml and then declined with elimination half-life calculated at 2.4 hr. Mean AUC of QHS was estimated at 2601 ng·h/ml, which was the highest AUC in comparison due to the highest oral dose taken. At 500 mg dosage regimen orally, the lag time in the parasitemia curve was 5.76 hr, which was longer than oral AS (2.81 hr) and DHA (4.03 hr) but was better than AM and AE trials (figure 11, bottom), indicating that fast effect of QHS capsules was not as good as oral AS and DHA even given the higher doses [197, 260, 266]. The patients treated with oral QHS showed a 13.95 hr of PC_{50} and the 1464.4 %·h/µl. of AUEC (table 17).

The absorption of QHS capsules with 1.21 hr half-life was slower than the absorptions of AS and DHA drugs, suggesting that the slow reduction of parasitemia may have resulted from the slow absorption. Compared with oral AS and DHA study, oral QHS appeared to have very low bioavailability of 30% [267, 268] and low antimalarial potency [1-4].

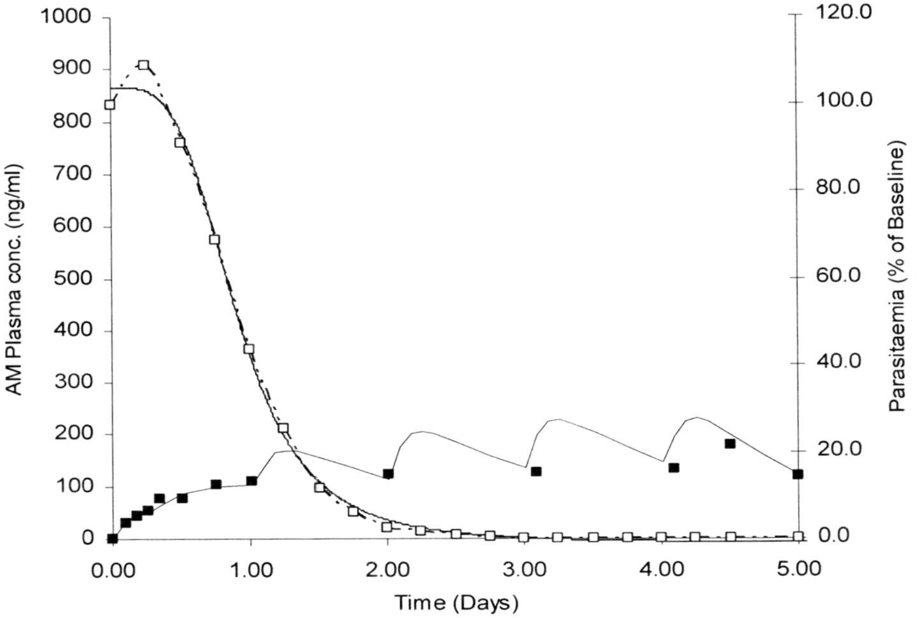

Figure 15. Pharmacokinetic/pharmacodynamic profiles are in plasma following arteether (AE) intramuscular administration of 4.8 mg/person at 0 hr and 1.6 mg/kg at 6 hr on day 1 and then daily 1.6 mg at day 2-5 in sesame oil. AE measured by HPLC-ECD (diamonds) and computer fitted curves (solid-line) [200]. Mean parasite densities versus time measured by microscopy (empty squares) and computer fitting curve (dashed line) [22, 200] are from malaria human trials. The parasitemia was counted 100% at zero while the first dosing time.

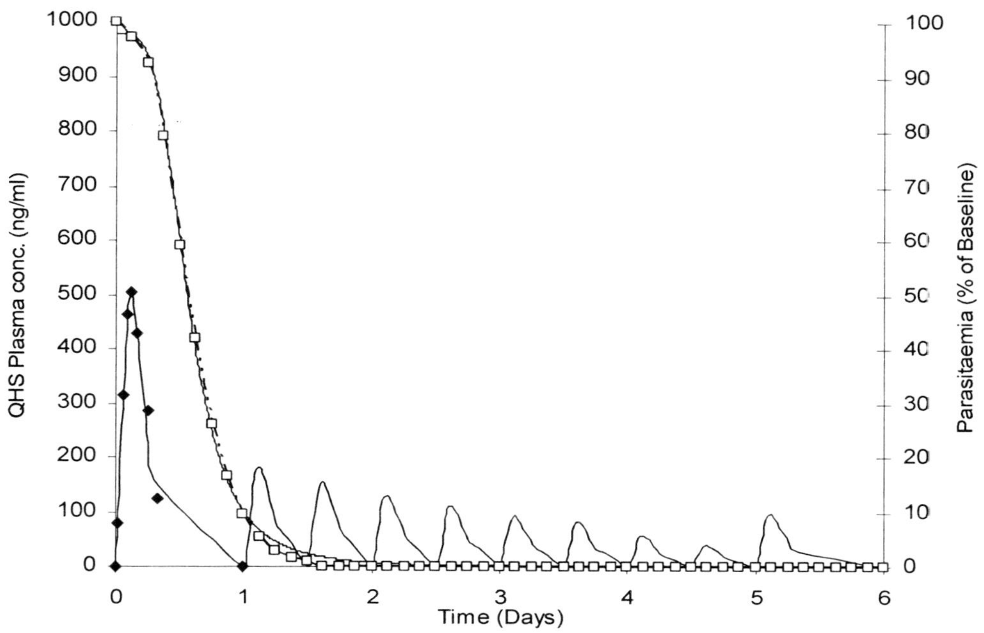

Figure 16. Pharmacokinetic/pharmacodynamic profiles are in plasma following artemisinin (QHS) oral administration of 500 mg/person on first day followed by 250 mg twice daily for 4 days and then another 500 mg on 6th day. QHS measured by HPLC-ECD (solid diamond) and computer fitted curves (solid-line), which was simulated by declining metabolism of QHS in humans [197, 266]. Mean parasite densities versus time measured by microscopy (empty squire) and computer fitting curve (dashed line) are from malaria human trials [260]. The parasitemia was counted 100% at zero while the first dosing time.

The relationships of PK and PD have been evaluated for the five-artemisinin drugs above, and the impressive inputs for each drug with the regimen could be summarized as follows:

1. Without intravenous PK/PD data, oral AS is the fastest killer in the malaria treatments out of the other four artemisinins. Oral AS can provide the highest peak concentration and very short exposure time (figure 12-15); the former as the role to eliminate parasites rapid (figure 11, bottom) and the latter to avoid fatal neurotoxicity (Section 3.5.) and to prevent resistance.
2. Although DHA has similar efficacy to AS in vitro [1-4], the agent does not have a rapid effect like that of AS even with double oral doses. The explanations include lower bioavailability [269, 270], slower absorption phase, and long lag time on effect activity. However, the principle reason is due to the lower peak concentration in the treated humans when compared to oral AS.
3. Intramuscular AM or AE reveals a low efficacy and slow parasite killing. Due to the sesame oil formulation, AM and AE have a very low and prolonged absorption from muscle injection sites [187]. In the beginning, parasitemia counts after dosing did not decrease due to the low and delayed peak concentrations (75-110 ng/ml) of AM and AE. The low peak concentration may be the reason why the lag time is longer for

7.2-8.9 hr without parasites killing after injection. Similarly, there is very slow clearance rate on parasites with mean PC_{50} time of 15.63-19.68 hr, which may have resulted in inadmissible failures in AE trials [200]. Although the drug exposure times of AM and AE are much longer than AS, DHA and QHS, the long exposure time did not assist efficacy. Instead, it induced neurotoxicity (Section 3.5.), therefore, the formulation would not be encouraged to use in humans to treat acute and severe malarias.

4. Oral artemisinin (QHS) does not show well in this PK/PD comparison probably due to the highest oral dose (500 mg/person). Although the high dose produced a higher plasma concentration (2601 ng·h/ml of AUC) and high peak concentration (588 ng/ml), the low relative antimalarial potency [1-4] and slow bioavailability [268] considerably limited the efficacy. It suggests that the artemisinin derivatives with lower antimalarial potency still can not produce rapid effects even at an increased dose level.

5.5. Rapid Efficacy Affected by Drug Peak Level and Antimalarial Potency

PK/PD evaluation indicates that the effect of parasitemia decrease appeared to be significantly slower (2.8-8.9 hours) than the decline of drugs, reflecting a sum mean of the lag phase time, stages effect time, and even body elimination time with the different compounds and dosage regimens, suggesting that PD effects are longer than PK outcomes. The elimination half lives in PK were in the range of 0.7-22.7 hr, whereas the PC_{50} in PD were in the range of 8.48-19.68 hr. In this evaluation, AS is pharmacokinetically and pharmacodynamically superior to other four artemisinins for the treatment of malaria, demonstrating the most rapid killing activities with greater E_{max} in the PD analysis after oral administration. AS showed the highest peak concentration, the fastest and most reliable oral absorption rate, and the most limited drug exposure time than other four artemisinins. Although AM and AE showed the longest half lives and the highest exposure level (high AUC values), they had the worst efficacy (the longest lag time, the greatest AUEC, and the longest PC_{50}) due to the slowest absorption rate and the lowest peak concentration (table 17). However, the inadmissible failure (48.0-86.8% curative rates) in those monotherapies led us to either re-assess their importance or seek alternative approaches (table 4):

1. In vitro, at dose range 10^{-7}-10^{-5} M (30 –3000 ng/ml), synchronous culture study shows that artemisinin is rapidly effective against both rings and schizonts, demonstrating 100% growth inhibition of these stages within 4-6 h. The inhibitory effects of AM are more gradual, requiring 8-10 hr of exposure time to achieve 70% growth inhibition of the ring and 40-50% inhibition of schizonts stages. DHA is found to be highly effective against all stages of the parasite, in most cases achieving 100% growth inhibition by 2-4 hr [5]. Concentration of 10^{-6}-10^{-5} M (280-2800 ng/ml) artemisinin shows a parasitical effect after only 3 hr of drug exposure, whereas 10^{-7} M (28 ng/ml) artemisinin requires 24 hr of exposure for a cidal effect [251]. It is clear that the low dose will increase the exposure time, and high dose will

shorten the treatment period. Therefore, the low dose range cannot be selected for artemisinin drugs in human treatments in malaria because i) the artemisinins have very short half-lives, and ii) longer exposure time of artemisinins is principle factor to induce the fatal neurotoxicity.

In addition, in treating patients with severe and complicated malaria, where the ultimate survival of the patient is the key; low effective doses cannot be used without an undue delay in the necessary treatment time [252]. There is no evidence that rapid parasite killing with high sufficient doses is harmful and that the therapeutic blood drug concentration should be achieved as quickly as possible without danger of toxicity [247]. Therefore, the plasma concentration of the artemisinin derivatives in human against *P. falciparum* should at least be in the range of 10^{-6}-10^{-5} (300-3000 ng/ml) or even higher for AS or DHA as the more potent compounds. AE or AM should have higher plasma concentrations (more than that of AS or DHA). AL, being the lowest potency agent in regards to the first drug exposure [1-4], should have the highest plasma concentration.

2. Artemisinins reliably reduce initial malaria parasitemia by a factor of 10^4 per 48 hour. Therefore, asexual cycle and modeling studies suggest that six days of treatment should cure parasite burdens of up to 10^{12} parasites [271]. This model is difficult to reconcile with the high recrudescence rates (10%–15%) seen with artemisinin monotherapy and is also difficult to recognize with a higher potency agent (AS or DHA) and with higher concentrations. This poor efficacy of cure in the monotherapy, which is not due to resistance [272], is usually attributed to the intrinsically lower peak concentration of artemisinins, which has been demonstrated in the above PK/PD evaluation.

The pharmacokinetic factors are not only focusing on the high peak concentration, but are also concentrating on tissue distribution in red blood cells of artemisinins [184]. More recently, the tissue distribution in rats and protein binding in human blood were conducted in WRAIR laboratory. Table 18 demonstrates the RBC/plasma ratios of five radiolabeled artemisinins in human whole blood at various concentrations [45, and our unpublished data]. For equal volumes of RBC and plasma, the fraction of the five artemisinins found in the RBC is lower than in the plasma in normal volunteer blood. The ratios are almost constant in human blood over a broad range of concentration. After correction for the 55:45 ratios of plasma and RBC volumes, the RBC/plasma ratios are 0.23 for ^{14}C-AE, 0.28 for ^{14}C-AM, 0.44 for ^{14}C-AL, 0.52 for ^{14}C-DHA, and 0.71 for ^{14}C-AS, indicating that the radioactivity remained in human RBC is the highest for AS and the lowest for AE.

The big advantage of DHA and AS is its readiness of entering human red blood cell (0.52 and 0.71 ratio of RBC/plasma, respectively) compared to AE and AM (0.23 and 0.28 ratio of RBC/plasma, respectively). It means that to reach same targets (RBC) the drug peak concentrations for AE and AM should be required to be two to three times higher than that of DHA and AS. In addition, the binding affinities are high for AE and AM radiolabels with 1945 and 1673 ng/ml of 50% bound concentration in human plasma (BC_{50}). Conversely, the binding affinities are low for AS and DHA radioactivities with 143 and 162 ng/ml of BC_{50}, indicating the free drug concentration can be much higher in human plasma with AS or DHA than that with AE and AM.

Table 18. The bound ratios of human red blood cells (RBC) and plasma with ^{14}C-AE, ^{14}C-AM, ^{14}C-AL, ^{14}C-DQHS, and ^{14}C-AS in human whole blood from low to high concentration with incubated dialysis method at 37°C [165]

Concentration (MW)	^{14}C-AE (312.4)	^{14}C-AM (298.4)	^{14}C-AL (418.5)	^{14}C-DHA (284.9)	^{14}C-AS (384.4)
0.125 nM	0.20 ± 0.01	0.28 ± 0.01	0.43 ± 0.01	0.52 ± 0.03	0.72 ± 0.05
0.25 nM	0.24 ± 0.03	0.27 ± 0.01	0.44 ± 0.02	0.53 ± 0.04	0.71 ± 0.03
0.5 nM	0.22 ± 0.02	0.28 ± 0.01	0.47 ± 0.02	0.52 ± 0.05	0.73 ± 0.05
1 nM	0.23 ± 0.02	0.27 ± 0.02	0.43 ± 0.03	0.51 ± 0.03	0.74 ± 0.04
2 nM	0.22 ± 0.01	0.26 ± 0.01	0.45 ± 0.02	0.50 ± 0.03	0.74 ± 0.06
4 nM	0.23 ± 0.01	0.29 ± 0.02	0.45 ± 0.01	0.51 ± 0.04	0.69 ± 0.06
8 nM	0.24 ± 0.03	0.27 ± 0.02	0.45 ± 0.02	0.53 ± 0.03	0.64 ± 0.04
16 nM	0.25 ± 0.03	0.29 ± 0.03	0.44 ± 0.02	0.51 ± 0.04	
Mean value	0.23 ± 0.02	0.28 ± 0.02	0.44 ± 0.02	0.52 ± 0.04	0.71 ± 0.08

All values represent mean ± SD for n = 4 individual samples, AE = arteether, AM = artemether, AL = artelinic acid, DHA = dihydroartemisinin; MW = molecular weight.

3. Although DHA tablets and AM intramuscular formulation have a similar AUC compared to AS tablets (table 17), their efficacies are much lower than that of AS tablets (figure 11, bottom). The initial killing of parasites do not appear to be done very well by the two drug regimens because they do not have enough high peak concentration to cover all red blood cells. The uptake of DHA in infected erythrocytes has been shown to be 300 times higher than in the uninfected erythrocytes, and the maximum uptake of the drug occurs after 1-2 hr [265]. In this case, as we discussed above, the plasma concentration of the artemisinin derivatives in human against *P. falciparum* should be much more than the range of 10^{-6}-10^{-5} (300-3000 ng/ml) for the first drug exposure in order to cover all RBC targets [251, 252]. In the report above, compared to oral AS, the other 4 artemisinins with oral and intramuscular formulations have a lower peak level, could not stop the parasite and cover all RBC in the initial several hours having greatly extended the lag and PC_{50} times.
4. High peak concentration (C_{max}) is also more important than high drug concentration (AUC) to cure malaria because sufficient drug is needed to cover all RBCs (including infected cells) in order to kill as many parasites as possible in the initial dosing. AUC concentration is counted during this period of time and very often lacks the necessary high peak concentrations. For example, in the AE clinical trial, the AUCs are higher than other four artemisinin drugs (table 17), but it has lower C_{max} value that results in poor efficacy. Therefore, the high concentration (AUC) without high peak level is not able to cover all RBCs; this could have given rise to some untreated RBCs, including infected cells. The untreated RBCs may be the reason for recrudescence in all monotherapy approaches with artemisinins. In addition, QHS is a low antimalarial potency agent [1-4]. Even though oral doses 5-fold higher than AS

have been given to patients in trials, QHS still demonstrates poor efficacy because its peak concentration is only a half of that of AS, suggesting that any artemisinin drug with lower antimalarial potency should not be used in malaria treatment.

In conclusion, the rapid efficacy of artemisinins is principally dependent on drug peak concentration (C_{max}) in the first drug exposure and drug relative antimalarial potency. The relative antimalarial potency is maintained by the capability for killing various stages of parasites, rapid oral absorption, high peak concentration, plasma protein binding, drug distribution in targets (RBCs), and membrane permeability of RBCs in infected subjects. Other factors of the pharmacokinetic parameters, such as drug exposure level (AUC) and drug exposure time (half-life), tend to be of minor significance when considering efficacy.

6. How to Maintain Rapid Efficacy and Avoid Lethal Toxicities

6.1. Deserting Some of the Artemisins

Artemisinin compounds have impressive parasiticidal properties in vitro, rapidly arresting parasite metabolism in concentrations within the lower nanomolar range and killing parasites more quickly than other antimalarial drugs [264]. These compounds have variously been formulated for oral, rectal, and parenteral administrations. AE was developed under the sponsorship of the World Health Organization despite lacking clear advantages over AM, for which a much larger clinical experience already exists; AE is no longer being investigated as an antimalarial agent because AE is not better than AM either in efficacy or in pharmacokinetic profiles in our PK/PD analysis (table 17) with a more slow absorption from muscle [22, 200] and therapeutic efficacy summary of the clinical trials (table 4). However, locally formulated intramuscular products are used in India (α and β arteether) and the Netherlands (β-arteether, Artemotil). Data from India showed that α and β–AE dissolved in peanut oil have good efficacy in uncomplicated and even severe malaria with 6.7-14.0% recrudescence (re-infection) and 8.5% mortality in the patients with severe malaria [39-43, 273-274]. Although pharmacokinetic results of α and β-AE are not available from humans, some animal studies (rats and monkeys) demonstrated that the C_{max} of α and β-AE with peanut oil could reach levels up to 160-360 ng/ml [275-277] suggesting that the C_{max} profile is better than β-AE alone dissolved in sesame oil with a C_{max} in the range of 78-161 ng/ml in rats and monkeys after first dosing (figure 2, 3, 6).

Artemisinin (QHS) itself is a highly crystalline compound that does not dissolve in oil or water; thus, QHS can only be given by the oral route. This may be the reason that the oral efficacy of QHS in humans is poor [260] and that the oral efficacy of QHS is also inferior with regards to pharmacokinetic benefit [197, 266]. Since humans were last reported to use QHS tablets in 1998 [278], no recent reports have been found for using QHS to treat malaria. For these derivatives, the sodium salts of AS and AL are used for parenteral administration. AL (a water soluble derivative) was at one time under development by the Walter Read Army Institute of Research. Although AL has not been further developed since 2003 (principally due to a 3-fold higher toxicity than AS [66, 179]), various formulations and combinations of AS with other antimalarials are under active development.

That these three artemisinins (AE, QHS, and AL) are paid less attention today with respect to further development is not a surprise. AE clinical trials with sesame oil in humans [200] have been pharmacokinetically inferior to other artemisinins demonstrated (table 17). In addition, QHS and AL have shown poor efficacy due to the lower relative antimalarial potency [1-4] – not to mention suffering the moderate toxicity of AL [66]. These results suggest that only AS, AM, and DHA are suitable for further advanced development and treatment in humans with the advent of artemisinin-based combination therapy for uncomplicated malaria or using monotherapy for severe and complicated malaria.

6.2. Artemisinin-Based Combination Therapy (ACT) for Uncomplicated Malaria

Artemisinin-based combination therapies (ACTs) hold considerable promise for both increased efficacy and for retardation in the rate of development of parasite resistance. Recently, WHO has endorsed ACTs as the "policy standard" for all malaria infections in areas where *P. falciparum* is the predominant infecting species [128]. ACT has been shown to improve cure rates, decrease malaria transmission and decrease antimalarial resistance on the north-west border of Thailand [126]. Also, enhanced cure rates and decreased gametocyte carriage has been confirmed in clinical trials in Africa as well [279-280].

Due to the rapid parasite clearance of artemisinin drugs in treating early cases of uncomplicated malaria, ACTs may both prevent the progression of malaria to severe disease and reduce severe cases as well as mortality. AM-Lumefantrine is the first registered, fixed, ACT treatment, which constitutes about 70% of all current clinically-used ACTs [129]. It is highly effective when given orally twice a day for three days (6-dose) with a small amount of fat [130, 131]. In the PK/PD evaluation above, intramuscular AM did not show exciting efficacy, pointing to pharmacokinetic disadvantages in humans. How could the AM reveal successful therapy after oral administration in the combination with lumefantrine?

A pharmacokinetic study exhibited that the oral administration of AM has greater pharmacokinetic advantage than that of intramuscular AM in humans. The antimalarial activity of AM following oral or intramuscular administration in the plasma of 15 adults with acute uncomplicated *P. falciparum* malaria was measured by bioassay. The peak concentrations (C_{max}) in plasma following oral administration were higher in patients in the acute phase (median, 541.8 ng/ml of DHA) than in patients in the convalescent phase (median, 271.6 ng/ml of DHA). Antimalarial activity in terms of the peak concentration in plasma (541.8 ng/ml) after oral administration was a median of 16 times higher than that after intramuscular administration (34.4 ng/ml). The ratio of the area under the plasma concentration-time curve during the first 24 h (AUC_{0-24}) after oral administration of AM to the AUC_{0-24} after intramuscular administration was a median of 3.3. In the acute phase, the time to C_{max} was significantly shorter after oral administration (median, 1 h) than after intramuscular administration (median, 8 h). Intramuscular AM is absorbed very slowly in patients with acute malaria [281]. Similar studies also reported that the oral AM produced

C_{max} from 406 to 818 ng/ml that are 5.5-11.2 folds higher than that of intramuscular AM [29, 46, 172, 282, 283].

Another commonly used ACT treatment, AS-mefloquine, has been distributed widely since 1994 as the first-line treatment in South-East Asian countries such as Thailand and Cambodia and remains highly effective for uncomplicated falciparum malaria. Under the WHO system of efficacy assessment, more than 95% of patients will remain free of malaria 28 days after such treatment (E2) [134, 135]. In uncomplicated malaria, when artemisinins are used orally, most pharmacokinetic information is now available for AS. In present report, the PK/PD evaluation demonstrated that oral AS is pharmacokinetically and pharmacodynamically superior to the other four artemisinins for the treatment of malaria. The absolute bioavailability of antimalarial activity after a single dose of oral AS in uncomplicated adult malaria is about 60% [91, 173]. Peak concentration (C_{max}) of DHA after oral AS can easily reach between 519 and 1309 ng/ml in many clinical trials [91, 173, 254, 269, 270, 284]. If the values of DHA and AS are included, the total C_{max} (624-1522 ng/ml) are significantly higher than that after oral AM (406-818 ng/ml) and that after oral DHA (466-1143 ng/ml) [269, 270, 282, 285, 286]. Although absolute bioavailability studies for oral AM and DHA are not possible given lack of intravenous formulations, pharmacodynamic activity (parasite clearance) after oral dosing of these derivatives is satisfactory but less than that of oral AS. Therefore, only four ACTs with AM and AS (without DHA) were recommended currently by a WHO Expert Consultative Group in 2001; there are AM-lumefantrine (Coartem), AS-mefloquine (Artequin), AS-amodiaquine, and AS-sulfadoxine/pyrimethamine [127].

In addition, oral formulation of AS and AM result in a great conversion of drugs to DHA in malaria patients. Actually, oral AS and AM are the prodrug of DHA with ratios of 1.4-8.6 for DHA/AM and 6.4-9.7 for DHA/AS (table 8) [161-173]. Following GI absorption (first-pass effects) and conversion (hydrolysis) of AS and AM, the concentration of DHA has a very large variability, from 248 to 8840 ng·h/ml (AUC values) in individual patients [161]. Four patients who were not cured by the oral AM regimen used in this study and had significantly lower plasma concentrations of DHA, the metabolite of AM [25]. Using same dose amount as AM, a much lower AUC (834 ng·h/ml) was detected in the four patients compared to the AUC (3684 ng·h/ml) in the other 46 patients. The low level of DHA present is likely responsible for the treatment failures.

However, these combinations still have some dosing difficulties. The AM-lumefantrine should ideally be given with food (preferably containing fat) to ensure adequate absorption and thus efficacy. In the initial study, the 4-dose AM-lumefantrine regimen showed a relatively high rate of late treatment failure (E1) [132]. In one study, the 6-dose AM-lumefantrine regimen was associated with a 28% treatment failure at 14 days in an area with high-grade mefloquine resistance (E3) [133]. Another commonly used ACT treatment, AS-mefloquine, has been used in South-East Asian countries such as Thailand and Cambodia quite widely since 1994 and remains highly effective for uncomplicated falciparum malaria. However, the failure rate of AS-mefloquine combination was up to 13% in Thailand and Cambodia [136], and the neuropsychiatric effects of mefloquine as well as its relative expense are problematic [137].

6.3. Injectable AS for Severe and Complicated Malaria

Peak concentration (C_{max}) is more important than plasma concentration (AUC) in producing the improved efficacy of antimalarial drugs that has been confirmed in the above PK/PD evaluation. Moreover, it is the antimalarial activity with high killing capability in blood in the first few hours following the first administration of a parenteral drug that is critical from a therapeutic standpoint, particularly in patients with severe malaria, in whom mortality can reach between 15% and 20%, despite appropriate antimalarial and supportive treatment [138].

When the peak concentration reaches 1052 ng/ml of DHA in plasma after a single 100 mg oral dose of AS [91, 260], it obtains the best efficacy in uncomplicated malaria compared to the other four-artemisinin drugs (figure 11 and table 17), and there is a total molecular number of DHA of 2.11 x 10^{12}/ml in plasma. This should be 0.87 x 10^{12}/ml in RBC (hematocrit =0.41), with the DHA molecular number at 94.5 in each erythrocyte in healthy subjects including other artemisinin derivatives that are mainly bound with RBC membranes [287]. This calculation is according to the data of DHA ratio of RBC/human plasma (table 18) and protein binding capacity of DHA at 1000 ng/ml (figure 17) in humans [288].

We know that the uptake of DHA in infected erythrocytes has been shown to be 300 times more than the uninfected erythrocytes *in vitro* [265], this is because the malaria parasite *P. falciparum* induces some unselective cation conductance in the RBC membrane that changes the permeability [289]. An in-patient who has 1% of erythrocyte infected malaria, with all drugs at C_{max} of 1052 ng/ml on average, the amount entering infected RBCs would be only 100 times higher than uninfected RBCs. In 5% or 20% RBC infected patients; the uptake of DHA in infected RBCs would be only 5 or 20 times higher than that in uninfected RBCs. Although we do not know the degree of DHA uptake by RBCs in malarial human, it is suggested that the high concentration (1052 ng/ml) in malaria patients is still not sufficient to distribute the drug to every erythrocyte (infected and uninfected) in each patient (from 1-20% infected RBC). Therefore, it is clear that the peak level at 1000 ng/ml in plasma is far from enough to cure the severe malaria with a hyperparasitemia. In this estimation, the minimum peak concentration for hyperparasitemia (> 5%) will be at least at 10,000-15,000 ng/ml.

Fortunately, the intravenous AS can provide sufficiently high peak concentration in the patients with a fast exposure time. In current clinical trials, the C_{max} was shown to be from 112 - 16149 ng/ml resulting from a dose of 120 mg/person or 2.4 mg/kg in various malaria including severe malaria [91, 173, 270, 290, 291]. Although those dose regimens are still not enough to cure severe and complicated malaria 100% of the time [91, 173, 270, 290, 291], there is now convincing evidence that for those who do develop severe malaria, intravenous AS will reduce the risk of death by approximately one-third [145, 146]. It is also encouraging is that intravenous AS is also safer and easier to use than injectable quinine [138].

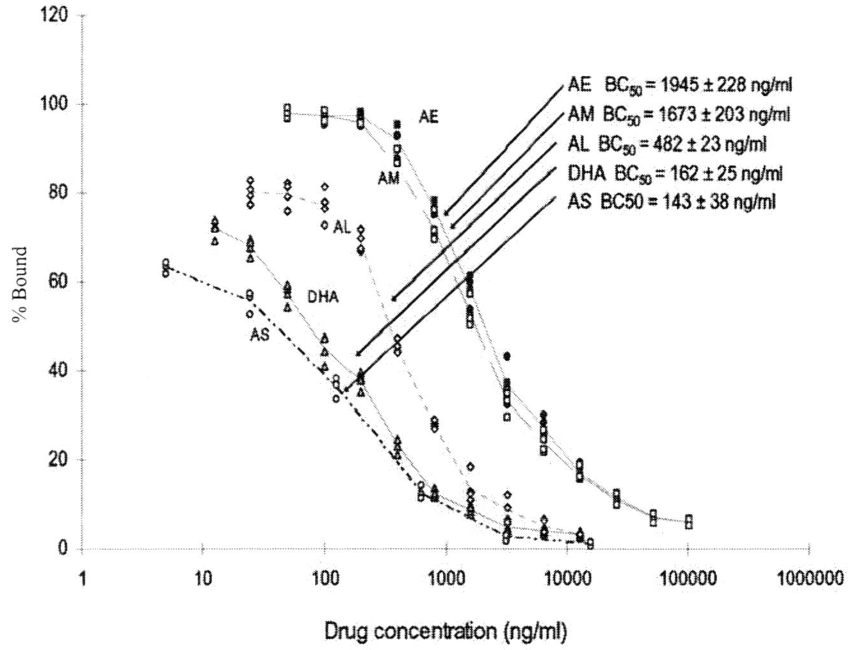

Figure 17. Comparison of 50% bound concentration (BC_{50}) of artemether (AM), arteether (AE), artelinic acid (AL), artesunate (AS) and dihydroartemisinin (DQHS) at varied concentration in human plasma samples by microdialysis equilibrium method at 37°C for 6 hours (n = 4).

Recently, there was a milestone clinical trial in the treatment development for severe malaria. Previous trials using intramuscular AM demonstrated less toxicity but no clear mortality benefit over quinine [141], most likely due to the erratic absorption of the intramuscularly administered oil-based preparation of AM [144]. More recent trials have used intravenous AS, a water-soluble derivative with a more favorable pharmacokinetic profile. The SEAQUAMAT trial, a multicentre randomized trial conducted in Bangladesh, Myanmar, Indonesia and India, recently reported a 34.7% reduction in mortality associated with intravenous AS compared with intravenous quinine [145, 146].

In this trial, AS with 5% $NaHCO_3$ buffer (Artesunate for Injection, Guilin) administered intravenously effectively clears parasites at or above 1 mg/kg administered daily or twice on the first day. Regimens using 2.4 mg/kg clear parasites and resolve fever more quickly than intravenous quinine with fewer side effects. Comparative studies to parenteral quinine demonstrated statistically significant reductions in parasite clearance times, yet most studies have not shown significant differences in coma resolution times. Clinical side effects in these efficacy trials have been rare but include rash (hives or a red rash) and possibly a higher incidence of blackwater fever. Minor side effects and laboratory abnormalities are often impossible to distinguish from the full array of pathophysiologic effects of severe malaria [145]. In SEAQUAMAT, intravenous AS was again well tolerated. There was a statistically ($p = 0.009$) significant reduction in hypoglycemia post study entry, which is a known side effect of quinine and quinidine. There were no differences in the incidence of hemodynamic shock, convulsions, dialysis or mechanical ventilation. There was a higher non-statistical rate of hemoglobinuria and neurological sequelae in the AS group among survivors, which may reflect the survival of severe cerebral cases who may have died in the quinine group. No other significant adverse events were attributed to AS [145, 146].

This is the largest trial ever performed in severe malaria and the first to demonstrate conclusively a mortality reduction over standard quinine therapy. This is good news for malaria-endemic areas in South-East Asia. The burden of malaria in this region is far worse than previously thought, with over 120 million cases each year in south/south-east Asia. The World Health Organization now advocates the use of ACT for uncomplicated malaria [137], a move that is likely to reduce the number of people who develop the severe disease. In making the case for WHO and the international physician community to accept injectable AS in the role of the preferred treatment for severe malaria, two proposals are offered here:

1) The monotherapy of intravenous AS should still be used.

To treat severe malaria, the monotherapy of injectable AS is needed in the first couple days in order to rapidly rescue lives and possibly reduce mortality. The TropNetEurop is recommending using intravenous AS to cure the patients with severe malaria [147] because they have been encouraged by the large and successful SEAQUAMAT trials in Asian. Unfortunately, there is currently no product available that is produced under good manufacturing practice (GMP) conditions.

Patients with malaria in rural areas may be obtunded or be experiencing bouts of vomiting, making them unable to take oral medications and leading to significant delay in treatment if facilities for parenteral treatment are unavailable. In such circumstances, the intravenous or rectal route of administration is attractive because rural healthcare workers can be trained to identify moderate and severe malaria and administer intravenous or rectal drugs before transfer of patients to hospital; of course, this assumes that the intravenous or rectal route of administration is culturally acceptable in these areas.

There are some cases, highlighted especially in patients with uncomplicated hyperparasitemic falciparum malaria (> 4% infected RBC), who are at risk of severe malaria and treatment failure. These infections require a three to five day course of treatment with oral agents. The only alternative is parenteral quinine, which is less effective (145, 146), more expensive, and less well tolerated [140]. In addition, in the second and third trimesters of pregnancy, injectable AS is also a better drug for uncomplicated malaria, but it needs to be given for long term oral treatment course with a dose adjustment because of the altered kinetics in pregnant women [112, 207]. Physicians would like to prescribe appropriate antimalarial therapy without the need for oral tablets but this is unlikely to be possible in the near future, especially for injectable AS [148, 149]. They also hope that some manufacturers will continue to supply injectable AS alone to be used in specific circumstances.

2) Loading dose of intravenous AS for severe and complicated malaria should be pursued.

All cases of falciparum malaria are potentially severe and life threatening, especially when managed inappropriately. A major reason for progression from mild through complicated to severe disease is missed or delayed diagnosis. Once diagnosed, the priority for treatment of complicated and severe disease is the parenteral administration of adequate, safe doses of an appropriate antimalarial, in the setting of the highest possible level of clinical care. Supportive management of complications such as coma, convulsions, metabolic acidosis, hypoglycemia, fluid and electrolyte disturbances, renal failure, secondary infections, bleeding disorders and anemia is also important. The most recent advance in decreasing mortality has been the use of intravenous AS instead of injection quinine [145. 146], which may very well revolutionize the management of severe disease [148]. However, recrudescence is still relatively high with monotherapy of intravenous AS alone [292]. Since recrudescence is not due to parasite resistance [78], one possible explanation of this parasitological failure may be a low peak concentration after first loading dose with the intravenous AS.

Currently, the therapeutic dosages of injectable AS to treat severe and complicated malaria are in the range of 2-2.4 mg/kg alone. The dose was designed in accordance with prior experience of physicians concerned with neurotoxicity, to reduce dose-dependent hemotoxicity, to prevent a submaximal antimalarial effect, and to keep a minimum curative rate (> 90%) during over twenty years of treatments [12, 161]. However, as this report describes in previous sections, this regimen will only produce 112 - 16149 ng/ml of C_{max} with great variability, which is a lower peak concentration than needed for patients with hyperparasitemia (ie. the C_{max} in the malaria patients with a high variability). In theory, the patients with severe malaria require 10,000-15,000 ng/ml peak concentration to cover each RBC, including infected cells, because the infected cell can concentrate 300-fold more DHA than normal RBC during the first 1-2 hr after dosing. The large variability in pharmacokinetics and pharmacodynamics by using AS should also be considered.

In an individual patient, several factors determine the profile of drug pharmacodynamics and pharmacokinetics. The stage and synchronicity of the infecting parasite population and the multiplication rate of sequestered mature stages (schizonts) determine the initial parasitemia time profile after drug administration [293]. If the patient is admitted to hospital at a time when a significant proportion of the parasites are undergoing schizogony, then parasitemia will rise following antimalarial drug treatment as schizonts rupture and release merozoites, which then invade new erythrocytes to produce circulating ring stages. These stages can be seen by the microscopist and counted, whereas the sequestered stages are not seen and therefore are not counted. The implication is that parasitemia will fall. If the majority of the parasites in the blood are young rings, and a drug which has little effect on the ring stage is used in treatment, then parasitemia will plateau and fall later as a result of sequestration [9, 293].

The overall individual parasitemia profile thus represents a hybrid of these different processes, and a population of patients provides a series of very different parasitemia profiles. As a result there is considerable inter-individual variance in parasite clearance profiles, although it is reasonable to assume that the distribution of parasite stages should be random in a patient population as there is no particular reason why a patient should present one level of parasite development – and not another – in the hospital. Thus, even before attempting to assess the effect of the drug in vivo, there is considerable inter-patient variance in the pharmacodynamic variables [68]. This means that the intravenous dose should be increased to a higher level (4-8 mg/kg) than current use for the loading dose. However, the question remains: is this intravenous dose safe for treatment of severe and complicated malaria?

Compared to oral AS, the injectable AS is superior in pharmacokinetics and pharmacodynamics to the oral AS and other four artemisinins in treating patients with severe malaria; injectable AS shows the highest peak concentration, the fastest effective time, rapid elimination, and a very short exposure moment compared to oral AS (table 5) [44]. As discussed in Section 3, the drug exposure time of artemisinins is the principle factor responsible for induction of neurotoxicity in animal species. Therefore, the active metabolites (DHA), the drug distributed in CNS, and/or the drug exposure level play relatively less important roles than the drug exposure time. The water-soluble artemisinins, AS in particular, have very short half-lives and produce limited exposure time in animal species and humans, indicating that once-daily oral or intravenous administration of AS is relatively safe. In fact, the animal experiments demonstrated that no neurotoxicity (pathologically or behaviourally) has been observed in animal species following intravenous administration at any repeated doses up to maximum tolerated doses (MTD). The MTD of AS was 240 mg/kg following intravenous injection daily in rats for 3 days, but no neurotoxicity was detected in these animals [66]. In another study, intravenous AS had no effect on neurotoxic scores at 120 mg/kg in sodium carbonate daily for 7 days (our unpublished data). After one intramuscular injection, a high dose of 420 mg/kg of AS did not produce any neuronal necrosis in the rats. Also, up to 200 mg/kg of AS used orally daily for 5-7 days did not exhibit neuronal changes or any specific clinical signs [56]. Therefore, the 4-8 mg/kg dose level with intravenous formulation should be safe with regards to neurotoxicity [152] and also safe with regards to hemotoxicity [16, 179]. One study used a high dose of oral AS, up to 6 mg/kg, with the AS being extremely well tolerated; to date, there is no convincing evidence that dose as high as this of oral AS have any significant toxicity [68]. In our current Phase I clinical trials, the 2-8 mg/kg doses have been exceedingly well tolerated following both single and multiple intravenous injections in volunteers with our new formulation (our unpublished data). In malaria patients, this dose offers a satisfactory margin of safety and would be unlikely to produce a submaximal antimalarial effect.

Angus et al., in order to characterize the *in vivo* dose-response relationship for AS (and thus, rationalize dosing), 47 adult patients with acute uncomplicated falciparum malaria and parasitemia >1% were randomized to receive a single oral dose of AS varying between 0 and 250 mg together with a curative dose of oral mefloquine. Acceleration of parasite clearance was used as the pharmacodynamic variable. An inhibitory sigmoidal maximum effect (E_{max}) pharmacodynamic model typical of a dose-response curve was fitted to the relationship between dose and shortening of parasite clearance time (PCT). The E_{max} was estimated as 28.6 h, and the 50% effective concentration was 1.6 mg/kg of body weight. These results imply that there is no reduction in PCTs with the use of single oral doses of artesunate higher than 2 mg/kg, effectively reflecting the average lower limit of the maximally effective dose [68]. It is suggested that the 2 mg/kg is a maximum effective dose in those selected patients. However, the author also pointed out that this dosage of 2 mg/kg would be the lowest to give maximum effects in an "average" patient. When taking into account the considerable variance between individuals in both pharmacokinetics and pharmacodynamics [68, 161, 294], a larger dose would be required to ensure that a maximum effect was obtained in all patients. Therefore, the loading dose of injection AS is reasonable to increase to another higher level (4-8 mg/kg) for the consideration of WHO experts and investigators in the further development and treatment.

After the first drug exposure to reduce parasitemia below 1%, the maintaining dose could be significantly cut or switch (sequentially) to another slower acting and low dose antimalarial agents (not artemisinins) in order to protect AS from recrudescence or resistance and to optimize antimalarial therapy in severe and complicated malaria [295]. Because these artemisinins have excellent intrinsic activity, which produce reductions in asexual parasite biomass of up to 10,000-fold per cycle, these drugs still need to be present in therapeutic concentrations during four asexual life cycles, or 8 days [271]. Previous studies have shown that once-daily administration with the artemisinin derivatives provides equivalent cure rates relative to more frequent administration [296, 297]. This suggests that exposure of the infecting parasite population to therapeutic concentrations of drug twice each life cycle is sufficient for maximum effect [293].

7. Conclusion

Artemisinins have been used empirically in the treatment of malaria for twenty years during which time their mechanism of action and pharmacokinetic properties has been gradually cleared. Empirical judgments of efficacy and optimal administration have been influenced by their undoubtedly impressive parasite clearance kinetics, which are superior to other commonly used antimalarials. Among the artemisinins, the pharmacodynamic and pharmacokinetic profiles of AS are relatively more superior to the other four artemisinins.

The mechanisms that affect neurotoxicity and reproductive toxicity are currently understandable. The artemisinins exposure time has an imperative role in the induction of neurotoxicity in animal species. Other factors of the pharmacokinetic parameters, such as drug distribution in the brain, toxicity of active metabolite (DHA), or drug exposure level, tend to be of minor importance. The neurotoxicity could be avoided in reduction of drug exposure time. For reprotoxicity, the high peak concentration is the major reason to induce the embryotoxicity in animals, and also in the days of marked sensitivity corresponding to the period of yolk sac hematopoiesis, which occurs during GD 9–14 in rats or GD 15 to week 6 in humans. The reproductive toxicity should be also avoided in lock of the exposure of artemisinins in these sensitive days (humans in first trimester), which the critical period for induction of embryo damage and resorption, to protect pregnant women from malaria with treatment of artemisinin derivatives, especially via intravenous agent. There is agreement that the artemisinin derivatives should not be withheld at any stage of pregnancy, in cases of severe and complicated malaria, if the life of the mother is at risk. It is considerable that the oral regimens of artemisinins are much safer than parenteral administrations in pregnant patients.

This report has also observed that the rapid efficacy of artemisinins is principally at the mercy of drug peak concentration (C_{max}) in the first drug exposure and drug relative antimalarial potency. Other factors of the pharmacokinetic parameters, such as drug exposure level (AUC) and drug exposure time (half-life), tend to be of minor significance. Some artemisinins (AE, AL, and QHS) that can not produce higher peak concentration with existing regimens or possess less antimalarial potency have been deserted in current development and treatment. The fundamental and reliable measures of efficacy in cure and mortality rates for uncomplicated and severe malaria demonstrated that current artemisinins (AS, AM, and DHA) perform in roles as ACT or monotherapy to provide a clear-cut advantage over other antimalarials in some geographical locations. The most recent advance in decrease of the mortality (34.7%) has been the use of intravenous AS, as opposed to injection quinine. Artemisinins are poorly efficacious at curing malaria as monotherapy, but the shortage has been overcome by ACTs (AM-lumefantrine, AS-mefloquine, AS-amodiaquine, and AS-sulfadoxine/pyrimethamine) and will be overcome by injection AS used in combination or sequential administration with a slower acting antimalarial drug. In any case, previous arguments for the long-term benefits of combination or sequential therapies in preventing the resistance and recrudescence still stand. When considering fast parasite killing and variance between individuals in both pharmacokinetics and pharmacodynamics, a monotherapy and larger loading dose of injection AS should be required to ensure that a maximum effect is obtained in all patients with severe and complicated malaria.

Acknowledgments

This study was supported by the United States Army Research and Materiel Command. The opinions or assertions contained herein are the private views of the author and are not to be construed as official, or as reflecting true views of the Department of the Army or the Department of Defense.

References

[1] Xie, HL; Gerena, L; Kyle, DE; Milhous, WK; Zhang, J; Li, QG. Development and validation of flow cytometric measurement for parasitemia in cultures of *P. falciparum* vitally stained with YOYO-1. *Parasitology*, 2006 (submitted)

[2] Bustos, MDG; Gay, F; Diquet, B. In vitro tests on Philippine isolates of Plasmodium falciparum against four standard antimalarials and four qinghaosu derivatives. *Bull. World Health Organization*, 1994, 72, 729-735.

[3] Basco, LK; Bras, JLe. In vitro activity of artemisinin derivatives against African isolates and clones of Plasmodium falciparum. *Am. J. Trop. Med Hyg*. 1993, 49, 301-307.

[4] China Cooperative Research Group on Qinghaosu and Its Derivatives as Antimalarials. Antimalarial efficacy and mode of action of qinghaosu and its derivatives in experimental models. *J. Trad. Chinese Med*, 1982, 2, 17-24.

[5] Skinner, TS; Manning, LS; Johnston, WA; Davis, TME. In vitro stage-specific sensitivity of Plasmodium falciparum to quinine and artemisinin drugs. *Int. J. Parasit.* 1996, 26, 519-525.

[6] China Cooperative Research Group on Qinghaosu and Its Derivatives as Antimalarials. The chemistry and synthesis of qinghaosu derivatives. *J. Trad. Chinese Med.* 1982, 2, 9-16.

[7] Gu, HM; Warhurst, DC; Peters, W. Rapid action of Qinghaosu and related drugs on incorporation of ^{3}H-isoleucine by Plasmodium falciparum in vitro. *Biochem. Pharmacol.* 1983, 32: 2463-2466.

[8] Caillard, VA; Beaute-Lafitte, A; Chabaud, AG; Landau, I. Plasmodium vinckei petteri: identification of the stages sensitive to arteether. *Exp. Parasit.* 1992, 75, 449-456.

[9] ter Kuile, FT; White, NJ; Holloway, P; Pasvol, G; Krishna, S. Plasmodium falciparum: In vitro Studies of the pharmacodynamic properties of drugs used for the treatment of severe malaria. *Exp. Parasit.* 1993, 76, 85-95.

[10] Dutta, GP; Bajpai, R; Vishwakarma, RA. Blood schizontocidal activity of artemisinin and arteether against Plasmodium berghei. *J. Parasit.* 1987, 11, 253-257.

[11] Dutta, GP; Bajpai, R; Vishwakarma, RA. Comparison of antimalarial efficacy of artemisinin and arteether against Plasmodium cynomolgi B infection in monkeys. *Trans. R. Soc. Trop. Med. Hug.* 1989, 83, 56-57.

[12] Barradell, LB; Fitton, A. Artesunate, A review of its pharmacology and therapeutic efficacy in the treatment of malaria. *Drugs.* 1996, 50: 714-741.

[13] Geary, TG; Divo, AA; Jensen, JB. Stage specific actions of antimalarial drugs on Plasmodium falciparum in culture. *Am. J. Trop. Med. Hyg.* 1989, 40: 240-244.

[14] Woerdenbag, HJ; Pras, N; Uden, W; Wallaart, TE; Beekman, AC; Lugt, CB. Progress in the research of artemisinin-related antimalarials: an update. *Pharm. World Sci.* 16, 169-180.

[15] Tripathi, R; Puri, SK;. Dutta, GP. Sodium beta-artelinate - a new potential gametocytocide. *Exp. Parasit*, 1996, 82, 251-254.

[16] Navaratnam, V; Mansor, SM; Sit, NW; Grace, J; Li, QG; Olliaro, P. Pharmacokinetics of artemisinin-type compounds. *Clin. Pharmacokinet.* 2000, 39, 255-270.

[17] Shmuklarsky, MJ; Klayman, DL; Milhous, W.K; Rossan, RN; Ager AL; Tang, Jr. DB; Heiffer, MH; Canfield, CJ; Schuster, BG. Comparison of ß-artemether and ß-arteether against malaria parasites in vivo and in vitro., *Am. J. Trop. Med. Hyg.*, 1993, 48, 377-384.

[18] Lin, AJ; Klayman, DL; Milhous, WK. Antimalarial activity of new water-soluble dihydroartemisinin derivatives. *J. Med. Chem*, 1987, 30, 2147-2150.

[19] Tripathi, R; Dutta, GP; Vishwakarma, RA. Comparison of antimalarial efficacy of α, ß, and α/ß arteether against Plasmodium cynomolgi B infection in monkeys. *Am. J. Trop. Med. Hyg.* 1991, 44, 560-563.

[20] Maeno, Y; Brown, AE; Smith, CD; Tegoshi, T; Toyoshima, T; Ockenhouse, CF; Corcoran, KD; Ngampochjana, M; Kyle, DE; Webster HK, et al.: A nonhuman primate model for human cerebral malaria: effects of artesunate (qinghaosu derivative) on rhesus monkeys experimentally infected with plasmodium coatneyi. *Am. J. Trop. Med. Hyg.* 1993. 49, 726-734.

[21] Looareesuwan, S; Wilairatana, P. The rational use of qinghaosu and its derivatives: what is the future of new compounds? *Med. Trop.* 1998, 58 (Suppl 3), 89S-92S.

[22] Looareesuwan, S; Oosterhuis, B; Schilizzi, BM; Sollie, FA; Wilairatana, P; Krudsood, S; Lugt, CB; Peeters, PA; Peggins, JO. Dose-finding and efficacy study for i.m. artemotil (beta-arteether) and comparison with i.m. artemether in acute uncomplicated P. falciparum malaria. *Br. J. Clin. Pharm.* 2002, 53, 492-500.

[23] van Hensbroek, MB; Onyiorah, E; Jaffar, S; Schneider, G; Palmer, A; Frenkel, J; Enwere, G; Forck, S; Nusmeijer, A; Bennett, S; Greenwood, B; Kwiatkowski, D. A trial of artemether or quinine in children with cerebral malaria. *N. Engl. J. Med.* 1996, 335, 69-75.

[24] Tran, TH; Day, NP; Nguyen, HP; Nguyen, TH; Tran, TH; Pham, PL; Dinh, XS; Ly, VC; Ha, V; Waller, D; Peto, TE; White, NJ. A controlled trial of artemether or quinine in Vietnamese adults with severe falciparum malaria. *N. Engl. J. Med.* 1996, 335, 76-83.

[25] Karbwang, J; Na-Bangchang, K; Thanavibul, A; Molunto, P. Plasma concentrations of artemether and its major plasma metabolite, dihydroartemisinin, following a 5-day regimen of oral artemether, in patients with uncomplicated falciparum malaria. *Ann. Trop. Med. Parasit.* 1998, 92, 31-36.

[26] Looareesuwan, S; Wilairatana, P; Viravan, C; Vanijanonta, S; Pitisutitithum, P; Kyle, DE. Open randomized trial of oral artemether alone and a sequential combination with mefloquine for acute uncomplicated falciparum malaria. *Am. J. Trop. Med. Hyg.* 1997, 56, 613-617.

[27] Mohamed, SS; Khalid, SA; Ward, SA; Wan, TSM; Tang, HPO; Zheng, M; Haynes, RK; Edwards, G, Simultaneous determination of artemether and its major metabolite dihydroartemisinin in plasma by gas chromatography-mass spectrometry-selected ion monitoring. *J. Chromatograph.* 1999, B 731, 251-260

[28] Murphy, S; English, M; Waruiru, C; Mwangi, I; Amukoye, E; Crawley, J; Newton, C; Winstanley, P; Peshu, N; Marsh, K. An open randomized trial of artemether versus quinine in the treatment of cerebral malaria in African children. *Trans. R. Soc. Trop. Med. Hyg.* 1996, 90, 298-301.

[29] Na-Bangchang, K; Karbwang, J; Thomas, CG; Thanavibul, A; Sukontason, K; Ward, SA; Edwards, G. Pharmacokinetics of artemether after oral administration to health Thai males and patients with acute, uncomplicated falciparum malaria. *Br. J. Clin. Pharm.* 1994, 37, 249-253.

[30] Salako, LA; Walker, O; Sowunmi, A; Omokhodion, SJ; Adio, R; Oduola, AM. Artemether in moderately severe and cerebral malaria in Nigerian children. *Trans. R. Soc. Trop. Med. Hyg.* 1994, 88 Suppl 1, S13-5.

[31] Sowunmi, A; Oduola, AMJ. Efficacy of artemether in severe falciparum malaria in African children. *Acta Tropica.* 1996, 61, 57-63.

[32] Walter, O; Salako, LA; Omokhodion, SI; Sowunmi, A. An open randomized comparative study of intramuscular artemether and intravenous quinine in cerebral malaria in children. *Trans. R. Soc. Trop. Med. Hyg.* 1993, 87, 564-566.

[33] de Vries, PJ; Dien, TK. Clinical pharmacology and therapeutic potential of artemisinin and its derivatives in the treatment of malaria. *Drugs.* 1996, 52, 818-836.

[34] Looareesuwan, S; Wilairatana, P; Vanijanonta, S; Pitisuttithum, P; Ratanapong, Y; Andrial, M. Monotherapy with sodium artesunate for uncomplicated falciparum malaria in Thailand: a comparison of 5- and 7-day regimens. *Acta Trop.* 1997, 67, 197-205.

[35] Li, GQ; Wang, XH; Guo, XB; Fu, LC; Jian, HX; Chen, PQ; Li, GQ. Dose finding of dihydroartemisinin in treatment of falciparum malaria. *Southeast Asian J. Trop. Med. Pub. Health.* 1999, 30, 17-19.

[36] Looareesuwan, S; Wilairatana, P; Vanijanonta, S; Pitisuttithum, P; Viravan, C. Treatment of acute, uncomplicated, falciparum malaria with oral dihydroartemisinin. *Ann. Trop. Med. Parasit.* 1996. 90, 21-28.

[37] Wilairatana, P; Chanthavanich, P; Singhasivanon, P; Treeprasertsuk, S; Krudsood, S; Chalermrut, K; Phisalaphong, C; Kraisintu, K; Looareesuwan, S. A comparison of three different dihydroartemisinin formulations for the treatment of acute uncomplicated falciparum malaria in Thailand. *Intern. J. Parasit.* 1998, 28, 1213-1218.

[38] Xu, C; Ding, Y; Qi, Z. Efficacy of dihydroartemisinin in treatment of 37 malaria cases. *Zhonghua Nei Ke Za Zhi.* 1997, 36, 187-189.

[39] Mishra, SK; Asthana, OP; Mohanty, S; Patnaik, JK; Das, BS; Srivastava, JS; Satpathy, SK; Dash, S; Rath, PK; Varghese, K. Effectiveness of alpha, beta-arteether in acute falciparum malaria. *Trans. R. Soc. Trop. Med. Hyg.* 1995, 89, 299-301.

[40] Mohanty, S; Mishra, SK; Satpathy, SK; Dash, S; Patnaik, J. Alpha, beta-arteether for the treatment of complicated falciparum malaria. *Trans. R. Soc. Trop. Med. Hyg.* 1997, 91, 328-330.

[41] Mohapatr, PK; Khan, AM; Prakash, A; Mahanta, J; Srivastava, VK. Effect of arteether alpha/beta on uncomplicated falciparum malaria cases in Upper Assam. *Indian J. Med. Res* 1996, 104, 284-287.

[42] Singh N, Shukla MM, Asthana OP, Sharma VP, 1998. Effectiveness of alpha-beta arteether in clearing Plasmodium falciparum parasitemia in central India (Madhya Pradesh). *Southeast Asian J. Trop. Med. Pub. Health.* 29: 225-227.

[43] Valecha, N; Gupta, S; Usha, D; Biswas, S; Sharma, A; Adak, T; Asthana, OP; Sharma, VP. Efficacy of alpha, beta-arteether in acute uncomplicated *P. Falciparum* malaria. *Inter. J. Clin. Pharm. Res.* 1997, 17, 11-15.

[44] Li, QG; Peggins, JO; Fleckenstein, L; Masonic, K; Heiffer, MH; Brewer, TG. Bioavailability and pharmacokinetics of dihydroartemisinin, arteether, artemether, artesunic acid and artelinic acid in rats. *J. Pharm. and Pharm.* 1998, 50, 173-182.

[45] Li, QG; Peggins, JO; Lin, AJ; Masonic, K; Trotman KM; Brewer, TG. Pharmacology and toxicology of artelinic acid: Preclinical investigation on pharmacokinetics, metabolism, protein and RBC binding, acute and anorectic toxicities. *Tran. Roy. Soc. Trop. Med. Hyg.* 1998, 92, 332-340.

[46] Teja-Isavadharm, P; Nosten, F; Kyle, DE; Luxemburger, C; Ter Kuile, F; Peggins, JO; Brewer, TG; White, NJ. Comparative bioavailability of oral, rectal, and intramuscular artemether in healthy subjects: use of simultaneous measurement by high performance liquid chromatography and bioassay. *Br. J. Clin. Pharmac.* 1996, 42, 599-604.

[47] Zhao, KC; Song, ZY. Pharmacokinetics of dihydroqinhaosu given orally to rabbits and dogs. *Yao Hsueh Hsueh Pao.* 1990, 25, 147-149.

[48] Benakis, A; Schopfer, C; Paris, M; Plessas, ChT; Karayannakos, PE; Dondas, I; Kotsarelis, D; Plessas, ST; Skalkeas, G. Pharmacokinetics of arteether in dog. *Eur. J. Drug Metab. Pharmacokin.* 1991, 16, 325-328.

[49] Titulaer, HA; Eling, WM; Zuidema, J. Pharmacokinetic and pharmacodynamic aspects of artelinic acid in rodents. *J. Pharm. Pharmacol.* 1993, 45, 830-835.

[50] van Vianen, PH; Klayman, DL; Lin, AJ; Lugt, CB; van Engen, AL; van der Kaay, HJ; Mons, B. Plasmodium berghei: the antimalarial action of artemisinin and sodium artelinate in vivo and in vitro, studied by flow cytometry. *Exp. Parasitol.* 1990, 70, 115-123.

[51] Grace, JM; Skanchy, DJ; Aguilar, AJ. Metabolism of artelinic acid to dihydroqinhaosu by human liver cytochrome P4503A. *Xenobiotica.* 1999, 29: 703-717.

[52] Brewer, TG; Grate, SJ; Peggins, JO; Weina, PJ; Petras, JM; Levine, BS; Heiffer, MH; Schuster, BG. Fatal neurotoxicity of arteether and artemether. *Am. J. Trop. Med. Hyg.* 1994, 51, 251-259.

[53] Genovese, RF; Petras, JM; Brewer, TG. Arteether neurotoxicity in the absence of deficits in behavioural performance in rats. *Ann. Trop. Med. Parasitol.* 1995, 89, 447-449.

[54] Kamchonwongpaisan, S; McKeever, P; Hossler, P; Ziffer, H; Meshnick, SR. Artemisinin neurotoxicity: Neuropathology in rats and mechanistic studies in vitro. *Am. J. Trop. Med. Hyg.* 1997, 56, 7-12.

[55] Petras, JM; Kyle, DE; Ngampochjana, M; Young, GD; Bauman, RA; Webster, HK; Corcoran, JD; Peggins, JO; Vane, MA; Brewer, TG. Arteether: Risks of two-week administration in macaca mulatta. *Am. J. Trop. Med. Hyg.* 1997, 57, 390-396.

[56] Dayan, AD. Neurotoxicity and artemisinin compounds do the observations in animals justify limitation of clinical use? *Med. Trop.* 58, 32S-37S.

[57] Brewer, TG; Peggins, JO; Grate, SJ; Petras, JM; Levine, BS; Weina, PJ; Swearengen, J; Heiffer, MH; Schuster, BG. Neurotoxicity in animals due to arteether and artemether. *Trans. R Soc. Trop. Med. Hyg.* 1994, 88 (Suppl, 1), 33-36.

[58] Davidson, DE. Role of arteether in the treatment of malaria and plans for further development. *Trans. R Soc. Trop. Med. Hyg.* 1994, 88 (Suppl, 1): S51-52.

[59] Genovese, RF; Newman, DB; Li, QG; Peggins, JO; Brewer, TG. Dose-dependent brainstem neuropathology following repeated arteether administration in rats. *Brain Res. Bull.* 1998, 45, 199-202.

[60] Meshnick, SR. Artemisinin: mechanisms of action, resistance and toxicity. *Int. J. Parasitol.* 2002, 32, 1655-1660.

[61] Si, YZ; Li, QG; Mog, SR; Upadhyay, R; Wong, E; Xie, LH; Weina, PJ. Toxicokinetics and neurotoxicity evaluation following oral administration of artelinic acid in rats. *Am. J. Trol. Med. Hyg.* 2000, 67, 255.

[62] Nontprasert, A; Pukrittayakamee, S; Nosten-Bertrand, M; Vanijanonta, S; White, NJ. Studies of the neurotoxicity of oral artemisinin derivatives in mice. *Am. J. Trop. Med. Hyg.* 2000, 62, 409-412.

[63] Nontprasert, A; Pukrittayakamee, S; Prakongpan, S; Supanaranond, W; Looareesuwan, S; White, NJ. Assessment of the neurotoxicity of oral dihydroartemisinin in mice. *Trans. R. Soc. Trop. Med. Hyg.* 2002, 96, 99-101.

[64] Nontprasert, A; Nosten-Bertrand, M; Pukrittayakamee, S; Vanijanonta, S; Angus, BJ; White, NJ. Assessment of the neurotoxicity of parenteral artemisinin derivatives in mice. *Am. J. Trop. Med. Hyg.* 1998, 59, 519-522.

[65] Classen, W; Altmann, B; Gretener, P; Souppart, C; Skelton-Stroud, P; Krinke, G. Differental effects of orally versus parenterally administered qinghaosu derivatives artemether in dogs. *Exp. Toxic. Pathol.* 1999, 51, 507-516.

[66] Li,QG; Xie, LH; Johnson, TO; Si, YZ; Haeberle, AS; Weina, PJ. Toxicity evaluation of artesunate and artelinate in *Plasmodium berghei*-infected and uninfected rats. *Trans. R. Soc. Trop. Med. Hyg.* 2006 Jul 19; [Epub ahead of print]

[67] Karbwang, J; Na-Bangchang, K; Wattanakoon, Y; Thanavibul, A; Harinasuta, T. Artemether 5 versus 7 day regimen for severe falciparum malaria. *Southeast Asian J. Trop. Med. Public. Health.* 1994, 25, 702-706.

[68] Angus, BJ; Thaiaporn, I; Chanthapadith, K; Suputtamongkol, Y; White, NJ. Oral artesunate dose-response relationship in acute falciparum malaria. *Antimicrob Agents Chemother.* 2002, 46, 778-782.

[69] Wilairatana, P; Krudsood, S; Treeprasertsuk, S; Chalermrut, K; Looareesuwan, S. The future outlook of antimalarial drugs and recent work on the treatment of malaria. *Arch. Med. Res.* 2002, 33, 416-421.

[70] Price, R; van Vugt, M; Phaipun, L; Luxemburger, C; Simpson, J; McGready, R; ter Kuile, F; Kham, A; Chongsuphajaisiddhi, T; White, NJ; Nosten, F. Adverse effects in patients with acute falciparum malaria treated with artemisinin derivatives. *Am. J. Trop. Med. Hyg.* 1999, 60, 547-555.

[71] Hien, TT. An overview of the clinical use of artemisinin and its derivatives in the treatment of falciparum malaria in Viet Nam. *Trans. R. Soc. Trop. Med. Hyg.* 1994, 88 Suppl 1, S7-8.

[72] Kar, K; Shankar, G; Bajpai, R; Dutta, GP; Vishwakarma, RA. Artemisinin: a potent antimalarial agent, general pharmacological properties. *Ind. J. Parasitol.* 1988, 12, 209-212.

[73] Li, GQ; Guo, XB; Fu, LC; Jian, HX; Wang, XH. Clinical trials of artemisinin and its derivatives in the treatment of malaria in China. *Trans. Royal Soc. Trop. Med. Hyg.* 1994, 88 (Suppl. 1), S1/5-6.

[74] Meshinick, S.R; Taylor, TE; Kamchonwongpaisan, S. Artemisinin and the antimalarial endoperroxides: from herbal remedy to targeted chemotherapy. *Microbil. Rev.* 1996, 60, 301-315.

[75] Myint, PT; Shwe, T. The efficacy of artemether (qinghaosu) in Plasmodium falciparum and P. vivax in Burma. *Southeast Asian J. Trop. Med. Public Health.* 1986, 17, 19-22.

[76] Myint, PT; Shwe, T. A controlled clinical trial of artemether (qinghaosu derivative) versus quinine in complicated and severe falciparum malaria. *Trans. R. Soc. Trop. Med. Hyg.* 1987, 81, 559-561.

[77] Afolabi, BB; Okoromah, CN. Intramuscular arteether for treating severe malaria. *Cochrane Database Syst. Rev.* 2004. 18, CD004391.

[78] Yeates RA. Artemotil Artecef. *Curr. Opin. Investig. Drugs.* 2002. 3, 545-549.

[79] White, NJ. Artemisinin: current status. *Trans. Royal Soc. Trop. Med. Hyg.* 1994, 88 (Suppl. 1), S1/3-4.

[80] Miller, LG; Planosian, CB. Ataxia and slurred speech after artesunate treatment for falciparum malaria. *New Engl. J. Med.* 1997, 336, 1328.

[81] Causer, LM; Filler, S; Wilson, M; et al. Evaluation of reported malaria chemoprophylatic failure among travelers in a US university exchange program, 2000. *Clin. Infect. Dis.* 2004, 39, 1583-1588.

[82] Keystone, JS. The sound of hoof beats does not always mean that it is a zebra. *Clin. Infect. Dis.* 2004, 39, 1589-1590.

[83] Franco-Paredes, C; Dismukes, R; Nicholls, D; Kozarsky, PE. Neurotoxicity due to antimalarial therapy associated with misdiagnosis of malaria [letter]. *Clin. Infect. Dis.* 2005, 40, 1710-1711.

[84] Newton, PN; Day, NPJ; White, NJ. Misattribution of central nervous system dysfunction to artesunate. *Clin. Infect. Dis.* 2005, 41, 1687-1688.

[85] Gachot, B; Eliaszewicz, M; Dupont, B. Artesunate and cerebellar dysfunction in falciparum malaria. *N. Engl. J. Med.* 1997, 337, 792-793.

[86] Miller, LG; Panosian, CB. Artesunate and cerebellar dysfunction in falciparum malaria-reply. *N. Engl. J. Med.* 1997, 337, 793.

[87] Ribeiro, IR; Olliaro, P. Safety of artemisinin and its derivatives. A systematic review of published and unpublished clinical trials. *Med. Trop. (Mars*), 1998, 58 (Suppl 3); S50-53.

[88] Toovey, S; Jamieson, A. Audiometric changes associated with the treatment of uncomplicated falciparum malaria with co-artemether. *Trans. R. Soc. Trop. Med. Hyg.* 2004, 98, 261-269.

[89] Toovey, S. Effects of weight, age, and time on artemether-lumefantrine associated ototoxicity and evidence of irreversibility. *Travel Med. Infect. Dis.* 2006 (in press)

[90] Hutagalung, R; Htoo, H; Nwee, P; Arunkamomkiri, J; Zwang, J; Carrara, VI; Ashley, E; Singhasivanon, P; White, NJ; Nosten, F. A case-control auditory evaluation of patients treated with artemether-lumefantrine. *Am. J. Trop. Med. Hyg.* 2006, 74, 211-214.

[91] Newton, P; Suputtamongkol, Y; Teja-Isavadharm, P; Pukrittayakamee, S; Navaratnam, V; Bates, I; White, N. Antimalarial bioavailability and disposition of artesunate in acute falciparum malaria. *Antimicrob Agents Chemother.* 2000, 44, 972-977.

[92] Karbwang, J; Na-Bangchang, K; Thanavibul, A; Bunnag, D; Chongsuphajaisiddhi, T; Harinasuta, T. Comparison of oral artesunate and quinine plus tetracycline in acute uncomplicated falciparum malaria. *Bull. World Health Organization* 1994, 72, 233-238.

[93] Kager, PA; Schultz, MJ; Zijlstra, EE; van Berg, B; van Boxtel, Ch.J. Arteether administration in humans: preliminary studies of pharmacokinetics, safety and tolerance. *Trans. R. Soc. Trop. Med. Hyg.* 1994, 88 (suppl 1), 53-54.

[94] Hoffman, SL. Artemether in severe malaria – still to many deaths. *New Engl. J. Med.* 1996, 335, 124-125.

[95] Park, BK; O'Neill, PN; Maggs, JL; Pirmohamed, M. Safety assessment of peroxide antimalarials: clinical and chemical perspectives. *Br. J. Clin. Pharmacol.* 1998, 46, 521-529.

[96] China Cooperative Research Group on qinghaosu and its derivatives as antimalarials. Studies on the toxicity of qinghaosu and its derivatives. *J. Tradit. Chin. Med.* 1982, 2, 31-38.

[97] Chen, LJ; Wang, MY; Sun, WK; Liu, MZ. Embryotoxicity and teratogenicity studies on artemether in mice, rats and rabbits. *Zhongguo Yao Li Xue Bao*. 1984, 5, 118-122.

[98] Li, ZL. Teratogenicity of sodium artesunate. *Zhong Yao Tong Bao*, 1988, 13, 42–44, 63–64.

[99] Si, YZ; Zeng, Q; Zhang, J; Johnson, TO; Xie, LH; Weina, PJ; Milhous, WK; Li, QG. Evaluation of the embryonic toxicity of artesunate in rats. *Am. J. Trop. Med. Hyg.* 2004, 71, 260.

[100] Xu, JH; Zhang, YP. Contragestational effects of dihydroartemisinin and artesunate. *Yao Xue Xue Bao*. 1996, 31, 657-661.

[101] Clark, RL; White, TE; Clode, SA; Gaunt, I; Winstanley, P; Ward, SA. Developmental toxicity of artesunate and an artesunate combination in the rat and rabbit. *Birth Defects Res. B. Dev. Reprod. Toxicol.* 2004, 71, 380-394.

[102] Longo, M; Zanoncelli, S; Torre, PD; Riflettuto, M; Cocco, F; Pesenti, M; Giusti, A; Colombo, P; Brughera, M; Mazue, G; Navaratman, V; Gomes, M; Olliaro, P. In vivo and in vitro investigations of the effects of the antimalarial drug dihydroartemisinin (DHA) on rat embryos. *Reprod Toxicol.* 2006 Aug 14; [Epub ahead of print]

[103] Ejiofor, JI; Kwanashie, HO; Anuka, JA. Some Pregnancy-Related Effects of Artemether in Laboratory Animals. *Pharmacology*. 2006, 77, 166-170.

[104] Longo, M; Zanoncelli, S; Manera, D; Brughera, M; Colombo, P; Lansen, J; Mazue, G; Gomes, M; Taylor, WR; Olliaro, P. Effects of the antimalarial drug dihydroartemisinin (DHA) on rat embryos in vitro. *Reprod. Toxicol.* 2006, 21, 83-93.

[105] Chen, HH; Zhou, HJ; Wu ,GD; Lou, XE. Inhibitory effects of artesunate on angiogenesis and on expressions of vascular endothelial growth factor and VEGF receptor KDR/flk-1. *Pharmacology*. 2004, 71, 1-9.

[106] Lou, XE; Zhou, HJ. Effects of artesunate on progesterone estrogen content and decidua in rats. *Yao Xue Xue Bao*. 2001, 36, 254-257.

[107] Lou, XE; Zhou, HJ; Huang, HB. Lipid-peroxidantion damage of embryo and placenta induced by artesunate in rats. *Zhejiang Da Xue Xue Bao Yi Xue Ban*. 2003, 32, 41-45.

[108] World Health Organization. Assessment of the safety of artemisinin compounds in pregnancy. Report of two informal consultations convened by WHO in 2002 (RBM and TDR). WHO/CDS/MAL/2003.1094.

[109] Li, GQ; Guo, XB; Jin, R; Wang, ZC; Jian, HX; Li, ZY. Clinical trials on qinghaosu and its derivatives: *Guangzhou College of Traditional Chinese Medicine*, 1990.

[110] Wang, TY. Follow-up observation on the therapeutic effects and remote reactions of artemisinin (Qinghaosu) and artemether in treating malaria in pregnant woman. *J. Tradit. Chin. Med.* 1989, 9, 28-30.

[111] Deen, JL; von Seidlein, L; Pinder, M; Walraven, GE; Greenwood, BM. The safety of the combination artesunate and pyrimethamine-sulfadoxine given during pregnancy. *Trans. R. Soc. Trop. Med. Hyg.* 2001, 95, 424-428.

[112] McGready, R; Cho, T; Keo, NK; Thwai, KL; Villegas, L; Looareesuwan, S; White, NJ; Nosten, F. Artemisinin antimalarials in pregnancy: a prospective treatment study of 539

episodes of multidrug-resistant Plasmodium falciparum. *Clin. Infect. Dis*. 2001, 33, 2009-2016.

[113] Adam, I; Ali, DM; Abdalla, MA. Artesunate plus sulfadoxine-pyrimethamine in the treatment of uncomplicated Plasmodium falciparum malaria during pregnancy in eastern Sudan. *Trans. R. Soc Trop. Med. Hyg*. 2006 Jan 24 (ahead of print)

[114] Bounyasong, S. Randomized trial of artesunate and mefloquine in comparison with quinine sulfate to treat P. falciparum malaria pregnant women. *J. Med. Assoc. Thai*. 2001, 84, 1289-1299.

[115] McGready, R; Brockman, A; Cho, T; Cho, D; van Vugt, M; Luxemburger, C; Chongsuphajaisiddhi, T; White, NJ; Nosten, F. Randomized comparison of mefloquine-artesunate versus quinine in the treatment of multidrug-resistant falciparum malaria in pregnancy. *Trans. R. Soc. Trop. Med. Hyg*. 2000, 94, 689-693.

[116] McGready, R; Cho, T; Samuel; Villegas, L; Brockman, A; van Vugt, M; Looareesuwan, S; White, NJ; Nosten, F. Randomized comparison of quinine-clindamycin versus artesunate in the treatment of falciparum malaria in pregnancy. *Trans. R. Soc. Trop. Med. Hyg*. 2001, 95, 651-656.

[117] McGready, R; Keo, NK; Villegas, L; White, NJ; Looareesuwan, S; Nosten, F. Artesunate-atovaquone-proguanil rescue treatment of multidrug-resistant Plasmodium falciparum malaria in pregnancy: a preliminary report. *Trans. R. Soc. Trop. Med. Hyg*. 2003, 97, 592-594.

[118] McGready, R; Stepniewska, K; Edstein, MD; Cho, T; Gilveray, G; Looareesuwan, S; White, NJ; Nosten, F. The pharmacokinetics of atovaquone and proguanil in pregnant women with acute falciparum malaria. *Eur. J. Clin. Pharmacol*. 2003, 59, 545-552.

[119] McGready, R; Ashley, EA; Moo, E; Cho, T; Barends, M; Hutagalung, R; Looareesuwan, S; White, NJ; Nosten, F. A randomized comparison of artesunate-atovaquone-proguanil versus quinine in treatment for uncomplicated falciparum malaria during pregnancy. *J. Infect. Dis*. 2005, 192, 846-853.

[120] Orton, L; Garner, P. Drugs for treating uncomplicated malaria in pregnant women. *Cochrane Database Syst. Rev*. 2005, 20, CD004912.

[121] Brabin, BJ; Ramagosa, C; Abdelgalil, S; Menendez, C; Verhoeff, FH; McGready, R; Fletcher, KA; Owens, S; d'Alessandro, U; Nosten, F; Fischer, PR; Ordi, J; The sick placenta: the role of malaria. *Placenta*. 2004, 25, 359-378.

[122] Price, RN. Artemisinin drugs: novel antimalarial agents. Expert Opin. Investig. *Drugs*. 2000, 9, 1815–1827.

[123] White, NJ; Olliaro, P. Artemisinin and derivatives in the treatment of uncomplicated malaria. *Med. Trop. (Mars.)* 1998, 58 (Suppl.3), 54–56.

[124] White, NJ. Antimalarial drug resistance and combination chemotherapy. *Philos. Trans. R. Soc. Lond. B. Biol. Sci*. 1999, 354, 739–749.

[125] White, NJ. Delaying antimalarial drug resistance with combination chemotherapy. *Parasitologia*. 1999, 41, 301–308.

[126] Nosten, F; vanVugt, M; Price, RN; Luxemburger, C; Thway, KL; Brockman, A; McGready, R; ter Kuile, F; Looareesuwan, S; White, NJ. Effects of artesunate-mefloquine combination on incidence of Plasmodium falciparum malaria and

mefloquine resistance in western Thailand: a prospective study. *Lancet.* 2000, 356, 297–302.

[127] World Health Organization. Antimalarial Drug Combination Therapy: *Report of a Technical Consultation.* 2001, WHO, Geneva.

[128] Roll-Back Malaria. The RBM partnership's global response; a programmatic strategy 2004–2008. Available at: http://rbm.who.int/partnership/ board/meetings/docs/ strategy_rev.pdf (accessed November 2004).

[129] Haynes, RK. From artemisinin to new artemisinin antimalarials: biosynthesis, extraction, old and new derivatives, stereochemistry and medicinal chemistry requirements. *Curr. Top Med. Chem.* 2006, 6, 509-537.

[130] White, NJ; van Vugt, M; Ezzet, F. Clinical pharmacokinetics and pharmacodynamics of artemether lumefantrine. *Clin. Pharmacokinet.* 1999, 37, 105–125.

[131] van Vugt, M; Looareesuwan, S; Wilairatana, P; McGready, R; Villegas, L; Gathmann, I; Mull, R; Brockman, A; White, NJ; Nosten, F. Artemether-lumefantrine for the treatment of multidrug-resistant falciparum malaria. *Trans. R. Soc. Trop. Med. Hyg.* 2000, 94, 545–548.

[132] Omari, AA; Gamble, C; Garner, P. Artemether-lumefantrine for uncomplicated malaria: a systematic review. *Trop. Med. Int. Health.* 2004, 9, 192-199.

[133] Poravuth, Y; Socheat, D; Fandeur, T; et al. Efficacy and safety of six dose regimen of Coartem® in the treatment of acute uncomplicated falciparum malaria in Cambodia 2002. In: Gay F, editor. Proceedings of Mekong Malaria Symposium, 2002, Siem Reap, Angkor Wat, Kingdom of Cambodia. (Mekong Malaria Forum, RMCP-EC): 54.

[134] Hien, TT; Dolecek, C; Mai, PP; et al. Dihydroartemisinin-piperaquine against multidrug-resistant Plasmodium falciparum malaria in Vietnam: randomized clinical trial. *Lancet.* 2004, 363, 18-22.

[135] Guthmann, JP; Cohuet, S; Rigutto, C; Fortes, F; Saraiva, N; Kiguli, J; Kyomuhendo, J; Francis, M; Noel, F; Mulemba, M; Balkan, S. High efficacy of two artemisinin-based combinations (artesunate + amodiaquine and artemether + lumefantrine) in Caala, Central Angola. *Am. J. Trop. Med. Hyg.* 2006, 75, 143-145.

[136] Khim, N; Bouchier, C; Ekala, MT; Incardona, S; Lim ,P; Legrand, E; Jambou, R; Doung, S; Puijalon, OM; Fandeur, T. Countrywide survey shows very high prevalence of Plasmodium falciparum multilocus resistance genotypes in Cambodia. *Antimicrob. Agents Chemother.* 2005, 49, 3147-3152.

[137] Davis, TM; Karunajeewa, HA; Ilett, KF. Artemisinin-based combination therapies for uncomplicated malaria. *Med. J. Aust.* 2005, 21, 182, 181-185.

[138] Anstey, NM; Price, RN; White, NJ. Improving the availability of artesunate for treatment of severe malaria. Artesunate reduces mortality and should now be the treatment of choice in severe malaria in adults: good news for countries in our region, but registration in Australia must wait. *Med. J. Aust.* 2006, 184, 3-4.

[139] Malik, EM; Mohamed, TA; Elmardi, KA; Mowien, RM; Elhassan, AH; Elamin, SB; Mannan, AA; Ahmed, ES. From chloroquine to artemisinin-based combination therapy: The Sudanese experience. *Malar. J.* 2006, 5, 65.

[140] Luxemburger, C; Nosten, F; Raimond, SD; Chongsuphajaisiddhi, T; White, NJ. Oral artesunate in the treatment of uncomplicated hyperparasitemic falciparum malaria. *Am. J. Trop. Med. Hyg.* 1995, 53, 522-525.

[141] Artemether-Quinine Meta-analysis Study Group. A meta-analysis using individual patient data of trials comparing artemether with quinine in the treatment of severe falciparum malaria. *Trans. R. Soc. Trop. Med. Hyg.* 2001, 95, 637-650.

[142] Whitty, CJ; Ansah, E; Reyburn, H. Treating severe malaria. *BMJ.* 2005, 330, 317-318.

[143] Davis, TM; Phuong, HL; Ilett, KF; et al. Pharmacokinetics and pharmacodynamics of intravenous artesunate in severe falciparum malaria. *Antimicrob. Agents Chemother.* 2001, 45, 181-186.

[144] Hien, TT; Davis, TM; Chuong, LV; et al. Comparative pharmacokinetics of intramuscular artesunate and artemether in patients with severe falciparum malaria. *Antimicrob. Agents Chemother.* 2004, 48, 4234-4239.

[145] Dondorp, A; Nosten, F; Stepniewska, K; Day, N; White, N. South East Asian Quinine Artesunate Malaria Trial (SEAQUAMAT) group. Artesunate versus quinine for treatment of severe falciparum malaria: a randomised trial. *Lancet.* 2005, 366, 717-725.

[146] Ashley, EA; White, NJ. Artemisinin-based combinations. *Curr. Opin. Infect. Dis.* 2005, 18, 531-536.

[147] Jelinek, T. Intravenous artesunate recommended for patients with severe malaria: position statement from TropNetEurop. *Euro Surveill.* 2005, 10, E051124.5.

[148] Pasvol, G. The treatment of complicated and severe malaria. *Br. Med. Bull.* 2006, 75-76, 29-47.

[149] Nosten, F; Ashley, E; McGready, R; Price, R. We still need artesunate monotherapy. *BMJ.* 2006, 333, 45.

[150] Weina, PJ; Haeberle, AS; Lowe, MC; Cantilena, L; Milhous, WK. Intravenous artesunate: New product for the treatment of severe and complicated malaria. *Am. J. Trop. Med. Hyg.* 2005, 73, 32.

[151] Gordi, T; Lepist, EI. Artemisinin derivatives: toxic for laboratory animals, safe for humans? *Toxicol. Lett.* 2004, 147, 99-107.

[152] Li, QG; Mog, SR; Si, YZ; Kyle, DE; Gettayacamin, M; Milhous, WK. Neurotoxicity and efficacy of arteether related to its exposure times and exposure levels in rodents. *Am. J. Trop. Med. Hyg.* 2002, 66, 516-525.

[153] McLean, WG; Ward, SA. In vitro neurotoxicity of artemisinin derivatives. *Med. Trop. (Mars).* 1998, 58(3 Suppl), 28-31.

[154] Fishwick , J; McLean, WG; Edwards, G; Ward, SA. The toxicity of artemisinin and related compounds on neuronal and glial cells in culture. *Chem. Biol. Interact.* 1995, 96, 263-271.

[155] Li, QG; Brewer, TG; Peggins, JO. Anorectic toxicity of dihydroartemisinin, arteether and artemether in rats following multiple intramuscular doses. *International. J. Toxicol.* 1998, 17, 663-676.

[156] Wesche, DL; DeCoster, MA; Tortella, FC; Brewer, TG. Neurotoxicity of artemisinin analogs in vitro. *Antimicrob Agents Chemother.* 1994, 38, 1813-1819.

[157] Benakis, A; Binh, TQ; Keundjian, A; Scheiwe, MW. Pharmacokinetics/ Pharmacodynamics findings after repeated administration of ARTESUNATE

thermostable suppositories (RECTOCAPS) in Vietnamese patients with uncomplicated malaria. *Eur. J. Drug. Metab. Pharmacokinet.* 2006, 31, 41-45.

[158] Batty, KT; Le, AT; Ilett, KF; Nguyen, PT; Powell, SM; Nguyen, CH; Truong ,XM; Vuong, VC; Huynh, VT; Tran,QB; Nguyen, VM; Davis, TM. A pharmacokinetic and pharmacodynamic study of artesunate for vivax malaria. *Am. J. Trop. Med. Hyg.* 1998, 59, 823-827.

[159] Li, QG; Bossone, CA; Ohrt, C; Chung, H; Harris, D; Harre, J; Lee, P; Kathcart, AK; Brueckner, RP. Early signs and biomarkers of the neurotoxicity: toxicokinetic and toxicodynamic evaluation following 15-mg/kg arteether daily intramuscular injections for two weeks in beagle dogs. *Am. J. Trol. Med. Hyg.* 2000, 62, 142.

[160] Li, QG; Carpenter, C; Trotman, C; Kathcart, AK; Donahue, R; Milhous, WK. Pharmacokinetic comparison of artesunate and dihydroartemisinin in beagle dogs. *Am. J. Trol. Med. Hyg.* 1999, 61: 274.

[161] Kyle, DE; Teja-Isavadharm, P; Li, Q; Leo, K. Pharmacokinetics and pharmacodynamics of qinghaosu derivatives: how do they impact on the choice of drug and the dosage regimens? *Med. Trop. (Mars).* 1998, 58(3 Suppl), 38-44.

[162] Karbwang, J; Na-Bangchang, K; Tin, T; Sukontason, K; Rimchala, W; Harinasuta, T. Pharmacokinetics of intramuscular artemether in patients with severe falciparum malaria with or without acute renal failure. *Br. J. Clin. Pharmacol.* 1998, 45, 597-600.

[163] van Agtmael, MA; Van Der Graaf, CA; Dien, TK; Koopmans, RP; van Boxtel, CJ. The contribution of the enzymes CYP2D6 and CYP2C19 in the demethylation of artemether in healthy subjects. *Eur. J. Drug Metab. Pharmacokinet.* 1998, 23, 429-436.

[164] Karbwang, J; Na-Bangchang, K; Congpuong, K; Thanavibul, A; Wattanakoon, Y; Molunto, P. Pharmacokinetics of oral artemether in Thai patients with uncomplicated falciparum malaria. *Fundam. Clin. Pharmacol.* 1998, 12, 242-244.

[165] Mordi, MN; Mansor, SM; Navaratnam, V; Wernsdorfer, WH. Single dose pharmacokinetics of oral artemether in healthy Malaysian volunteers. *Br. J. Clin. Pharmacol.* 1997, 43, 363-365.

[166] Thomas, CG; Ward, SA; Edwards, G. Selective determination, in plasma, of artemether and its major metabolite, dihydroartemisinin, by high-performance liquid chromatography with ultraviolet detection. *J. Chromatogr.* 1992, 583, 131-136.

[167] van Agtmael, MA; Butter, JJ; Portier, EJ; van Boxtel, CJ. Validation of an improved reversed-phase high-performance liquid chromatography assay with reductive electrochemical detection for the determination of artemisinin derivatives in man. *Ther. Drug Monit.* 1998, 20, 109-116.

[168] van Agtmael, MA; Gupta, V; van der Wosten, TH; Rutten, JP; van Boxtel, CJ. Grapefruit juice increases the bioavailability of artemether. *Eur. J. Clin. Pharmacol.* 1999, 55, 405-410.

[169] Navaratnam, V; Mansor, SM; Chin, LK; Mordi, MN; Asokan, M; Nair, NK. Determination of artemether and dihydroartemisinin in blood plasma by high-performance liquid chromatography for application in clinical pharmacological studies. *J. Chromatogr. B. Biomed. Appl.* 1995, 669, 289-294.

[170] Karbwang, J; Na-Bangchang, K; Molunto, P; Banmairuroi, V; Congpuong, K. Determination of artemether and its major metabolite, dihydroartemisinin, in plasma

using high-performance liquid chromatography with electrochemical detection. *J. Chromatogr. B. Biomed. Sci. Appl.* 1997, 690, 259-265.

[171] van Agtmael, MA; Gupta, V; van der Graaf, CA; van Boxtel, CJ. The effect of grapefruit juice on the time-dependent decline of artemether plasma levels in healthy subjects. *Clin. Pharmacol. Ther.* 1999, 66, 408-414.

[172] Tan-ariya, P; Na-Bangchang, K; Ubalee, R; Thanavibul, A; Thipawangkosol, P; Karbwang, J. Pharmacokinetic interactions of artemether and pyrimethamine in healthy male Thais. *Southeast Asian J. Trop. Med. Public Health.* 1998, 29, 18-23.

[173] Batty, KT; Thu, LT; Davis, TM; Ilett, KF; Mai, TX; Hung, NC; Tien, NP; Powell, SM; Thien, HV; Binh, TQ; Kim, NV. A pharmacokinetic and pharmacodynamic study of intravenous vs oral artesunate in uncomplicated falciparum malaria. *Br. J. Clin. Pharmacol.* 1998, 45, 123-129.

[174] Benakis, A; Paris, M; Loutan, L; Plessas, CT; Plessas, ST. Pharmacokinetics of artemisinin and artesunate after oral administration in healthy volunteers. *Am. J. Trop. Med. Hyg.* 1997, 56, 17-23.

[175] Navaratnam, V; Mansor, SM; Mordi, MN; Akbar, A; Abdullah, MN. Comparative pharmacokinetic study of oral and rectal formulations of artesunic acid in healthy volunteers. *Eur. J. Clin. Pharmacol.* 1998, 54, 411-414.

[176] Navaratnam, V; Mordi, MN; Mansor, SM. Simultaneous determination of artesunic acid and dihydroartemisinin in blood plasma by high-performance liquid chromatography for application in clinical pharmacological studies. *J. Chromatogr. B. Biomed. Sci. Appl.* 1997, 692, 157-162.

[177] Genovese, RF; Newman, DB; Brewer, TG. Behavioral and neural toxicity of the artemisinin antimalarial, arteether, but not artesunate and artelinate, in rats. *Pharmacol. Biochem. Behav.* 2000, 67, 37-44.

[178] Li, Q; Xie, LH; Si, Y; Wong, E; Upadhyay, R; Yanez, D; Weina, PJ. Toxicokinetics and hydrolysis of artelinate and artesunate in malaria-infected rats. *Int. J. Toxicol.* 2005, 24, 241-250.

[179] Xie, LH; Johnson, TO; Weina, PJ; Si, Y; Haeberle, A; Upadhyay, R; Wong, E; Li, Q. Risk assessment and therapeutic indices of artesunate and artelinate in Plasmodium berghei-infected and uninfected rats. *Int. J. Toxicol.* 2005, 24, 251-264.

[180] China Cooperative Research Group on Qinghaosu and Its Derivatives as Antimalarials. Metabolism and pharmacokinetics of qinghaosu and its derivatives. *J. Tradit. Chin. Med*, 1982, 2, 25-30.

[181] Niu, XY; Ho, LY; Ren, ZH; Song, ZY. Metabolic fate of Qinghaosu in rats; a new TLC densitometric method for its determination in biological material. *Eur. J. Drug Metab. Pharmacokinet.* 1985, 10, 55-59.

[182] Zhao, KC; Song, ZY. Distribution and excretion of artesunate in rats. *Proc. Chin. Acad. Med. Sci. Peking Union Med. Coll.* 1989, 4, 186-188.

[183] Jiang, JR; Zou, CD; Shu, HL; Zeng, YL. Assessment of absorption and distribution of artemether in rats using a thin layer chromatography scanning technique. *Zhongguo Yao Li Xue Bao.* 1989, 10, 431-434.

[184] Li, QG; Xie, LH; Haeberle, A; Zhang, J; Weina, PJ. The evaluation of radiolabeled artesunate on tissue distribution in rats and protein binding in humans. (accepted May 23, 2006, ASTMH, in press)

[185] Kearney, BP; Aweeka, FT. The penetration of anti-infectives into the central nervous system. *Neurol Clin.* 1999, 17, 883-900.

[186] Davis, TM; Binh, TQ; Ilett, KF; Batty, KT; Phuong, HL; Chiswell, GM; Phuong, VD; Agus, C. Penetration of dihydroartemisinin into cerebrospinal fluid after administration of intravenous artesunate in severe falciparum malaria. *Antimicrob. Agents Chemother.* 2003, 47, 368-370.

[187] Li, QG; Brueckner, RP; Peggins, JO; Trotman, KM; Brewer, TG. Arteether toxicokinetics and pharmacokinetics in rats after 25 mg/kg/day single and multiple doses. *Eur. J. Drug Metab. Pharmacokinet.* 1999, 24, 213-223.

[188] Kager, PA; Schultz, MJ; Zijlstra, EE; van den Berg, B; van Boxtel, CJ. Arteether administration in humans: preliminary studies of pharmacokinetics, safety and tolerance. *Trans R. Soc. Trop. Med. Hyg.* 1994, 88 Suppl 1, S53-S54.

[189] Brewer, TG; Genovese, RF; Newman, DB; Li, Q. Factors relating to neurotoxicity of artemisinin antimalarial drugs "listening to arteether". *Med. Trop. (Mars).* 1998, 58(3 Suppl), 22-27.

[190] Rowland, M; Tozer, TN. Clinical Pharmacokinetics: Concepts and applications, Malcolm Rowland and Thomas N. Tozer (Ed.), Willianms and Wilkins, Baltimore, 1995, USA, 83.

[191] Mayer, PR. Absorption, metabolism, and other factors that influence drug exposure in toxicology studies. *Toxicol. Pathol.* 1995, 23, 165-169.

[192] Shargel, L; Yu, ABC. Applied Biopharmaceutics and Pharmacokinetics, Leon Shargel and Andrew B.C (Ed.), YU. *Appleton and Lange,* 1993, Norwalk, CN, 353.

[193] Li, QG; Peggens, JO; Brown, LD; Brewer, TG. Pharmacokinetics and hydrolysis of sodium artelinate in dogs. *AM. J. Trop. Med. Hyg.* 1994, 51, 260.

[194] Noker, P; Lin, TT. Toxicity dose range study of 14 days oral administration of artelinic acid in dogs. Contract Research Reports, Southern Research Institute, Birmingham, USA, 2000. (Contract Report, unpublished data)

[195] Li, QG; Xie, LH; Peggins, JO. Pharmacokinetics and tolerant dose range studies of AL and AS following daily intramuscular dosing for 7 days in rats. *Am. J. Trol. Med. Hyg.* 2001, 65, 214.

[196] Ashton, M; Hai, TN; Sy, ND. Artemisinin pharmacokinetics is time-dependent during repeated oral administration in healthy male adults. *Drug Metab. Dispos.* 2998. 26, 2601-2605.

[197] Ashton, M; Sy, ND; Gordi, T; Hai, TN. Thach, DC; Huong, NV; Johansson, M; Coeng, LD. Evidence for time-dependence artemisinin kinetics in adults with uncomplicated malaria. *Pharm. Pharmacol. Lett.* 1996. 6, 127-130.

[198] van Agtmael, MA; Xiungquing, J; Koopmans, RP; Degen, P; Royce, CM. van Boxtel, CJ. Multiple dose pharmacokinetics of artemether in Chinese patients treated for falciparum malaria. *Acta Pharmacol. Ther. Latinoam.* 1996, 46, 244.

[199] Khanh, NX; de Vries, PJ; Ha, LD; van Boxtel, CJ; Koopmans, R; Kager, PA. Declining concentrations of dihydroartemisinin in plasma during 5-day oral treatment with artesunate for falciparum malaria. *Antimicro. Agent Chemtherap.* 1999, 43, 690-692.

[200] Li, Q; Lugt, CB; Looareesuwan, S; Krudsood, S; Wilairatana, P; Vannaphan, S; Chalearmrult, K; Milhous, WK. Pharmacokinetic investigation on the therapeutic potential of artemotil (beta-arteether) in Thai patients with severe Plasmodium falciparum malaria. *Am. J. Trop. Med. Hyg.* 2004, 71, 723-731.

[201] Klaassen, CD; Rozman, K. Chapter 3, Absorption, distribution, and excretion of toxicants, In. Casarett and Doull's Toxicology, The Basic Science of Poisons, Mary O. Amdur, John Doull, and Cortis D (Ed.). 1993, Klaassen. McGraw-Hill, Inc. Press. 53.

[202] Li, QG; Milhous, WK; Weina, PJ. Regimen strategy to decrease artemisinin agents related failure and recrudescence in severe and complicated malaria treatment. *Medicine and Health in the Tropics* (Marseille-France) 2005, Abstract Book, 131.

[203] Geyer, HJ; Scheuntert, I; Rapp, K; Kettrup, A; Korte, F; Greim, H; Rozman, K. Correlation between acute toxicity of 2,3,7,8-tetrachlorodibenzo-p-dioxin (TCDD) and total body fat content in mammals. *Toxicology.* 1990, 65, 97-107.

[204] Kimbrough, RD. How toxic is 2,3,7,8-tetrachlorodibenzodioxin to humans? *J. Toxicol. Environ. Health.* 1990, 30, 261-271.

[205] Culotta, E; Koshland, DE Jr. DNA repair works it works its way to the top. *Science.* 1994, 266, 1926-1929.

[206] Dawes, M; Chowienczyk, PJ. Drugs in pregnancy. Pharmacokinetics in pregnancy. *Best Pract. Res. Clin. Obstet. Gynaecol.* 2001. 15, 819-826.

[207] McGready, R; Stepniewska, K; Ward, SA; Cho, T; Gilveray, G; Looareesuwan, S; White, NJ; Nosten, F. Pharmacokinetics of dihydroartemisinin following oral artesunate treatment of pregnant women with acute uncomplicated falciparum malaria. *Eur. J. Clin. Pharmacol.* 2006. 62, 367-371.

[208] Clyde, DF. Clinical problems associated with the use of primaquine as a tissue schizontocidal and gametocytocidal drug. *Bull. World Health Organ.* 1981, 59, 391-395.

[209] Salako, LA. Pharmacokinetics of antimalarial drugs: their therapeutic and toxicological implications. *Ann. Ist. Super Sanita.* 1985. 21, 315-325. .

[210] Nosten, F; McGready, R; d'Alessandro, U; Bonell, A; Verhoeff, F; Menendez, C; Mutabingwa, T; Brabin, B. Antimalarial Drugs in Pregnancy: *Current Drug Safety*, Volume 1, Number 1, January 2006, pp. 1-15(15)

[211] Colwell, EJ; Hickman, RL; Kosakal, S. Tetracycline treatment of chloroquine-resistant falciparum malaria in Thailand. *JAMA.* 1972. 220, 684-686.

[212] Cohlan, SQ; Bevelander, G; Tiamsic, T. Growth inhibition of prematures receiving tetracycline. *Am. J. Dis. Child.* 1963. 105, 453-461.

[213] Manson, JD. Tetracyclines and the teeth. *Lancet.* 1966. 1(7446), 1104.

[214] Krejci, L; Brettschneider, I. Congenital cataract due to tetracycline. *Ophthal. Paediat. Genet.* 1983. 3, 59-60.

[215] Schiffer, MA. Fatty liver associated with administration of tetracycline in pregnant and nonpregnant women. *Am. J. Obstet. Gynecol.* 1966. 96, 326-332.

[216] Allen, ES; Brown, WE. Hepatic toxicity of tetracycline in pregnancy. *Am. J. Obstet. Gynecol.* 1966, 95, 12-18.

[217] Fakeye, TO; Fehintola, FA; Ademowo, OG; Walker, O. Therapeutic monitoring of chloroquine in pregnant women with malaria. *West Afr. J. Med.* 2002, 21, 286-287.

[218] Massele, AY; Kilewo, C; Aden Abdi, Y; Tomson, G; Diwan, VK; Ericsson, O; Rimoy, G; Gustafsson, LL. Chloroquine blood concentrations and malaria prophylaxis in Tanzanian women during the second and third trimesters of pregnancy. *Eur. J. Clin. Pharmacol.* 1997. 52, 299-305.

[219] Na Bangchang, K; Davis, TM; Looareesuwan, S; White, NJ; Bunnag, D; Karbwang, J. Mefloquine pharmacokinetics in pregnant women with acute falciparum malaria. *Trans. R. Soc. Trop. Med. Hyg.* 1994. 88, 321-323.

[220] McGready, R; Stepniewska, K; Seaton, E; Cho, T; Cho, D; Ginsberg, A; Edstein, MD; Ashley, E; Looareesuwan, S; White, NJ; Nosten, F. Pregnancy and use of oral contraceptives reduces the biotransformation of proguanil to cycloguanil. *Eur. J. Clin. Pharmacol.* 2003. 59, 553-557.

[221] Na-Bangchang, K; Manyando, C; Ruengweerayut, R; Kioy, D; Mulenga, M; Miller, GB; Konsil, J. The pharmacokinetics and pharmacodynamics of atovaquone and proguanil for the treatment of uncomplicated falciparum malaria in third-trimester pregnant women. *Eur. J. Clin. Pharmacol.* 2005. 61, 573-582.

[222] Menendez C. Malaria during pregnancy. *Curr. Mol. Med.* 2006. 6, 269-273.

[223] Akintonwa, A; Meyer, MC; Yau, MK. Placental transfer of chloroquine in pregnant rabbits. *Res. Commun. Chem. Pathol. Pharmacol.* 1983. 40, 443-455.

[224] Si, YZ; Xie, LH; Young-Sun, Y; Melendez, V; Weina, P; Milhouse, WK; Li, QG. Pharmacokinetic comparison of artesunate in rats following Intravenous, intramuscular and subcutaneous administration. *Experimental Biology.* 2004 (Annual Meeting of ASPET) in Washington, DC, April 17-21, 2004.

[225] Si, YZ; Li, QG; Haeberle, A; Milhouse, WK; Weina, P. [14C] artesunate tissue distribution in pregnant rats following a single intravenous dose with whole-body autoradiography. *Am. J. Trop. Med. Hyg.* 2006, 75 (5), 18.

[226] Potchoiba, MJ; West, M; Nocerini, MR. Quantitative comparison of autoradioluminographic and radiometric tissue distribution studies using carbon-14 labeled xenobiotics. *Drug Metab. Dispos.* 1998. 26, 272-277.

[227] Schweitzer, A; Fahr, A; Niederberger, W. A simple method for the quantitation of 14C-whole-body autoradiograms. *Int. J. Rad. Appl. Instrum. [A]* 1987. 38, 329-333.

[228] Solon, EG; Kraus, L. Quantitative whole-body autoradiography in the pharmaceutical industry. Survey results on design, methods, and regulatory compliance. *J. Pharmacol. Toxicol. Methods.* 2001. 46, 73-81.

[229] Chen, HH; Zhou, HJ; Wang, WQ; Wu, GD. Antimalarial dihydroartemisinin also inhibits angiogenesis. *Cancer Chemother. Pharmacol.* 2004. 53, 423-432.

[230] Anfosso, L; Efferth, T; Albini, A; Pfeffer, U. Microarray expression profiles of angiogenesis-related genes predict tumor cell response to artemisinins. *Pharmacogenomics J.* 2006. 6, 269-278.

[231] Efferth, T. Mechanistic perspectives for 1,2,4-trioxanes in anti-cancer therapy. *Drug Resist. Updat.* 2005. 8, 85-97.

[232] Dell'Eva, R; Pfeffer, U; Vene, R; Anfosso, L; Forlani, A; Albini, A; Efferth, T. Inhibition of angiogenesis in vivo and growth of Kaposi's sarcoma xenograft tumors by the anti-malarial artesunate. *Biochem. Pharmacol.* 2004. 68, 2359-2366.

[233] Huan-huan, C; Li-Li, Y; Shang-Bin, L. Artesunate reduces chicken chorioallantoic membrane neovascularisation and exhibits antiangiogenic and apoptotic activity on human microvascular dermal endothelial cell. *Cancer Lett.* 2004. 211, 163-173.

[234] Chen, HH; Zhou, HJ. Inhibitory effects of artesunate on angiogenesis. *Yao Xue Xue Bao.* 2004. 39, 29-33.

[235] Chen, HH; Zhou, HJ; Fang, X. Inhibition of human cancer cell line growth and human umbilical vein endothelial cell angiogenesis by artemisinin derivatives in vitro. *Pharmacol. Res.* 2003. 48, 231-236.

[236] Zon, LI. Developmental biology of hematopoiesis. *Blood.* 1995. 8, 2876–2891.

[237] Choe, H; Hansen, JM; Harris, C. Spatial and temporal ontogenesis of glutathione peroxidase, and glutathione disulfide reductase during development of the prenatal rat. *J. Biochem. Mol. Toxicol.* 2001, 15, 197–206.

[238] Phillips-Howard, PA; Wood, D. The safety of antimalarial drugs in pregnancy. *Drug Saf.* 1996. 14, 131-145.

[239] Adam, I; Ali, DM; Abdalla, MA. Artesunate plus sulfadoxine-pyrimethamine in the treatment of uncomplicated Plasmodium falciparum malaria during pregnancy in eastern Sudan. *Trans. R. Soc. Trop. Med. Hyg.* 2006. 100, 632-635.

[240] Steketee, RW; Wirima, JJ; Campbell, CC. Developing effective strategies for malaria prevention programs for pregnant African women. *Am. J. Trop. Med. Hyg.* 1996. 55(1 Suppl), 95-100.

[241] Steketee, RW; Nahlen, BL; Parise, ME; Menendez, C. The burden of malaria in pregnancy in malaria-endemic areas. *Am. J. Trop. Med. Hyg.* 2001. 64(1-2 Suppl), 28-35.

[242] Newman, RD; Parise, ME; Slutsker, L; Nahlen, B; Steketee, RW. Safety, efficacy and determinants of effectiveness of antimalarial drugs during pregnancy: implications for prevention programmes in Plasmodium falciparum-endemic sub-Saharan Africa. *Trop. Med. Int. Health.* 2003. 8, 488-506.

[243] Kumar, N; Zheng, H. Stage-specific gametocytocidal effect in vitro of the antimalaria drug qinghaosu on *Plasmodium falciparum. Parasitol. Res.* 1990. 76, 214-218.

[244] Mehra, N; Bhasin, VK. In vitro gametocytocidal activity of artemisinin and its derivatives on *Plasmodium falciparum. Jpn. J. Med. Sci. Biol.* 1993. 46, 37-43.

[245] Dutta, GP; Mohan, A; Tripathi, R. Study of the gametocytocidal/sporontocidal action of qinghaosu (artemisinin) by electron microscopy. *J. Parasitol.* 1990. 76, 849-852.

[246] Ding, Y; Qi, Z; et al.: Efficacy of dihydroartemisinin in treatment of 37 malaria cases. *Chin. J. Intern. Med.* 1997. 36, 187-189.

[247] White, NJ. Antimalarial pharmacokinetics and treatment regimens. *Br. J. Clin. Pharmacol.* 1992. 34, 1-10.

[248] Klayman, DL. An antimalarial drug from China. *Science.* 1985. 228, 1049-1055.

[249] Hien, TT; White, NJ. Qinghaosu. *Lancet.* 1993. 341, 603-608.

[250] Thu, LTA; Davis, TME; Binh, TQ; van Phuong, N; Anh, TK. Delayed parasite clearance in a Splenectomized patients with falciparum malaria who was treated with artemisinin derivatives. *Clin. Infect. Dis.* 1997. 25, 923-925.

[251] Alin, MH; Bjorkman, A. Concentration and time dependence of artemisinin efficacy against Plasmodium falciparum in vitro. *Am. J. Trop. Med. Hyg.* 1994. 50, 771-776.

[252] White, NJ; Krishna, S. Treatment of malaria: some considerations and limitations of the current methods of assessment. *Trans. Roy .Soc. Trop. Med. Hug.* 1989. 83, 767-777.

[253] Sharma, P; Swarup, D; Saxena, GN; Bhandari, S; Sharma, UB; Tuteja, R. An open study to evaluate the efficacy of artemether in severe falciparum malaria. *J. Assoc. Physicians India.* 1999. 47, 883-885.

[254] Suputtamongkol, Y; Newton, PN; Angus, B; Teja-Isavadharm, P; Keeratithakul, D; Rasameesoraj, M; Pukrittayakamee, S; White, NJ. A comparison of oral artesunate and artemether antimalarial bioactivities in acute falciparum malaria. *Br. J. Clin. Pharmacol.* 2001. 52, 655-661.

[255] Marsh, K; Forster, D; Waruiru, C; Mwangi, I; Winstanley, M; Marsh, V; Newton, C; Winstanley, P; Warn, P; Peshu, N. et al. Indicators of life-threatening malaria in African children. *N. Engl. J. Med.* 1995. 332, 1399-1404.

[256] Looareesuwan, S. Overview of clinical studies on artemisinin derivatives in Thailand. *Trans. Roy. Soc. Trop. Med. Hyg.* 1994. 88 (Suppl 1), 9-11.

[257] Ambroise-Thomas, P. Intra-muscular artemether in the treatment of severe malaria: synthesis of current results. *Med. Trop. (Mars).* 1997. 57, 289-293..

[258] Bhatt, KM; Samia, BM; Bhatt, SM; Wasunna, KM. Efficacy and safety of an artesunate/mefloquine combination, (artequin) in the treatment of uncomplicated P. falciparum malaria in Kenya. *East Afr. Med. J.* 2006. 83, 236-242.

[259] Kaiwa, S; Kano, S; Suzuki , M. Morphologic effects of artemether on Plasmodium falciparum in Aotus trivirgatus. *Am. J. Trop. Med. Hyg.* 1993. 49, 812-818.

[260] Hassan, Alin M; Ashton, M; Kihamia, CM; Mtey, GJ; Bjorkman, A. Multiple dose pharmacokinetics of oral artemisinin and comparison of its efficacy with that of oral artesunate in falciparum malaria patients. *Trans. R. Soc. Trop. Med. Hyg.* 1996. 90, 61-65.

[261] Na-Bangchang, K; Tippawangkosol, P; Thanavibul, A; Ubalee, R; Karbwang, J. Pharmacokinetic and pharmacodynamic interactions of mefloquine and dihydroartemisinin. *Int. J. Clin. Pharmacol. Res.* 1999. 19, 9-17.

[262] Titulaer, HAC; Zuidema, J; Lugt, CB. Formulation and pharmacokinetics of artemisinin and its derivatives. *Intern. J. Pharmaceui.* 1991. 69, 83-92.

[263] Murphy, S; Watkins, WM; Bray, PG; Lowe, B; Winstanley, PA; Peshu, N; Marsh, K. Parasite viability during treatment of severe falciparum malaria: differential effects of artemether and quinine. *Am. J. Trop. Med. Hyg.* 1995. 53, 303-305.

[264] White, NJ. Clinical pharmacokinetics and pharmacodynamics of artemisinin and derivatives. *Trans. R. Soc. Trop. Med. Hyg.* 1994. 88(Suppl 1), S41–S43.

[265] Gu, H.M; Warhurst, DC; Peters, W. Uptake of [3H]-dihydroartemisinin by erythrocytes infected with plasmodium falciparum in-vitro. *Trans. R. Soc. Trop. Med. Hyg.* 1984. 78, 265-270.

[266] Ashton, M; Hai, TN; Sy, ND; Huong, DX; Van Huong, N; Nieu, NT; Cong, LD. Artemisinin pharmacokinetics is time-dependent during repeated oral administration in healthy male adults. *Drug Metab. Dispos.* 1998. 26, 25-27.

[267] Zhao, KC; Song, ZY. Pharmacokinetics of dihydroqinghaosu in human volunteers and comparison with qinghaosu. *Yao Xue Xue Bao.* 1993, 28, 342-346.

[268] Koopmans, R; Ha, LD; Duc, DD; Dien, TK; Kager, PA; Khanh, NX; van Boxtel, CJ; De Vries, PJ. The pharmacokinetics of artemisinin after administration of two different suppositories to healthy Vietnamese subjects. *Am. J. Trop. Med. Hyg.* 1999. 60, 244-247.

[269] Na-Bangchang, K; Krudsood, S; Silachamroon, U; Molunto, P; Tasanor, O; Chalermrut, K; Tangpukdee, N; Matangkasombut, O; Kano, S; Looareesuwan, S. The pharmacokinetics of oral dihydroartemisinin and artesunate in healthy Thai volunteers. *Southeast Asian J. Trop. Med. Public Health.* 2004. 35, 575-582.

[270] Binh, TQ; Ilett, KF; Batty, KT; Davis, TM; Hung, NC; Powell, SM; Thu, LT; Thien, HV; Phuong, HL; Phuong, VD. Oral bioavailability of dihydroartemisinin in Vietnamese volunteers and in patients with falciparum malaria. *Br. J. Clin. Pharmacol.* 2001. 51, 541-546.

[271] White, NJ. Antimalarial drug resistance. *J. Clin. Invest.* 2004. 113, 1084-1092.

[272] Ittarat, W; Pickard, AL; Rattanasinganchan, P; Wilairatana, P; Looareesuwan, S; Emery, K; Low, J; Udomsangpetch, R; Meshnick, SR. Recrudescence in artesunate-treated patients with falciparum malaria is dependent on parasite burden not on parasite factors. *Am. J. Trop. Med. Hyg.* 2003. 68, 147-152.

[273] Pareek, A; Nandy, A; Kochar, D; Patel, KH; Mishra, SK; Mathur, PC. Efficacy and safety of beta-arteether and alpha/beta-arteether for treatment of acute Plasmodium falciparum malaria. *Am. J. Trop. Med. Hyg.* 2006. 75, 139-142.

[274] Asthana, OP; Srivastava, JS; Pandey, TK; Vishwanathan, KA; Dev, V; Mahapatra, KM; Nayak, NC; Balsara, AB; Mandal, OP; Gupta, N; Mishra, SK; Mohanty, S; Sathpathy, S; Das, BS; Patnaik, JK; Sathpathy, SK; Dash, B. Multicentric clinical trials for safety and efficacy evaluation of alpha;beta arteether in complicated P. falciparum malaria. *J. Assoc. Physicians India.* 2001. 49, 1155-1160.

[275] Rajanikanth, M; Madhusudanan, KP; Gupta, RC. An HPLC-MS method for simultaneous estimation of alpha,beta-arteether and its metabolite dihydroartemisinin, in rat plasma for application to pharmacokinetic study. *Biomed. Chromatogr.* 2003. 17, 440-446.

[276] Sabarinath, S; Rajanikanth, M; Madhusudanan, KP; Gupta, RC. A sensitive and selective liquid chromatographic/electrospray ionization tandem mass spectrometric assay for the simultaneous quantification of alpha-,beta-arteether and its metabolite dihydroartemisinin in plasma, useful for pharmacokinetic studies. *J. Mass Spectrom.* 2003. 38, 732-742.

[277] Rajanikanth, M; Madhusudanan, KP; Gupta, RC. Liquid chromatographic-mass spectrometric method for the determination of alpha-, beta-arteether in rat serum. *J. Chromatogr. B. Analyt. Technol. Biomed. Life Sci.* 2003. 783, 391-399.

[278] Ashton, M; Nguyen, DS; Nguyen, VH; Gordi, T; Trinh, NH; Dinh, XH; Nguyen, TN; Le, DC. Artemisinin kinetics and dynamics during oral and rectal treatment of uncomplicated malaria. *Clin. Pharmacol. Ther.* 1998. 63, 482-493.

[279] von Seidlein, L; Milligan, P; Pinder, M; Bojang, K; Anyalebechi, C; Gosling, R; Coleman, R; Ude, JI; Sadiq, A; Duraisingh, M; Warhurst, D; Alloueche, A; Targett, G; McAdam, K; Greenwood, B; Walraven, G; Olliaro, P; Doherty, T. Efficacy of artesunate plus pyrimethamine-sulphadoxine for uncomplicated malaria in Gambian children: a double-blind, randomised, controlled trial. *Lancet.* 2000. 355, 352-357.

[280] Adjuik, M; Babiker, A; Garner, P; Olliaro, P; Taylor, W; White, N. International Artemisinin Study Group. Artesunate combinations for treatment of malaria: meta-analysis. *Lancet.* 2004. 363, 9-17.

[281] Silamut, K; Newton, PN; Teja-Isavadharm, P; Suputtamongkol, Y; Siriyanonda, D; Rasameesoraj, M; Pukrittayakamee, S; White, NJ. Artemether bioavailability after oral or intramuscular administration in uncomplicated falciparum malaria. *Antimicrob. Agents Chemother.* 2003. 47, 3795-3798.

[282] Le, NH; Na-Bangchang, K; Le, TD; Thrinh, KA; Karbwang, J. Pharmacokinetics of a single oral dose of dihydroartemisinin in Vietnamese healthy volunteers. *Southeast Asian J. Trop. Med. Public Health.* 1999. 30, 11-16.

[283] Karbwang, J; Na-Bangchang, K; Congpuong, K; Molunto, P; Thanavibul, A. Pharmacokinetics and bioavailability of oral and intramuscular artemether. *Eur. J. Clin. Pharmacol.* 1997. 52, 307-310.

[284] Chanthap, L; Tsuyuoka, R; Na-Bangchang, K; Nivanna, N; Suksom, D; Sovannarith, T; Socheat, D. Investigation of bioavailability, pharmacokinetics and safety of new pediatric formulations of artesunate and mefloquine. *Southeast Asian J. Trop. Med. Public Health.* 2005. 36, 34-43.

[285] Newton, PN; van Vugt, M; Teja-Isavadharm, P; Siriyanonda, D; Rasameesoroj, M; Teerapong, P; Ruangveerayuth, R; Slight, T; Nosten, F; Suputtamongkol, Y; Looareesuwan, S; White, NJ. Comparison of oral artesunate and dihydroartemisinin antimalarial bioavailabilities in acute falciparum malaria. *Antimicrob Agents Chemother.* 2002. 46, 1125-1127.

[286] Na-Bangchang, K; Thanavibul, A; Tippawangkosol, P; Karbwang, J. Pharmacokinetics of the four combination regimens of dihydroartemisinin/mefloquine in acute uncomplicated falciparum malaria. *Southeast Asian J. Trop. Med. Public Health.* 2005. 36, 23-33.

[287] Asawamahasakda, W; Benakis, A; Meshnick, SR. The interaction of artemisinin with red cell membranes. *J. Lab. Clin. Med.* 1994. 123, 757-762.

[288] Li, QG; Xie, LH; Barcus, M; Wellington, S; Brueckner, RP; Weina, P. Binding evaluation of new artemisinin analogs to plasma proteins and red blood cell of human and animal species in vitro and in vivo. (*unpublished data*)

[289] Brand, VB; Sandu, CD; Duranton, C; Tanneur, V; Lang, KS; Huber, SM; Lang, F. Dependence of Plasmodium falciparum in vitro growth on the cation permeability of the human host erythrocyte. *Cell Physiol. Biochem.* 2003. 13, 347-356.

[290] Nealon, C; Dzeing, A; Muller-Romer, U; Planche, T; Sinou, V; Kombila, M; Kremsner, PG; Parzy, D; Krishna, S. Intramuscular bioavailability and clinical efficacy of

artesunate in gabonese children with severe malaria. *Antimicrob Agents Chemother.* 2002. 46, 3933-3939.

[291] Ilett, KF; Batty, KT; Powell, SM; Binh, TQ; Thu le, TA; Phuong, HL; Hung, NC; Davis, TM. The pharmacokinetic properties of intramuscular artesunate and rectal dihydroartemisinin in uncomplicated falciparum malaria. *Br. J. Clin. Pharmacol.* 2002. 53, 23-30.

[292] Rehwagen, C. WHO ultimatum on artemisinin monotherapy is showing results. *BMJ.* 2006. 332(7551), 1176.

[293] White, NJ. Assessment of the pharmacodynamic properties of antimalarial drugs in vivo. *Antimicrob. Agents Chemother.* 1997. 41, 1413–1422.

[294] Newton, PN; Barnes, KI; Smith, PJ; Evans, AC; Chierakul, W; Ruangveerayuth, R; White, NJ. The pharmacokinetics of intravenous artesunate in adults with severe falciparum malaria. *Eur. J. Clin. Pharmacol.* 2006. 62, 1003-1009.

[295] White, NJ; Nosten, F; Looareesuwan, S; Watkins, WM; Marsh, K; Snow, RW; Kokwaro, G; Ouma, J; Hien, TT; Molyneux, ME; Taylor, T; Newbold, CI; Ruebush II, TK; Danis, M; Greenwood, BM; Anderson, RM; Olliaro, P. Averting a malaria disaster. *Lancet.* 1999. 353, 1965–1967.

[296] Bunnag, D; Viravan, C; Looareesuwan, S; Karbwang, J; Harinasuta, T. Double blind randomised clinical trial of oral artesunate at once or twice daily dose in falciparum malaria. *Southeast Asian J. Trop. Med. Public Health* 1991. 22, 539–543.

[297] Luxemburger, C; ter Kuile, FO; Nosten, F; Dolan, G; Bradol, JH; Phaipun, L; Chongsuphajaisiddhi, T; White, NJ. Single day mefloquine- artesunate combination in the treatment of multi-drug resistant falciparum malaria. *Trans. R. Soc. Trop. Med. Hyg.* 1994. 88, 213–217.

In: Progress in Malaria Research
Editor: Lee O. Koning, pp. 99-126

ISBN: 978-1-60021-590-2

Chapter II

The Role of Antibodies in Protection Against Complications of *Plasmodium Falciparum* Malaria

Michael Eisenhut
University of Liverpool, Institute of Child Health,
United Kingdom

Abstract

Transfer experiments of immunoglobulin from donors immune to *Plasmodium (P.) falciparum* malaria to patients symptomatic with *P. falciparum* malaria lead to a reduction in parasitemia and demonstrated the importance of immunoglobulines in anti-plasmodial immunity. Subsequent immunoepidemiological studies demonstrated that antibodies against *P. falciparum* bloodstage antigens are in addition to their antiparasitic effect essential in protection against complications of *P. falciparum* infection like severe anemia, placental malaria in pregnancy and possibly cerebral malaria which account for the majority of malaria related morbidity and mortality worldwide. Comparison of antibody levels between patients with complicated and uncomplicated *P. falciparum* malaria have shown that it is not the global quantity of antiplasmodial antibodies indicating previous exposure to the parasite which is associated with protecion from complications. Studies showed that antibodies against specific blood stage antigens on the surface of parasitized red blood cells and merozoites are most closely associated with protection from complications of *P. falciparum* malaria. Targets for antibodies which were found to be protective against complications of *P. falciparum* infection include in merozoites: merozoite surface proteins (MSP) 1 and 2, glutamate rich protein on the merozoite surface and apical merozoite antigen-1 and rhoptry protein-1. On the erythrocyte surface *P. falciparum* membrane protein-1, which is involved in cytoadherence, induces antibodies protective against complications. Antibodies against glycosylphosphatidylinositol (GPI) anchors of proteins on the merozoite surface, which may prevent cytoadherence promoting induction of endothelial adhesion molecules by tumor necrosis factor, have also been associated with clinical immunity.

Within the antigens mentioned only specific regions elicited protective antibodies like the C-terminal 19kDa fragment or block 2 of MSP-1 or the acylated phosphoinositol portion of GPI. Protective antibodies were found to be of the subclasses IgG-1 and IgG-3 for protein antigens involved. This may be partially due to their ability to bind to Fc receptors on monocytes promoting antibody dependent cellular inhibiton.

Future research needs to aim at a comprehensive analysis of antigens eliciting a protective antibody response. This could be achieved by using 2-dimensional immunoblotting of bloodstage antigens comparing immunoglobulin subclass responses to the full profile of parasite proteins identified by proteomics and mass spectrometry between patients with clinical immunity to *P. falciparum* and patients with complicated *P. falciparum* malaria. The relative importance of the various different antigens involved in inducing a protective response needs to be quantified.

1. Introduction

Clinical symptoms in *Plasmodium falciparum* malaria like pyrexia are associated with the development of blood stages of this parasite in patients. Clinical immunity to malaria has been defined as the presence of bloodstages in an asymptomatic individual [1]. In areas of intense transmission of this parasite development of clinical immunity to complications of *P. falciparum* malaria like anemia, metabolic acidosis and cerebral malaria is associated with an increasing pyrogenic threshold of parasite density (that is the levels of parasitemia in peripheral blood at which pyrexia occurs) over several years of continuous exposure (See figure 1) [2]. Immunity to blood stage parasites cannot be mediated by cytotoxic T-cells because red blood cells don't carry MHC class I required for T-cell dependent cytotoxicity [3]. The focus of research into immune mechanisms against blood stages of *P. falciparum* has therefore been directed to antibody-mediated immunity. Motivating for early researchers to explore the role of antibodies in induction of immunity was also the observation that infants within the first 3-4 months of life appear to be protected against the symptoms of malaria, which lead to speculations that a substance which is transferable through the placenta like IgG antibodies may mediate protection. In this chapter I tried to summarize what is known about the role of antibodies in preventing and reducing the symptoms of *P. falciparum* malaria in humans. Similar to the approach of a systematic review both studies with positive as well as those with negative results were included and the methodology critically analysed.

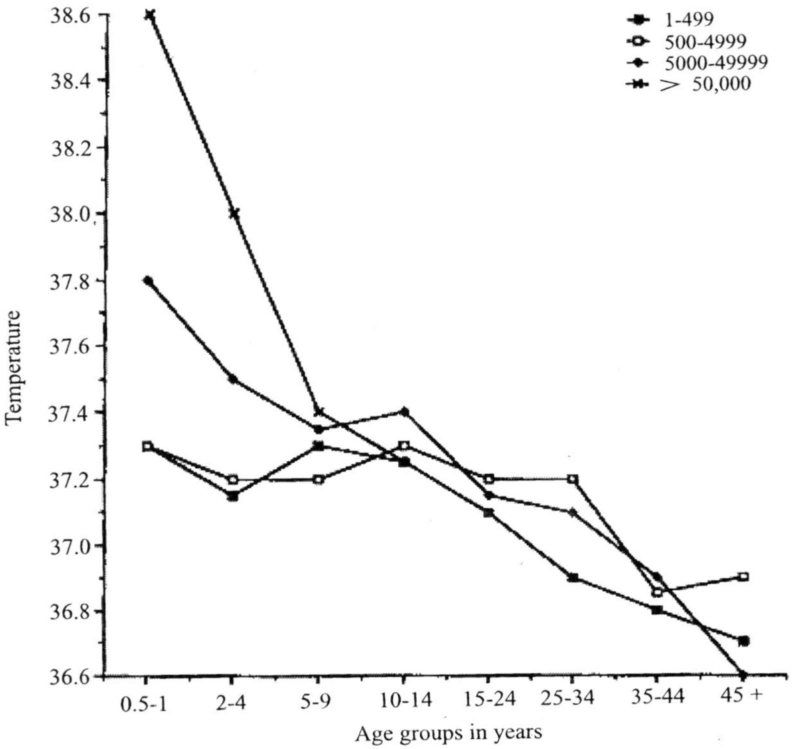

Figure 1. Results of body temperature measurements and peripheral blood stage counts from a cross sectional study in 1622 randomly selected individuals from 10 villages in Liberia from an area of continuous transmission [2].

2. The Role of Immunoglobulins in Protection Against Complications of *Plasmodium Falciparum* Malaria

2.1. Lessons from Immunoglobulin Transfer Experiments

The role of antibodies in antiplasmodial immunity was first investigated by Coggeshall et al. [4] who showed that protection against *P. knowlesi* could be transferred to non-immune rhesus monkeys through serum obtained from monkeys previously immunized against this species. Subsequently early experiments in humans showed that gamma-globulin transfer equivalent to 10 to 20 percent of the recipients own gamma-globulin. from apparently immune Gambian adults to 12 children aged 4 months to 2.5 years with symptomatic parasitemia (10 000 to 230 000/microliter) with *P. falciparum* resulted in a parasite count of <1% of the initial values with trophozoites being undetectable in 8/12 patients and a maximum count of 80/ microliter (figure 2). Gametocyte development was not affected. Decrease in parasitemia was accompanied by a progressive reduction of clinical symptoms

[5]. Gamma-globulin synthesis was found to be generally increased in patients exposed continuously to infection with *P. falciparum* but this increase did not extend to IgA or IgD levels. Treatment with antimalarial drugs and stay outside areas endemic for *P. falciparum* malaria was found to be associated with a reduction of gamma-globulin synthesis. The results were found to be reproducible in transfer studies using gamma-globulin from West African adults in children from East Africa symptomatic with *P. falciparum* malaria [6] in transfer experiments of immunoglobulin from adults to children with malaria in Nigeria [7] and in transfer studies using gamma globulin from adults from Cote d'Ivoire in Thai patients with *P. falciparum* malaria [8] (see figure 3).

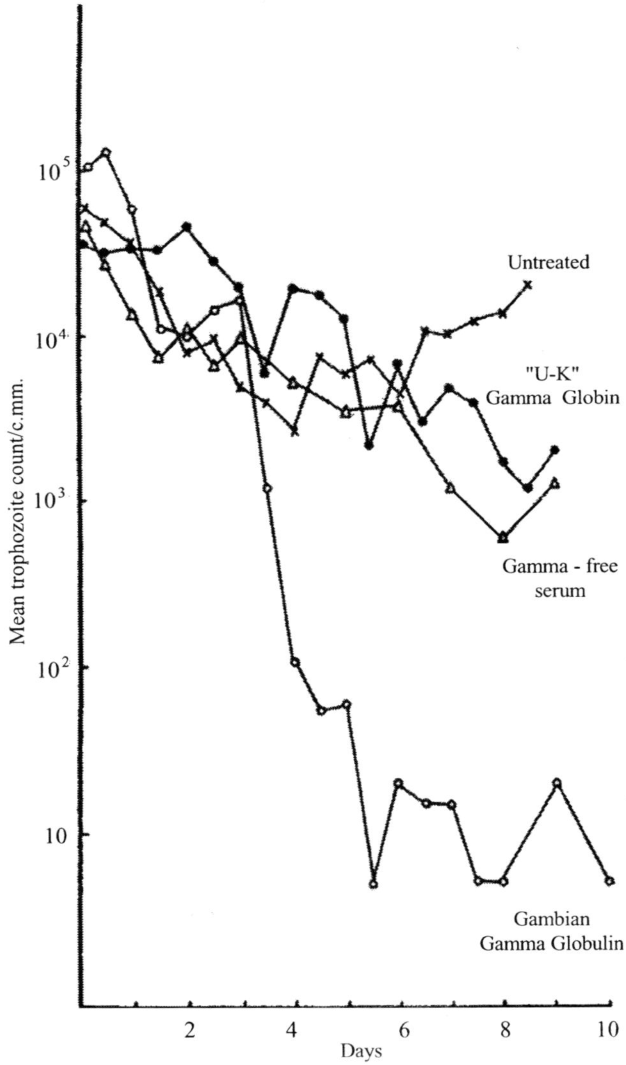

Figure 2. Mean trophozoite counts (logarithmic scale) in four groups of children with acute *Plasmodium falciparum* malaria. The treated children received either (i) γ-globulin prepared from blood donors in Great Britain, or (ii) serum prepared from Gambian adults γ-free and (iii) γ-globulin prepared from Gambian adults [5].

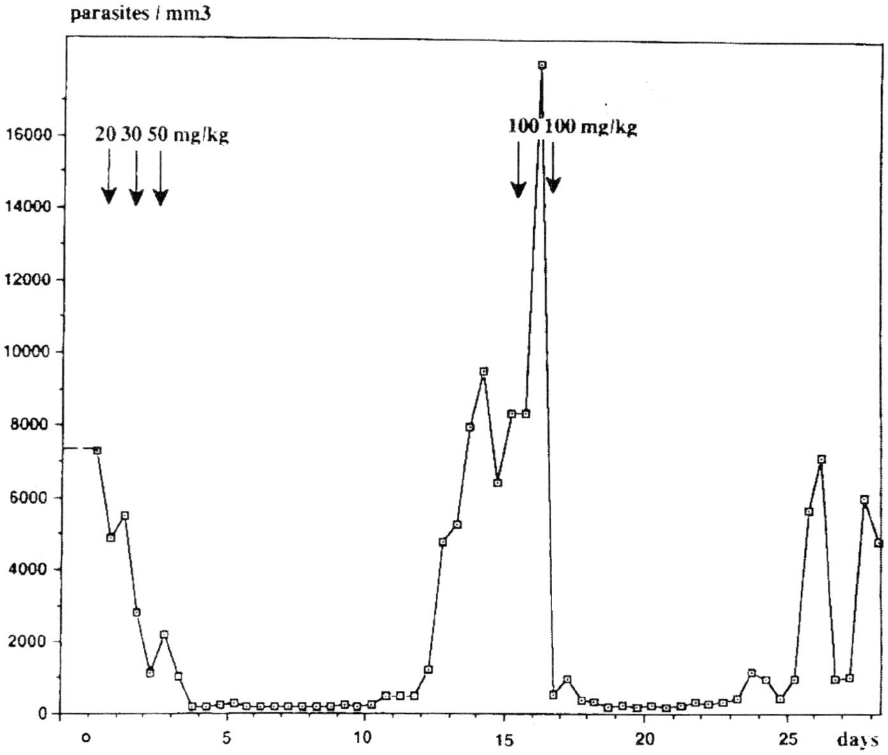

Figure 3. Development of blood stage count in a Thai patient after injections of immunoglobulin from adults from an area with continuous transmission in Cote d'Ivoire [8].

2.2. Association of Levels of Antiplasmodial Immunoglobulin Against Unfractionated Blood Stage Antigen Mixtures with Protection Against Symptoms of *P. Falciparum* Infection

On the basis of promising results of immunoglobulin transfer experiments cross sectional and prospective studies investigating the association of levels of antiplasmodial antibodies with antiparasitic and clinical immunity have been undertaken. A detailed prospective study of 76 children in Gabon found that children with symptomatic (pyrexia) parasitemia had significantly lower IgG levels against unfractionated schizont preparations compared to children with asymptomatic parasitemia over a period of about a year [9]. Children with asymptomatic parasitemia were however significantly older (mean 11.5 vs. mean 9.6 years) than symptomatic children. A cross sectional study found no difference in levels of IgG or IgM against unfractionated schizont antigen between children of the same age and area or residence with mild or severe malaria [10]. These early studies illustrated the importance of age dependency of antiplasmodial immunoglobulin levels and the necessity to correct effects of immunoglobulin levels for age.

2.3. The Role of Cytophilic Immunoglobulin Subclasses

The results reported above lead investigatior to explore whether a specific type of immunoglobulin in terms of either antigen specificity or subclass was effective against *P. falciparum* blood stages.

Bouharoun-Tayoun et al [11] noted that the antibodies used in a previous successful transfer experiment [8] had no detectable inhibitory effect on either penetration of merozoites or intra-erythrocytic development of the parasite in vitro but sometimes increased parasite growth. The transferred gamma globulin was however found to enable antibody-dependent cellular inhibition (ADCI) of *P. falciparum* by monocytes indicating that its activity may be related to the ability to collaborate with this cell population. This phenomenon had been described by other groups before [12, 13] and was found to be associated with the IgG fraction of the immunoglobulins, was not present in individuals recovering from their first *P. falciparum* infection and was directed against a mixture of trophozoites and schizonts but not against ring forms [13]. Antibodies collaborating with monocytes (therefore called "cytophilic" antibodies) were found to be IgG3 and to a slightly lesser extent IgG1. It was demonstrated that ADCI is dependent on monocyte generated TNF [14]. The same antibody subclass has also been labelled as "opsonizing" because it can mediate phagocytosis of cells with antigen on the surface including parasitized red blood cells. The first study investigating the association of cytophilic antiplasmodial antibodies with protection from infection was conducted in French Guinea where a cross-sectional study investigated the levels of opsonizing antibodies comparing persons living in endemic areas without parasitemia and persons from endemic areas with acute malaria. They found that opsonization promoting antibody levels were significantly higher in patients without parasitemia despite their global antibody titres to parasitized red blood cells detected by immunofluorescence assay not being significantly different. Opsonizing antibodies were found to be of IgG1 and IgG3 subclass and antiplasmodial IgG2 and IgG4 antibodies were found to inhibit the opsonizing activity of IgG1 and 3 [15]. A study from Burkina Faso found a dominance of ADCI causing antibodies in hyperimmune adults, which were predominantly of IgG3 and IgG1 subclass. Sera from nonimmune persons were found to reduce ADCI [16]. This was confirmed in a study in Ivory Coast in which clinically immune adults had higher IgG1 and 3 antibodies against total blood stage antigens than nonimmune subjects with an acute malaria attack. This study also confirmed again the increase in antiplasmodial IgG1 and 3 levels in patients with age, which illustrated that studies attempting to prove the protective efficiency of an immunoglobulin subclass need to correct any effect for age [17]. Taking age into account was a subsequent prospective study in 145 individuals of all age groups conducted in Senegal. It found that corrected for age IgG3 antibody levels against unfractionated schizont antigen were the only subclass associated with a reduced incidence of clinical malaria attacks over a 2-year period. IgG3 levels were found to account for 35.2% of the age-associated protective effect in the 3-6-years-old age group and 5.8% in the older inhabitants [18].

IgG3 levels to an unfractionated *P. falciparum* blood stage antigen extract were significantly associated with survival in a group of 41 patients (14 deaths) on an intensive care unit in Senegal [19]. A cross-sectional study comparing IgG subclass levels against unfractionated schizont antigen between age matched patients with complicated and uncomplicated malaria in the Amazon region in Brazil found significantly higher IgG1 levels in patients with uncomplicated malaria.with no significant difference in other subclasses [20].

2.4. The Role of Antigen and Epitope Specific Antibody Responses

2.4.1. Merozoite Antigens

Rhoptry-Associated Protein-1

Rhoptries are intracellular organelles of malaria parasites involved in the invasion of red blood cells by *Plasmodium* merozoites. Antibodies against rhoptry-associated protein-1 (RAP-1) have inhibitory effects on *P. falciparum* growth in vitro.

Antibody levels (ELISA) to (RAP-1) peptide 202-210 were higher in children with asymptomatic parasitemia compared to children who were pyrexial with parasitemia in Gabon [9]. This result was confirmed in another cross-sectional study in children (1-4 years) in Tanzania where children with asymptomatic parasitemia had significantly higher levels of antibodies against the RAP-1 peptides 23-486 and 293-608 [21].

Merozoite Surface Protein-1

Plasmodium falciparum merozoite surface protein-1 (PfMSP-1) is synthesized during schizogony and postsynthetic processing gives rise to multiple fragments. Its gene is divided into 17 distinct blocks. Proteins encoded by block 17 (the C-terminal 19-kDa fragment) and block 2 have been investigated for their relevance for immunity to *P.falciparum* blood stages.

A)The C-Terminal 19-kDa Fragment

The C-terminal 19-kDa fragment (PfMSP-1_{19kD}) comprises of two epidermal growth factor (EGF)-like motifs, which may be involved in attachment of the parasite to specific red cell surface receptors. Antibodies to PfMSP-1 can block parasite invasion of red blood cells in vitro [3]. Studies addressing the protective properties of anti-PfMSP-1_{19kD} antibodies however yielded contradictory results:

An early prospective study in Papua New Guinea investigated the correlation of levels of PfMSP-1 antibodies to the N and the C-terminal area (then called BVp42) and incidence rate of clinical malaria in 0.5-15 year old children [22]. When age and past exposure (antibody levels to a schizont extract) were corrected for only antibodies to the C-terminal area were significantly associated with a reduced incidence of clinical malaria and severe parasitemia.

In a prospective study in Sierra Leone and the Gambia antibodies to PfMSP-1_{19kD} EGF 2/MAD20 domain (recombinant and expressed in bacteria) were associated with asymptomatic (11% were positive for this antibody) as opposed to symptomatic parasitemia (0 % were positive) in Gambian children but not in children from Sierra Leone after correction for age. Most of the children were older than 1 year of age. 4 children from Sierra Leone with antibodies to this domain experienced clinical infection. This study demonstrated that most of the protection is due to the antibody response to other antigens and that this antigen is poorly immunogenic [23].

A prospective study in Kenya investigated PfMSP-1_{19kD} antibody prevalence and levels in 144 infants comparing afebrile and febrile parasitemic children matched by age [24]. This study included a prospective study of neonates assessing the predictive value of maternal antibodies to this antigen in cord blood. Prevalence and levels of antibodies were significantly higher in the afebrile group compared to the febrile group one month prior to the first infection. The loss of hemoglobin with the first infection was significantly less in antibody positive infants. Untreated infants, who went on to clear their parasitemias without requiring treatment had significantly higher levels one month prior to their first detected infection. A prospective study in Gambian children investigating anti-MSP-1_{19kD} IgG levels in patients recovering from chloroquine resistant falciparum malaria while treated with chloroquine noted that parasitemia resolved more quickly in anti-MSP-1_{19kD} IgG positive children than in children without this antibody [25]. Two prospective studies, one in Tanzanian infants and one in 3 to 15 year old children from Ghana, did not find an association of MSP-1_{19kD} antibody levels or prevalence and absence of clinical malaria episodes [26, 27]. These studies could however not exclude exposure confounding i.e. whether the lack of malaria episodes was due to lack of infection as they did not investigate for asymptomatic parasitemia. The same applies to a prospective study conducted in 337 children in The Gambia where prevalence of antibodies to MSP-1_{19kD} was not associated with a reduced incidence of clinical malaria. This study found however that antibody levels against this antigen were associated with a reduced incidence of malaria [28]. The conclusion of the authors was that antibody levels significantly higher than the cut-off for detection were important for protection. The lack of protection associated with anti MSP-1_{19kD} antibodies was however confirmed in a prospective study in which exposure bias was probably excluded as 278/280 of children (3-15 years of age) included in this study were always parasitemic on monthly checks over the 17 months surveillance period of this study [29]. A crossectional study including mainly adult gold miners from Brazil found no association of MSP1_{19kD} antibodies and lack of symptoms comparing asymptomatic and symptomatic parasite carriers [30].

Possible reasons for the contradictory results of the studies listed (See table 1) fall into 3 categories:

a) Exposure confounding: Individuals found to be symptomatic with parasitemia may have had more antibodies because of higher exposure and the low levels of antibodies in asymptomatic individuals may have been due to lack of infections.
b) Presence of variable amounts of "blocking" MSP-1_{19kD} antibodies interfering with the inhibitory effect of MSP-1_{19kD} antibodies (31, 32).
c) Antibodies to this antigen are predominantly IgG-1. IgG-1may be more important for protection than IgG-3 in infancy because of its longer lifespan facilitating persistence of protective maternal antibodies. In older individuals the protective responses to other antigens more likely to elicit IgG-3 subclass responses predominate.

A possible resolution to the contradictory results of immunoepidemiological studies mentioned above was reported recently from Kenya [33] where a treatment time to infection study over a 10-week period was conducted in 76 people (age 1-80). Using a neutralization assay based on transgenic *P. falciparum* expressing the *P.chabaudi* MSP-119 ortologue, individuals with high level MSP-1_{19kD} –specific invasion inhibitory antibodies (IIA) (>75th percentile) had a significantly prolonged time to infection after controlling for age, blood-stage *P.falciparum* infection before drug administration, and pre-existing anti-MSP-1_{19} antibodies. Total IgG as well as IgG1 and IgG3 MSP-1_{19} antibody levels were not associated with a prolonged time to infection. This group also noted that the protective effect appeared to be limited to individuals in the highest quartile of MSP-1_{19}-specific IIA. This may indicate that only high levels of this antibody are protective.

B) Block 2 of MSP-1

The block 2 region is located within the N-terminal half of MSP-1. All block-2 sequences belong to one of three main polymorphic repeat sequence types labelled K1, MAD20 and RO33.

Based on a population genetic study Conway et al [28] identified block 2 as under most intense selection with the lowest interpopulation variance. Antibody positivity against K1 and MAD-like block 2 was independently and corrected for age associated with a reduced incidence of clinical malaria in a prospective study over 5 months on 337 children (3-7 years of age) in The Gambia. Antibodies to sequences flanking the main sequence types were not found to be protective and the effect of antibodies to the polymorphic repeat sequences was found to be additive [34]. This result was confirmed in a prospective study including 280 children 3-15 years of age in Ghana [29]. Another recent study in Brazilian gold miners [30] investigating a small subgroup of 40 participants comparing symptomatic and asymptomatic parasite carriers however found no difference in proportion of participants not recognizing any of the block 2 antigens.

Merozoite Surface Protein 2

Merozoite surface protein 2 (MSP 2) is an integral membrane protein associated with the merozoite surface of *P. falciparum*. Research has focused on the genetically variable central region which contains the group-specific sequences of serogroup A (3D7-type) and serogroup B (FC27-type). MSP 2 specific monoclonal antibodies have been shown to inhibit in vitro parasite invasion and growth. The protective efficacy of anti-MSP 2 antibodies was investigated in a prospective study in 230 children (age 0.5-15 years) in Papua New Guinea. There were less episodes of symptomatic *P. falciparum* infection in children who had higher titres of antibodies against serogroup A but not against serogroup B [35]. Antibody levels (ELISA) to merozoite surface antigen-2 peptide 213-220 were higher in children with asymptomatic parasitemia compared to children who were pyrexial with parasitemia in Gabon [9].

Apical Membrane Antigen-1

A study on individuals of all age groups (n=1071) in Kenya revealed that antibodies against the full length ectodomain (both FVO and 3D7 allele constructs) prior to malaria transmission season were significantly associated with protection from malaria in the following 6 months after adjusting for age and antibody reactivity to whole parasite (schizont) extract. [36].

2.4.2. Trophozoite Antigens

Ring-Infected Erythrocyte Surface Antigen

Ring-infected erythrocyte surface antigen (Pf/155RESA) is present in the organelles of merozoites and, from its location within the dense granules, it is released into the parasitophorus vacuole space shortly after merozoite invasion and then translocated to the erythrocyte membrane. RESA-defective *P. falciparum* strains induce lower levels of TNF after schizont rupture and peptides of RESA induced TNF secretion in vitro [37]. A prospective study in the Gambia revealed that IgG against the peptide 963-986 of Pf155/ring-infected erythrocyte surface antigen (RESA) was significantly more prevalent (18.4% vs. 7.3%) in children (3-8 years old) who had asymptomatic parasitemia compared to children with fever plus high parasitemia [38]. Children in another study in Burkina Faso who had lower levels of antibodies to repeat amino acid seqences of RESA had at least one malaria attack during the subsequent prospective study during the transmission period [39]. The reduction in malaria episodes with anti-RESA antibodies was confirmed in a prospective study in Papua New Guinea [35]. Longitudinal studies in Madagaskar and Malawi revealed an absence of malaria attacks during the transmission season in adults with higher levels of antibodies to the Pf155/RESA peptides $(EENV)_4$, $(EENVEHDA)_4$ and $(DDEHVEEPTVA)_3$ [40].

Glutamate Rich Protein

The glutamate-rich protein (GLURP) is present in all stages of *P. falciparum* development: the parasitophorous vacuole, erythrocytic schizonts and the surface of newly released merozoites. In a prospective study of 115 children (3-15 years) in Ghana children who remained asymptomatic with parasitemia over more than a year of surveillance were compared with children with symptomatic parasitemia [41]. It was found that IgG levels against the R0 region of GLURP were significantly higher in asymptomatic children. In another prospective study in The Gambia the presence of anti-$GLURP_{489-1271}$ IgG was found to be significantly associated with asymptomatic infection when compared to clinical malaria in 218 children. The association was only significant for children aged 5-8 years [42].

2.4.3. Schizont Antigens

Variant Surface Antigen on the Surface of Infected Red Blood Cells

Variant surface antigens (VSA) are a class of molecules expressed on the surface of *P. falciparum*-infected erythrocytes in the so-called knob structures. VSA are organized in families, which include the well characterized *Plasmodium falciparum* erythrocyte membrane proteins 1 (PfEMP 1), rifins and stevors. They are responsible for the sequestration of parasitized erythrocytes to the walls of postcapillary venules in organs including the brain and the placenta. The mechanisms of sequestration is by binding of these proteins to endothelial receptors such as intercellular adhesion molecule 1 (ICAM1), vascular CAM1, CD 36, thrombospondin, E-selectin, chondroitin sulphate A, hyaluronic acid, CD 51 and CD 31 [1]. In addition these proteins are involved in the formation of rosettes (see below).

The first study to suggest an involvement of antibodies to surface antigens of trophozoite and schizont carrying red blood cells (RBC's) in protection from symptomatic *P. falciparum* infection was conducted in 134 children (1-11 years of age) in The Gambia.

Antibodies against antigens on the unfixed RBC surface were measured by a micro-agglutination assay and were associated with a reduction of symptomatic parasitemia [43].

The incidence of clinical malaria was also increased in individuals in a prospective study in Sudan who had no antibodies to PfEMP 1 before the transmission season [44].

A prospective cohort study in 118 children (3 to 15 years of age) in Ghana compared children with symptomatic and asymptomatic (no pyrexia) parasitemia and found that children with asymptomatic parasitemia had after correction for age significantly higher antibodies to variant surface antigens but not to a conserved peptide (Mcvar-1 amino acids 183 to 194) of this antigen [45]. Clinical immunity involved specific antibodies against the PfEMP 1 of the infecting parasite strain only [46, 47].

2.4.4. Glycosylphosphatidylinositol

The search for antigens inducing production of the cytokine tumor necrosis factor (TNF), which has been involved in generation of pyrexia and induction of endothelial expression of intercellular adhesion molecules associated with cytoadherence and sequestration of parasitized red blood cells e.g. in brain in cerebral malaria, identified lipid-carbohydrate glycoconjugates as important inducers [48]. A hypothesis was put forward that clinical immunity characterized by asymptomatic parasitemia is due to immunity against this component of the parasite. Further investigation of TNF inducing lipid-carbohydrate glycoconjugates revealed that they are identical with glycosylphosphadylinositol (GPI) which forms the molecular structure anchoring MSP-1, MSP-2, MSP-4, MSP-5, MSP-10, CSP, rhoptry organelle proteins and gamete surface antigens to the cell membrane [49, 50]. Supportive evidence for the role of anti-GPI immunity in protection from symptoms and complications of malaria was found in children in Kenya where in a prospective nonbiased cohort study children's anti GPI antibody levels correlated over 4 years with protection against malaria attributable hemoglobin loss and pyrexia. The target of anti-GPI antibodies was found to be the acylated phosphoinositol portion [51]. Another group however identified the carbohydrate domain as the dominant epitope [1]. Against a role of GPI antibodies in clinical immunity was evidence that anti-phosphatidylinositol IgM antibodies were higher in patients with severe compared to patients with mild malaria [52] and IgG antibodies were not significantly different. There was no association between plasma TNF levels and titres of anti-phospholipid antibodies. Anti-phosphatidylinositol IgG antibodies were not significantly higher in children with mild versus cerebral malaria in another study in East Africa (age 1-5) [53]. Antiphosphatidylinositol antibodies were higher in patients with symptomatic versus asymptomatic *P.falciparum* infection [54]. In a study in The Gambia anti-GPI antibody levels in all age groups (6 months to >75 years) was documented. A comparison between levels in patients (n=233, age 3-8 years) with symptomatic and asymptomatic parasitemia was also made. No anti-GPI antibodies were observed in children <2 years of age and the peak of antibody prevalence was in the age group 15 to 20 years of age. Patients with cerebral malaria (n=84) or severe anemia (n=22) had anti-GPI antibody levels, which were not significantly different from patients with mild malaria with or without adjustment for age

[55]. The lack of IgG antibodies to GPI in children under 2 years of age raised the possibility that the predominant form of malarial GPI responsible for inducing anti-GPI antibodies is free glycolipid rather that protein-GPI complexes. The lack of importance of anti-GPI antibodies in young children was confirmed in a study of anti-GPI IgG and IgM levels in children 1-4 years of age where anti GPI IgG antibodies were found in 1/19 of clinically immune asymptomatic parasitemic children (56). In a prospective study in Papua, Indonesia, a strong antibody response to GPI was associated with a subsequently reduced risk of symptomatic *P.falciparum* malaria in children (6-12 years) but not in adults [57]. There has been no association of anti-GPI antibody levels and placental TNF-alpha levels or the presence of acute or chronic placental malaria [58]. Some of the contradictory results of the studies quoted above may result from the fact that the studies conducted so far mostly used as antigen for assays native GPI prepared in an one-step HPLC protocol. This protocol is known to be associated with significant contamination of the resultant GPI preparation, both from phospholipids as well as possibly *P. falciparum* peptides [1]. Another reason is that due to the poor immunogenicity of this compound in early childhood an antibody response with protective properties may in areas without continuous transmission only evolve in older children or adulthood.

2.4.5. The Role of IgM Antibodies

IgM has been involved in rosette formation, which is the binding of parasitized red blood cells to 2 or more uninfected red blood cells (RBC) [59]. The rosetting process has been involved in the pathogenesis of sequestration in the microvasculature. In Burkina Faso IgM but not IgG levels to an unfractionated schizont extract were significantly higher in children who had asymptomatic parasitemia only compared to children with symptomatic parasitemia in a prospective study during the transmission season [60].

In a prospective study in Kenya [24] PfMSP-1_{19} IgM prevalence or level was not different in infants with afebrile versus febrile parasitemia.

2.4.6. The Role of IgE Antibodies

Significantly higher IgE levels have been found in patients with cerebral malaria compared to age matched children with uncomplicated malaria [61]. This was confirmed in other studies showing higher IgE levels in patients with severe versus uncomplicated malaria [62]. Subsequently it has been demonstrated that IgE can efficiently activate monocytes to kill parasites by inducing surface expression and cross-linking of CD23, the low affinity receptor for IgE. This cross-linking leads to activation of inducible nitric oxide synthase, accumulation of cGMP and cAMP, activation of the transcription factor NF-kappaB and through this of the genes coding TNF. Comparison of IgE and TNF concentrations in the blood of patients with malaria showed an increase in parallel with severity of disease.

Sera from malaria immune persons induced significantly less TNF in monocytes after exposure to *P. falciparum* antigen if IgE depleted [63]. In adult Thai patients IgE and not IgG anti-plasmodial (unfractionated schizont antigen) antibodies were higher in patients with severe compared to uncomplicated disease [64]. Another prospective study in 700 individuals (1-84 years) in a holoendemic area in Tanzania however found that high anti-*P.falciparum* (lysates of infected erythrocytes) IgE levels were associated with a reduced risk of acute malaria after adjustment for age and total IgE [65]. The contradictory role of antiplasmodial IgE was further investigated in a large (n=647) prospective study and it was found that in 0.5 –4.0 year old children anti-schizont IgE levels were higher in patients with uncomplicated compared to severe malaria but in 5-15 year old patients, individuals with severe malaria had significantly higher IgE levels. The authors hypothesized that with increasing age antiplasmodial IgE levels exceed a threshold above which the pathogenic effects outweigh the beneficial effects [66].

2.4.7. Antibody Responses Not Associated with Immunity to P.Falciparum in Previous Studies

Antibodies against total schizont extract measured by ELISA were not associated with less clinical malaria [43]. Antibodies against unfractionated P. falciparum antigen, the tetrapeptide Asn-Ala-Asn-Pro ($(NANP)_{40}$), residues 188-363 from the N-terminal part of MSP-1, central or C terminal regions of Pf155/RESA peptide and microagglutinating antibodies against infected erythrocytes were not lower in patients with severe versus mild malaria [10] and for anti $(NANP)_{40}$ antibodies there was no association with a reduced incidence of clinical malaria between children with high titers of this antibody in a prospective study of 391 children in The Gambia [67].

Antibody levels to the circumsporozoite protein of *P. falciparum* were not higher in children with mild versus severe malaria in a crossectional study [10]. Protection from episodes of clinical malaria in a prospective study in The Gambia was not associated antibodies against the conserved sequence of the circumsporozoite protein [43]. The same applied to the peptide antigens 188-363 and 1147-1287 of the MSP 1 antigen or the C terminal or central repeat regions of Pf155/RESA. In other prospective studies antibody responses to the Block 1 and RQ33-like block 2 of MSP-1 were not associated with a reduced incidence of malaria episodes in children in The Gambia and Ghana [27, 28].

Antibodies against Ag44 (134-residue C-terminal fragment of rhoptry protein) were not associated with lack of infection in a prospective study in Vietnam. [68] There was no difference in antibody levels against erythrocyte binding antigen 175 of *P. falciparum*, which is located in the apical micronemes of merozoites between groups with and without clinical malaria in children (n=284, 3-9 years of age) in The Gambia [69]. There was no significant difference in levels of anti-phosphatidyl cholin IgG between non-cerebral and fatal cerebral malaria patients [70].

2.4.8. Subclass Responses to Specific Antigens

More recent studies have attempted to define the subclass type of antibodies to antigens found to be protective. One study investigated factors directing antigen specific class switching in vivo in 1000 inhabitants (all age groups) of Tanzanian villages. It found that $MSP\text{-}1_{19kD}$ and AMA-1 preferentially induce class switching to IgG1, with the degree of polarization of the response being influenced by the intensity of antigen exposure, whereas MSP-2, and to a lesser extent GPI preferentially induce class switching to IgG3, with the degree of polarization being influenced by both the intensity of antigen exposure and the age of the individual. The data also suggested that inherent characteristics of antigens have a major influence on the molecular events leading to class switching, and secondly, that young children may be relatively defective in the ability to produce IgG3. The gradual polarization of the antibody subclass response also implied an ongoing influence of antigen on the maturing immune response. Polarized IgG1 responses have also been found to Pf1155/RESA, crude schizont lysate, RAP-1, and MSP-6, while IgG3 responses were reported for polymorphic C-terminal region (block 2) of MSP-1, MSP-3, MSP-4 and MSP-7 [71]. The authors commented that there was a striking correlation between the presence of amino acid sequences that are simultaneously polymorphic and repetitive in the antigens that induce predominantly IgG3 and the absence of such polymorphic repeats in the IgG1-inducing antigens.

Analysis of the subclass response to GLURP [41] revealed that the ratio of IgG1 + IgG3 over IgG2 + IgG4 was significantly higher in asymptomatic parasitemic children compared to symptomatic children. Another study found that lack of clinical malaria in a 12 month cohort study in Myanmar was in 30 villagers associated with significantly higher IgG3 levels against GLURP or MSP-3 [72]. The responses to GLURP and MSP-3 were found to be mutually exclusive.

A longitudinal survey of 355 children (3-8 years of age) in The Gambia found that children who had asymptomatic parasitemia (n=28) had a significantly higher prevalence of IgG3 antibodies against the serogroup A of MSP 2 and IgG1 antibodies against serotype B compared to symptomatic children (n=25). IgG2 and 4 antibody prevalence was not associated with asymptomatic parasitemia [73].

In a prospective study in 248 inhabitants in Burkina Faso IgG2 responses to the epitope (EENV)4 of the C-terminal part of RESA, the 27-34 amino acid sequence of the N-terminal conserved region of MSP 2 and the epitope MSP2 Ct1 (199-206 amino acid sequence of the C-terminus conserved region of MSP-2) were associated with a reduced risk of infection [74]. IgG2 antibodies to the 277 to 287-amino acid sequence of MSP 1or amino acid sequences of the C-terminal conserved region of MSP-2 (Ct 2) were found not to be associated with a reduced risk of malaria. IgG4 anti RESA antibodies were associated with an increased risk of infection. IgG3 against MSP2-Ct2 was associated with a reduced risk of a malaria attack.

In a prospective study in 329 children (3-7 years) in The Gambia, after adjustment for potentially confounding factors like age and presence of parasitemia, presence of IgG3 against the C-terminal region of MSP 2 was associated with a reduced incidence of malaria during a 5 month period [75].

In a prospective study in Vietnam IgG3 subclass antibodies but not total IgG against the rhoptry associated membrane antigen (RAMA) was associated with a reduced incidence of infection [68].

2.5. The Role of Antibodies in Prevention of Complications Associated with Malaria in Pregnancy

Pregnancy-associated malaria (PAM) is characterized by accumulation of parasitized red blood cells in the placental intervillous space and is a major cause of low birthweight and maternal anemia. Placental malaria appears to have a profound influence on development of antiplasmodial antibodies in infancy: A prospective study in Kenya compared antibody levels to seven different epitopes in 50 children born to a mother with placental malaria (PM) to 50 infants without and found reduced levels for antibodies to epitopes on CSP, RAP-1 and EBA-175 in children 4-12 months of age born to mothers with PM [76] There was no significant difference in antibody levels for most of the antigens in the first 4 months indicating that transferred antibodies are not involved in this reduction in antibody development. It has been proposed that the exposure of the fetus to plasmodial antigens, which may be more likely with PM and has been demonstrated by the presence of antiplasmodial IgM in cord blood [77], may induce a degree of immune tolerance.

Infected red blood cells from the placenta of women with malaria are unique in their ability to adhere to chondroitin sulfate A (CSA) in vitro and in their absence of adhesiveness to other receptors normally used by parasitized red blood cells. This special property explains the fact that otherwise clinically immune women can develop PAM. The tendency to develop PAM is lost during subsequent pregnancies suggesting a development of immunity. The *P. falciparum* antigen mediating adhesion to the syncytiotrophoblast of placental tissue has been identified as belonging to the PfEMP-1 family of variant surface antigens. The PfEMP1 antigen involved, as evident from detectable antibodies against it, is only found in women about half way during their first pregnancy and antibodies against this antigen prior to pregnancy are associated with protection against placental parasitemia [78]. Serum inhibition of parasite adhesion in vitro to CSA has been related to reduced prevalence and reduced density of placental parasitemia [79].In a cross-sectional study in 477 Kenyan women chronic pregnancy-associated malaria with low or absent anti-placenta adhering PfEMP1 IgG had lower haemoglobin and delivered smaller babies than did corresponding women with high titers of this antibody [80].This result was confirmed by an independent study in Kenya in which secundigravid women with antiadhesion antibodies delivered babies that were on average 398 g heavier and 2 weeks more mature that women without [81]. The process of antibody mediated protection by anti CSA adhering PfEMP 1 antibodies was defined further in a study in pregnant women in Cameroon and found that they appear at around 20 weeks of gestation in primigravid women about 5 weeks after the peak of parasitemia and correlate negatively with placental parasitemia [78]. Another receptor for syncytiotrophoblast binding PfEMP 1 was found to be hyaluronic acid (HA) which is expressed at low levels in normal placenta and higher levels in inflammatory conditions such as pre-eclamptic toxemia [82, 83]. Another mechanism by which parasitized red blood cells bind to the syncytiotrophoblast of the placenta was detected in women from Cameroon: It involved the binding of the Fab fragment of nonimmune IgG to PfEMP-1 which then forms a bridge for attachment to the Fc-receptors in the placenta. This mechanism was independent of CSA [84]. This result has been reported by one group and requires further confirmation in other studies. Other components of antiplasmodial immunity have also been associated with a reduction of placental malaria: Maternal anti-MSP-1_{19kD} antibodies at the time of delivery were associated with a reduced incidence and mean parasite density of placental malaria in a prospective study in Kenya [24]. Antibodies against adhesive PfEMP 1 antigens appear to be of IgG1 and 3 subclass [85].

2.6. Vertical Transfer of Antiplasmodial Antibodies and Protection of Infants from Complications of *P. Falciparum* Infection

Direct evidence of maternal-fetal transmission of antiplasmodial antibodies was found by comparison of titres in maternal and cord blood [86]. Immunoglobulin subclasses binding to infected red blood cells detected included IgG1,2 and 3 and to a lesser extent IgG4. No difference in antigen specificity between maternal and cord antibodies was detectable but cord blood immunoglobulin concentrations were generally lower.

The first study demonstrating the antiplasmodial activity of transplacentally transferred antibodies was an immunoglobulin transfer experiment in which a gammaglobulin fraction extracted from cord blood was transferred to a 12 month old child with symptomatic parasitemia. The trophozoite count dropped from 83700/microliter to 7750 by the 4th day and no trophozoites were seen from the 5th day onwards [7]. An early review revealed that the presence of antiplasmodial antibodies in infants was not associated with a reduced risk of infection [87]. A subsequent investigations of antibody subclasses responses to unfractionated late trophozoite and schizont antigen in umbilical cord blood in Cameroon revealed that newborns who had *P.falciparum*-specific IgG2 detected in cord blood were less likely to present with a *P.falciparum* infection during the first 6 months of life [88]. Investigations of antibodies against unfractionated schizont antigen and MSP-1_{19kD} in infants at birth in Liberia correlated their levels prospectively with the probability of a future clinical malaria episode. There was a lower risk of developing an episode of clinical malaria during the first year of life in the infants with high levels of anti-MSP-1_{19kD} at birth [89]. Another study in 50 Kenyan infants found that increased anti-MSP-1 $_{19kD}$ IgG1levels was correlated with a lower mean parasite density [90]. A lack of association between the age of onset of clinical malaria and cord serum IgG to Pf155/RESA and specifically the C-terminal repeat region of this antigen ($(EENV)_6$) and a peptide from the circumsporozoite central repeat region ($(NANP)_6$) was found in a longitudinal study on 49 infants in Nigeria [91].

2.7. The Role of Antibodies in Malaria Induced Anemia

Severe malarial anemia is thought to result from suppression of erythropoiesis by cytokines (e.g. TNF) and an increased breakdown of non-parasitised red blood cells. In the latter process antibodies may be involved.

The Coombs direct antiglobulin test (DAT) is often positive during or after acute falciparum malaria but DAT results were found not to correlate with the severity or persistence of anemia or reticulocytosis [92]. Previous studies showed that these antibodies have schizont specificity [93]. An analysis of IgG-subclasses bound to RBC's in Gambian children with past or present malaria showed that only IgG1 but not IgG 2-4 subclasses were associated with anemia. This probably relates to complement fixation by the IgG1 molecules and the interaction of IgG1 with phagocytic cells [94].

Severe anemia in 56 adult patients with symptomatic *P. falciparum* infection without clinical immunity in Vietnam was found to be associated with high IgM erythrocyte antibody titers against parasite free red blood cells. The survival time of ^{51} Cr-tagged normal red cells was reduced in the majory of patients [95]. Anti-GPI antibody levels correlated with a reduction in haemoglobin loss in a previous prospective study [51]

2.8. The Ròle of Antibodies in Prevention of Cerebral Malaria

The first investigation into the role of immunoglobulins in cerebral malaria (CM) compared IgG and IgM levels detected by counter immune electrophoresis against unfractionated heat labile total *P. falciparum* antigen in Thai patients with (n=40) versus without (n=57) cerebral malaria. IgG antibodies were not significantly different between groups but IgM levels were significantly lower in the group of patients with CM [96]. A crossectional study comparing 24 children with cerebral and 22 children with uncomplicated malaria found that antibodies to unfractionated schizont antigen, MSP-1, 2 and RESA were not significantly different between groups. Antibodies against the 3D7 genotype of MSP-2 were associated with a better prognosis among children with cerebral malaria but this was attributed to the decreased virulence of this genotype [97].

Sera from patients with CM were also found to have less antibodies able to disrupt rosetting of red blood cells and more antibodies causing microagglutination of parasitized and non parasitized red blood cells than patients with non-cerebral malaria [98, 99].

The target antigen of anti-rosetting antibodies is unknown.

Based on results of in vitro studies showing that sequestration of parasitized red blood cells is important in the pathogenesis of CM and the fact that immune serum can inhibit and reverse cytoadherence between *P. falciparum*-parasitized erythrocytes and a variety of cell lines a randomized, double blind, placebo controlled trial of immunoglobulin from immune adults in patients with cerebral malaria was undertaken in Malawi. 31 children with cerebral malaria were enrolled. There was no difference in outcomes (death, parasite clearance, fever clearance and coma resolution) between the two groups. The study did not provide evidence that antibodies could reverse sequestration in vivo [100]. A possible cause was that the product may not have contained antibodies appropriate to the parasite variants causing the disease. Support for the hypothesis that antibodies against antigens, which may be directly or through induction of TNF involved in promoting cytoadherence in cerebral capillaries by induction of intercellular adhesion molecule-1, are protective against cerebral malaria was found in a cross sectional study in adults in Senegal. Comparing patients of similar age with mild and cerebral malaria it was found that while MSP-1_{19kD} antibodies were not significantly different between groups anti-GPI antibodies were significantly higher in patients with mild malaria [101].

2.9. Agenda for Future Research

Future research needs to clarify whether antiplasmodial IgG3, which appears to be required as the dominant subclass for the status of clinical immunity, requires the continuous presence of low-level parasitemia or antigen deposits throughout the year. The short half live of IgG3 of about 2 weeks [102] which also applies to transplacentally transferred IgG3 [103] suggests that antigen presence is required for the maintenance of an effective immune response. Investigations using sensitive PCR methods or gamma radiation emitting radioisotope labelled monoclonal antibodies to deposited antigens could address the question of persistent plasmodia or protein antigen. The importance of the type of antibody subclass in addition to antigen specificiy for clinical immunity means that vaccine development has to aim at differential induction of protective subclasses [104].

When investigating immunoglobulin subclasses in antiplasmodial immunity it may be better to screen purified native *P. falciparum* antigens, rather than nonglycosylated recombinant or synthetic peptides, as potential targets for naturally acquired cytophilic antibodies. Future studies need to aim at a comprehensive registry of immunorelevant antigens for a protective antibody response. Future strategies for vaccination against *P. falciparum* associated morbidity and mortality need to incorporate a complete set of protective immunoglobulin responses. To achieve this crude extracts from late trophozoite and schizont stages need to be subjected to 2-dimensional western blotting [105] in which the immunoglobulin subclasses can be visualized. The 2 dimensional isotype specific "immunomaps" of a comprehensive set of antigens for clinically immune patients with *P. falciparum* infection and those with complicated malaria need to be compared and could form the baseline for prospective studies. The now fully deciphered *P. falciparum* genome could form the basis of masspectrometric identification of antigens recognized in clinically immune but not in patients with complications. The pathogenicity of antigens (e.g. potential for TNF induction) revealed by this 2-dimensional approach can then be further elucidated by a monocyte Western blot [106].

Table 1. Antigen specific immunoglobulin responses associated with asymptomatic parasitemia. (- = no data)

Age range of study participants (years)	Country	Antigen	Protective immunoglobulin subclass	References
5-17	Gabon	RAP-1	-	[9]
1-4	Tanzania		-	[21]
< 1	Kenya	MSP-1_{19kD}	-	[24]
-	The Gambia	MSP-2	IgG3	[75]
3-8	The Gambia		IgG1+IgG3	[73]
-	Burkina Faso		IgG3	[74]
0.5-15	Papua New Guinea		-	[35]
3-8	The Gambia	RESA	-	[38]
-	Burkina Faso		-	[74]
3-15	Ghana	GLURP	IgG1+IgG3	[41]
5-8	The Gambia		-	[42]
1-11	Ghana	PfEMB-1	-	[45]

3. Conclusion

Antibody mediated clinical immunity to adverse effects of *P. falciparum* infection is associated with multiple antigens from schizont, trophozoite and merozoite blood stages (see table 1). Transfer experiments demonstrated that the effect of antibodies is also antiparasitic but that control of parasitemia is incomplete (see figure 3). Antibodies, which were protective against clinical manifestations of *P. falciparum* infection, were found to be of the IgG 1 or IgG3 subclass where investigated. Immunity to placental malaria is different from other forms of clinical immunity and specifically associated with protection from adhesion of parasitized red blood cells to the syncytiotrophoblast. Future research needs to aim at a complete picture of antigens and antibody subclasses, which are part of a protective immune response. This will provide the framework for a vaccine with the primary goal of reducing mortality and morbidity from complications of infection with *P. falciparum*.

References

[1] Schofield, L., and Mueller , I. (2006). Clinical immunity to malaria. *Curr. Mol. Med,* 6, 205-221.

[2] Petersen, E., Hogh, B., Marbiah, N.T., David, K.,and Hanson , A.P. (1991). Development of immunity against *Plasmodium falciparum* malaria: Clinical and parasitologic immunity cannot be separated. *J. Infect. Dis,* 164, 949-953.

[3] Yazdani, S.S., Mukherjee, P., Chauhan, V.S., and Chitnis, C.E. (2006). Immune responses to asexual blood-stages of malaria parasites. *Curr. Mol. Med,* 6, 187-203.

[4] Coggeshall, L.T., and Kumm, W.H. (1937). Demonstration of passive immunity in experimental monkey malaria. *J. Exp. Med,* 66, 177.

[5] Cohen, S., McGregor, I.A., and Carrington, S. (1961). Gamma-globulin and acquired immunity to human malaria. *Nature,* 192, 733-737.

[6] McGregor, I.A., Carrington, S.P., and Cohen, S. (1963). Treatment of East African *P. falciparum* malaria with West African human γ-globulin. *Trans. R. Soc. Trop. Med. Hyg,* 57, 170-175.

[7] Edozien, J.C., Gilles, H.M., and Udeozo, I.O.K. (1962). Adult and cord-blood gamma-globulin and immunity to malaria in Nigerians. *The Lancet,* 2, 951-955.

[8] Sabchareon, A., Burnouf , T., Ouattara, D., Attanath, P., Bouharoun-Tayoun, H., Chantavanich, P., Foucault, C., Chongsuphajaisiddhi, T., and Druilhe P. (1991). Parasitologic and clinical human response to immunoglobulin administration in falciparum malaria. *Am. J. Trop. Med. Hyg,* 45, 297-308.

[9] Migot-Nabias, F., Luty, A.J.F., Ringwald, P., Vaillant, M., Dubois, B., Renaut, A., Mayombo, J., Minh, T.N., Fievet, N., Mbessi, J.R., Millet, P., and Deloron, P. (1999). Immune responses against *Plasmodium falciparum* asexual blood-stage antigens and disease susceptibility in Gabonese and Cameroonian children. *Am. J. Trop. Med. Hyg,* 61, 488-494.

[10] Erunkulu, O.A., Hill, A. V. S., Kwiatkowski, D.P., Todd, J.E., Iqbal, J., Berzins, K., Riley, E.M., and Greenwood, B.M. (1992). Severe malaria in Gambian children is not due to lack of previous exposure to malaria. *Clin. Exp. Immunol,* 89, 296-300.

[11] Bouharoun-Tayoun, H., Attanath, P., Sabchareon, A., Chongsuphajaisiddhi, T. and Druilhe, P. (1990). Antibodies that protect humans against *Plasmodium falciparum* blood stages do not on their own inhibit parasite growth and invasion in vitro, but act in cooperation with monocytes. *J. Exp. Med,* 172, 1633-1641.

[12] Theander, T.G., Anderson, B.J., Pedersen, B.K., Jepsen, S., Bygbjerg, I.C., Hviid, L., Larson, P.B., and Kharazmi, A. (1988). Cell-mediated immunity to Plasmodium falciparum infection: evidence against the involvement of cytotoxic lymphocytes. *Scand. J. Immunol,* 28, 105.

[13] Celada, A., Cruchaud, A., and Perrin, L.H. (1982). Opsonic activity of human immune serum on in vitro phagocytosis of Plasmodium falciparum infected red blood cells by monocytes. *Clin. exp. Immunol,* 47, 635-644.

[14] Bouharoun-Tayoun, H., Oeuvray,C., Lunel, F., and Druilhe, P. (1995) Mechanisms underlying the monocyte-mediated antibody-dependent killing of Plasmodium falciparum asexual blood stages. *J. Exp. Med,* 182, 409-418.

[15] Groux, H., and Gysin, J. (1990). Opsonization as an effector mechanism in human protection against asexual blood stages of *Plasmodium falciparum*: functional role of IgG subclasses. *Res. Immunol,* 141, 529-542.

[16] Bouharoun-Tayoun, H., and Druilhe, P. (1992). Antibodies in falciparum malaria: What matters most, quantity or quality? *Mem. Inst.* Oswaldo Cruz, Rio de Janeiro, 87 (Suppl.III), 229-234.

[17] Bouharoun-Tayoun, H., and Druilhe, P. (1992). *Plasmodium falciparum* malaria: evidence for an isotype imbalance, which may be responsible for delayed acquisition of protective immunity. *Infect Immun,* 60, 1473-1481.

[18] Aribot, G., Rogier, C., Sarthou, J-L., Trape, J-F., Balde, A.T., Druilhe, P., and Roussilhon, C. (1996). Pattern of immunoglobulin isotype response to *Plasmodium falciparum* blood-stage antigens in individuals living in a holoendemic area of Senegal (Dielmo, West Africa). *Am. J. Trop. Med. Hyg,* 54, 449-457.

[19] Sarthou, J-L., Angel, G., Aribot, G., Rogier, C., Dieye, A., Balde, A.T., Diatta, B., Seignot, P., and Roussilhon, C. (1997). Prognostic value of anti-*Plasmodium falciparum*-specific immunoglobulin G3, cytokines, and their soluble receptors in West African patients with severe malaria. *Infect. Immun,* 65, 3271-3276.

[20] Ferreira, M.U., Kimura, E.A.S., Katzin, A.M., Santos-Neto, L.L., Ferrari, J.O., Villalobos, J.M., and De Carvalho, M.E. (1998). The IgG-subclass distribution of naturally acquired antibodies to *Plasmodium falciparum*, in relation to malaria exposure and severity. *Ann. Trop. Med. Parasitol,* 92, 245-256.

[21] Alifrangis, M., Lemnge, M.M., Moon, R., Theisen, M., Bygbjerg, I., Ridley, R.G., and Jakobsen, P.H. (1999). IgG reactivities against recombinant rhoptry-associated protein-1 (rRAP-1) are associated with mixed *Plasmodium* infections and protection against disease in Tanzanian children. *Parasitology,* 119, 337-342.

[22] Al-Yaman, F., Genton, B., Kramer, K.J., Chang, S.P., Hui, G.S, Baisor, M., and Alpers M.P. (1996). Assessment of the role of naturally acquired antibody levels to

Plasmodium falciparum merozoite surface protein-1 in protecting Papua New Guinean children from malaria morbidity. *Am. J. Trop. Med. Hyg,* 54, 443-448.

[23] Egan, A.F., Morris, J., Barnish, G., Allen, S., Greenwood, B.M., Kaslow, D.C., Holder, A.A., and Riley E.M. (1996). Clinical immunity to *Plasmodium falciparum* malaria is associated with serum antibodies to the 19-kDa C-terminal fragment of the merozoite surface antigen, PfMSP-1. *J. Infect. Dis,* 173, 765-769.

[24] Branch, O.H., Udhayakumar, V., Hightower, A.W., Oloo, A.J., Hawley, W.A., Nahlen, B.L., Bloland, P.B., Kaslow, D.C., and Lal, A.A. (1998). A longitudinal investigation of IgG and IgM antibody responses to the merozoite surface protein-1 19-kilodalton domain of *Plasmodium falciparum* in pregnant women and infants: associations with febrile illness, parasitemia, and anemia. *Am. J. Trop. Med. Hyg,* 58, 211-219.

[25] Pinder, M., Sutherland, C.J., Sisay-Joof, F., Ismaili, J., McCall, M.B., Ord, R., Hallett, R., Holder, A.A., and Milligan, P. (2006). Immunoglobulin G antibodies to merozoite surface antigens are associated with recovery from chloroquine-resistant *Plasmodium falciparum* in Gambian children. *Infect. Immun,* 74, 2887-2893.

[26] Kitua, A.Y., Urassa, H., Wechsler, M., Smith, T., Vounatsou, P., Weiss, N.A., Alonso, P.L., and Tanner, M. (1999). Antibodies against *Plasmodium falciparum* vaccine candidates in infants in an area of intense and perennial transmission: relationships with clinical malaria and with entomological inoculation rates. *Parasite Immunol,* 21, 307-317.

[27] Dodoo, D., Theander, T.G., Kurtzhals, J.A.L., Koram, K., Riley, E., Akanmori, B.D., Nkrumah, F.K., and Hviid, L. (1999). Levels of antibody to conserved parts of *Plasmodium falciparum* merozoite surface protein 1 in Ghanaian children are not associated with protection from clinical malaria. *Infection and Immunity,* 67, 2131-2137.

[28] Conway, D.J., Cavanagh, D.R., Tanabe, K., Roper, C., Mikes, Z.S, Sakihama, N., Bojang, K.A., Oduola, A.M.J., Kremsner, P.G., Arnot, D.E., Greenwood, B.M., and McBride, J.S. (2000) A principal target of human immunity to malaria identified by molecular population genetic and immunological analyses. *Nat. Med,* 6, 689-692.

[29] Cavanagh, D.R., Dodoo, D., Hviid, L., Kurtzhals, J.A.L., Theander, T.G., Akanmori, B.D., Polley, S., Conway, D.J., Koram, K., and McBride, J.S. (2004). Antibodies to the N-terminal block 2 of *Plasmodium falciparum* merozoite surface protein 1 are associated with protection against clinical malaria. *Infect. Immun,* 72, 6492-6502.

[30] Scopel, K.K.G., Fontes C..J.F., Ferreira M.U., and Braga, E.M. (2005). *Plasmodium falciparum*: IgG subclass antibody response to merozoite surface protein-1 among Amazonian gold miners, in relation to infection status and disease expression. *Exp. Parasitol,* 109, 124-134.

[31] Blackman, M.J., Scott-Finnigan, T.J., Shai, S., and Holder, A.A. (1994). Antibodies inhibit the protease-mediated processing of a malaria merozoite surface protein. *J. Exp. Med,* 180, 389-393.

[32] Patino, J.A., Holder, A.A., McBride, J.S., and Blackman, M.J. (1997). Antibodies that inhibit malaria merozoite surface protein-1 processing and erythrocyte invasion are blocked by naturally acquired human antibodies. *J. Exp. Med,* 186, 1689-1699.

[33] John, C.C., O'Donnell, R.A., Sumba, P.O., Moormann, A.M., De Koning-Ward, T.F., King C.L., Kazura, J.W., and Crabb, B.S. (2004). Evidence that invasion-inhibitory antibodies specific for the 19-kDa fragment of merozoite surface protein-1 ($MSP-1_{19}$) can play a protective role against blood-stage *Plasmodium falciparum* infection in individuals in a malaria endemic area of Africa. *J. Immunol,* 173, 666-672.

[34] Polley, S.D., Tetteh, K.K.A., Cavanagh, D.R., Pearce, R.J., Lloyd, J..M., Bojang, K.A., Okenu, D..M..N., Greenwood, B.M., McBride, J.S., and Conway, D.J. (2003). Repeat sequences in block 2 of *Plasmodium falciparum* merozoite surface protein 1 are targets of antibodies associated with protection from malaria. *Infect. Immun,* 71, 1833-1842.

[35] Al-Yaman, F., Genton, B., Anders, R., Taraika, J., Ginny, M., Mellor, S., and Alpers, M.P. (1995). Assessment of the role of the humoral response to *Plasmodium falciparum* MSP2 compared to RESA and SPf66 in protecting Papua New Guinean children from clinical malaria. *Parasite Immunol,* 17, 493-501.

[36] Polley, S.D., Mwangi, T., Kocken, C.H., Thomas, A.W., Dutta, S., Lanar, D.E., Remarque, E., Ross, A., Williams, T.N., Mwambigu, G., Lowe, B., Conway, D.J., and Marsh, K. (2004). Human antibodies to recombinant protein constructs of *Plasmodium falciparum* Apical Membrane Antigen 1 (AMA 1) and their association with protection from malaria. *Vaccine,* 23, 718-728.

[37] Picot, S., Peyron, F., Deloron, P., Boudin, C., Chumpitazi, B., Barbe, G.,l and Vuillez, J.P. (1993). Ring-infected erythrocyte surface antigen (Pf/155RESA) induces tumour necrois factor-alpha production. *Clin. Exp. Immunol,* 93,184-188.

[38] Riley, E.M., Allen, S.J., Troye-Blomberg, M., Bennett, S., Perlmann, H., Andersson, G., Smedman, L., Perlmann, P., and Greenwood, B.M. (1991). Association between immune recognition of the malaria vaccine candidate antigen Pf155/RESA and resistance to clinical disease: a prospective study in a malaria-endemic region of West Africa. *Trans. R. Soc. Trop. Med. Hyg,* 85, 436-443.

[39] Chumpitazi, B.F., Deloron, P., Peyron, F., Boudin, C., Picot, S., and Ambroise-Thomas, P. (1991). Relationships between clinical protection and antibodies to *Plasmodium falciparum* RESA (ring-infected erythrocyte surface antigen) peptides. *Int. J. Parasitol,* 21, 271-274.

[40] Astagneau, P., Roberts, J.M., Steketee, R.W., Wirima, J.J., Lepers, J-P., and Deloron, P. (1995) Antibodies to a *Plasmodium falciparum* blood-stage antigen as a tool for predicting the protection levels of two malaria exposed populations. *Am. J. Trop. Med. Hyg,* 53, 23-28.

[41] Dodoo, D., Theisen, M., Kurtzhals J.A.L., Akanmori, B.D., Koram, K.A., Jepsen, S., Nkrumah, F.K., Theander T.G., and Hviid, L. (2000). Naturally acquired antibodies to the glutamate-rich protein are associated with protection against *Plasmodium falciparum* malaria. *J. Infect. Dis,* 181, 1202-1205.

[42] Dziegiel, M., Rowe, P., Bennett, S., Allen, S.J., Olerup, O., Gottschau, A., Borre, M., and Riley, E.M. (1993). Immunoglobulin M and G antibody responses to *Plasmodium falciparum* glutamate rich protein: correlation with clinical immunity in Gambian children. *Infect. Immun,* 61, 103-108.

[43] Marsh, K., Otoo, L., Hayes, R.J., Carson, D.C., and Greenwood, B.M. (1989). Antibodies to blood stage antigens of *Plasmodium falciparum* in rural Gambians and

their relation to protection against infection. *Trans. R. Soc. Trop. Med. Hyg,* 83, 293-303.

[44] Giha, H.A., Staalsoe, T., Dodoo, D., Roper, C., Satti, G.M., Arnot, D.E., Hviid, L., and Theander, T.G. (2000). Antibodies to variable *Plasmodium falciparum*-infected erythrocyte surface antigens are associated with protection from novel malaria infections. *Immunol. Lett,* 71, 117-126.

[45] Dodoo, D., Staalsoe, T., Giha, H., Kurtzhals J.A.L., Akanmori B. D., Koram, K., Dunyo, S., Nkrumah, F.K., Hviid, L., and Theander, T.G. (2001) Antibodies to variant antigens on the surfaces of infected erythrocytes are associated with protection from Malaria in Ghanaian children. *Infect. Immun,* 69, 3713-3718.

[46] Bull, P.C., Pain, A., Ndungu, F.M., Kinyanjui, S.M., Roberts, D.J., Newbold, C.I., and Marsh, K. (2005). *Plasmodium falciparum* antigenic variation: relationships between in vivo selection, acquired antibody response, and disease severity. *J. Infect. Dis,* 192, 1119-1126.

[47] Bull, P.C., Lowe, B.S., Kortok, M., Molyneux, C.S., Newbold, C.I., and Marsh, K. (1998). Parasite antigens on the infected red cell surface are targets for naturally acquired immunity to malaria. *Nat. Med,* 4, 358-360.

[48] Bate, C.A.W., Taverne, J., Roman, E., Moreno, C., and Playfair, J.H.L. (1992). Tumor necrosis factor induction by malaria exoantigens depends upon phospholipid. *Immunology,* 75, 129-135.

[49] Schofield, L., Vivas, L., Hackett, F., Gerold, P., and Schwarz, R.T. (1993). Neutralizing monoclonal antibodies to glycosylphosphatidyl inositol, the dominant TNF alpha-inducing toxin of *Plasmodium falciparum*: prospects for the immunotherapy of severe malaria. *Ann. Trop. Med. Parasitol,* 87, 617-626.

[50] Gilson, P.R., Nebl, T., Vukcevic, D., Moritz, R.L., Sargeant, T., Speed, T.P., Schofield, L., and Crabb, B.S. (2006). Identification and stoichiometry of glycosylphosphatidylyinositol anchored membrane proteins of the human malaria parasite *Plasmodium falciparum*. *Mol. Cell Proteomics,* 5, 1286-1299.

[51] Naik, R.S., Branch, O.H., Woods, A.S., Vijaykumar, M., Perkins, D.J., Nahlen, B.L., Lal, A.A., Cotter, R.J., Costello, C.E., Ockenhouse, C.F., Davidson, E.A.and Gouda, D.C., (2000) Glycosyl phosphatidylinositol anchors of *Plasmodium falciparum*: Molecular characterization and naturally elicited antibody response that may provide immunity to malaria pathogenesis. *J. Exp. Med,* 192, 1563-1575.

[52] Jakobsen, P.H., Morris-Jones, S.D., Hviid, L., Theander, T.G., Hoier-Madsen, M., Bayoumi, R.A.L., and Greenwood, B.M. (1993). Antiphospholipid antibodies in patients with *Plasmodium falciparum* malaria. *Immunology,* 79, 653-657.

[53] Facer, C.A. and Agiostratidou, G. (1994). High levels of antiphospholipid antibodies in uncomplicated and severe *Plasmodium falciparum* and in *P. vivax* malaria. *Clin. Exp. Immunol,* 95, 304-309.

[54] Jakobsen, P.H., McKay, V., N`jie, R., Olaleye, B.O., D'Alessandro, U., Bendtzen, K., Schousboe, I., and Greenwood, B.M. (1996). Soluble products of inflammatory reactions are not induced in children with asymptomatic *Plasmodium falciparum* infections. *Clin. Exp. Immunol,* 105, 69-73.

[55] De Souza, J. B., Todd, J., Krishegowda, G., Gowda, D.C., Kwiatkowski, D., and Riley, E.M. (2002). Prevalence and boosting of antibodies to *Plasmodium falciparum* glycosylphosphatidylinositols and evaluation of their association with protection from mild and severe clinical malaria. *Infect. Immun,* 70, 5045-5051.

[56] Boutlis, C.S., Gowda, D.C., Naik, R.S., Maguire, G.P., Mgone, C.S., Bockarie, M.J., Lagog, M., Ibam, E., Lorry, K., and Anstey, N.M. (2002). Antibodies to *Plasmodium falciparum* glycosylphosphatidylinositols: Inverse association with tolerance of parasitemia in Papua New Guinean children and adults. *Infect. Immun,* 70, 5052-5057.

[57] Hudson Keenihan, S.N., Ratiwayanto, S., Soebianto, S., Krisin, Marwoto, H., Krishnegowda, G., Gowda, D.C., Bangs, M.J., Fryauff, D.J., Richie, T.L., Kumar, S., and Baird, J.K.(2003). Age-dependent impairment of IgG responses to glycosylphosphatidylinositol with equal exposure to *Plasmodium falciparum* among Javanese migrants to Papua, Indonesia. *Am. J. Trop. Med. Hyg,* 69, 36-41.

[58] Suguitan, A.L. Jr., Gowda, D.C., Fouda, G., Thuita, L., Zhou, A., Djokam, R., Metenou, S., Leke, R.G., and Taylor, D.W. (2004). Lack of an association between antibodies to *Plasmodium falciparum* glycosylphosphatidylinositols and malaria-associated placental changes in Cameroonian women with preterm and full-term deliveries. *Infect. Immun,* 72, 5267-5273.

[59] Somner, E.A., Black, J., and Pasvol, G. (2000). Multiple human serum components act as bridging molecules in rosette formation by *Plasmodium falciparum*-infected erythrocytes. *Blood,* 95, 674-682.

[60] Boudin, C., Chumpitazi, B., Dziegiel, M., Peyron, F., Picot, S., Hogh, B., and Ambroise-Thomas, P. (1993). Possible role of specific immunoglobulin M antibodies to *Plasmodium falciparum* antigens in immunoprotection of humans living in a hyperendemic area, Burkina Faso. *J. Clin. Microbiol,* 31, 636-641.

[61] Perlmann, H., Helmby, H., Hagstedt, M., Carlons, J. and Larsson, P.H. (1994) IgE elevation and IgE anti-malarial antibodies in *Plasmodium falciparum* malaria: association of high IgE levels with cerebral malaria. *Clin. Exp. Immunol,* 97, 284-292.

[62] Seka-Seka, J., Brouh, Y., Yapo-Crezoit, A.C., and Atseye, N.H. (2004). The role of serum immunoglobulin E in the pathogenesis of *Plasmodium falciparum* malaria in Ivorian children. *Scand. J. Immunol,* 59, 228-230.

[63] Perlmann, P., Perlmann, H., ElGhazali, G., and Blomberg, M.T. (1999). IgE and tumor necrosis factor in malaria infection. *Immunol. Lett,* 65, 29-33.

[64] Perlmann, P., Perlmann, H., Looareesuwan, S., Krudsood, S, Kano, S., Matsumoto, Y., Brittenham, G., Troye-Blomberg, M., and Aikawa, M. (2000). Contrasting functions of IgG and IgE antimalarial antibodies in uncomplicated and severe *Plasmodium falciparum* malaria. *Am. J. Trop. Med. Hyg,* 62, 373-377.

[65] Bereczky, S., Montgomery, S.M., Troye-Blomberg, M., Rooth, I., Shaw, M-A., and Faernert, A. (2004). Elevated anti-malarial IgE in asymptomatic individuals is associated with reduced risk for subsequent clinical malaria. *Int. J. Parasitol,* 34, 935-942.

[66] Calissano, C., Modiano, D., Sirima, B.S., Konate, A., Sanou, I., Sawadogo, A., Perlmann, H., Troye-Blomberg, M., and Perlmann, P. (2003). IgE antibodies to

Plasmodium falciparum and severity of malaria in children of one ethnic group living in Burkina Faso. *Am. J. Trop. Med. Hyg,* 69, 31-35.

[67] Riley, E.M., Allen, S.J., Bennett, S., Thomas, P.J., O'Donnell, A., Lindsay, S.W., Good, M.F., and Greenwood, B.M. (1990). Recognition of dominant T cell-stimulating epitopes from the circumsporozoite protein of *Plasmodium falciparum* and relationship to malaria morbidity in Gambian children. *Trans. R. Soc. Trop. Med. Hyg,* 84, 648-657.

[68] Topolska, A.E., Richie, T.L., Nhan, D.H., andCoppel, R.L. (2004). Association between responses to the rhoptry-associated membrane antigen of *Plasmodium falciparum* and immunity to malaria infection. *Infect. Immun,* 72, 3325-3330.

[69] Okenu, D.M.N., Riley, E.M., Bickle, Q.D., Agomo, P.U., Barbosa, A., Daugherty, J.R., Lanar, D.E., and Conway, D.J. (2000). Analysis of human antibodies to erythrocyte binding antigen 175 of *Plasmodium falciparum. Infect. Immun,* 68-5559-5566.

[70] Das, B.K., Parida, S., and Ravindran, B., (1996) Aprognostic role for anti-phosphatidyl choline antibodies in human cerebral malaria. *Clin. Exp. Immunol,* 103,442-445.

[71] Tongren, J.E., Drakeley, C.J., McDonald, S.L.R., Reyburn, H.G., Manjurano, A., Nkya, W..M. M., Lemnge, M. M., Gowda, C.D., Todd, J.E., Corran, P.H., and Riley, E. M. (2006). Target antigen, age, and duration of antigen exposure independently regulate immunoglobulin G subclass switching in malaria. *Infect. Immun,* 74, 257-264.

[72] Soe, S., Theisen, M., Roussilhon, C., Saw-Aye, K., and Druilhe, P. (2004). Association between protection against clinical malaria and antibodies to merozoite surface antigens in an area of hyperendemicity in Myanmar: Complementarity between responses to merozoite surface protein 3 and the 220-kilodalton glutamate-rich protein. *Infect. Immun,* 72, 247-252.

[73] Taylor, R.R., Allen, S.J., Greenwood, B.M., and Riley, E.M. (1998). IgG3 antibodies to *Plasmodium falciparum* merozoite surface protein 2 (MSP2): Increasing prevalence with age and association with clinical immunity to malaria. *Am. J. Trop. Med. Hyg,* 58, 406-413.

[74] Aucan, C., Traore, Y., Tall, F., Nacro, B., Traore-Leroux, T., Fumoux, F.and Rihet ,P. (2000). High immunoglobulin G2 (IgG2) and low IgG4 levels are associated with human resistance to *Plasmodium falciparum* malaria. *Infect. Immun,* 68, 1252-1258.

[75] Metzger, W.G., Okenu, D.M.N., Cavanagh, D.R., Robinson, J.V., Bojang, K.A., Weiss, H.A., McBride, J.S., Greenwood, B.M. and Conway, D.J. (2003). Serum IgG3 to the *Plasmodium falciparum* merozoite surface protein 2 is strongly associated with a reduced prospective risk of malaria. *Parasite Immunol,* 25, 307-312.

[76] Bonner, P.C., Zhou, Z., Mirel, L.B., Ayisi, J.G., Shi, Y.P., Van Ejik, A.M., Otieno, J.A., Nahlen, B.L., Steketee, R.W., and Udhayakumar, V. (2005) Placental malaria diminishes development of antibody responses to *Plasmodium falciparum* epitopes in infants residing in an area of Western Kenya where *P. falciparum* is endemic. *Clin. Diag. Lab. Immunol,* 12, 375-379.

[77] Xi, R., Leke, G., Thuita, L.W., Zhou, A., Leke, R.J., Mbu, R., and Taylor, D.W. (2003). Congenital exposure to *Plasmodium falciparum* antigens: prevalence and antigenic specificity of in utero-produced antimalarial immunoglobulin M antibodies. *Infect. Immun,* 71, 1242-1246.

[78] Staalsoe, T., Megnekou, R., Fievet, N., Ricke, C.H., Zornig, H.D., Leke, R., Taylor, D.W., Deloron, P., and Hviid, L. (2001). Acquisition and decay of antibodies to pregnancy-associated variant antigens on the surface of *Plasmodium falciparum* infected erythrocytes that are associated with protection against placental parasitemia. *J. Infect. Dis,* 184, 618-626.

[79] Fried, M., Nosten, F., Brockman, A., Brabin, B.J., and Duffy, P.E. (1998). Maternal antibodies block malaria. *Nature,* 395, 851-852.

[80] Staalsoe, T., Shulman C.E., Bulmer, J.N., Kawuondo, K., Marsh, K., and Hviid, L. (2004). Variant surface antigen-specific IgG and protection against clinical consequences of pregnancy-associated *Plasmodium falciparum* malaria. *The Lancet,* 363, 283-289.

[81] Duffy, P.E., and Fried, M. (2003). Antibodies that inhibit *Plasmodium falciparum* adhesion to chondroitin sulfate A are associated with increased birth weight and the gestational age of newborns. *Infect. Immun,* 71, 6620-6623.

[82] Beeson, J.G., Rogerson, S.J., Cooke, B.M. Reeder, J.C., Chai, W., Lawson, A.M., Molyneux, M.E., and Brown, G.V.. (2000). Adhesion of Plasmodium falciparum-infected erythrocytes to hyaluronic acid in placental malaria. *Nat. Med.* 6, 86-90.

[83] Matejevic, D., Neudeck, H., Graf, R., Muller, T., and Dietl, J. (2001). Localization of hyaluronan with a hyaluronan-specific hyaluronic acid binding protein in the placenta in preeclampsia. *Gynecol. Obstet. Invest,* 52, 257-259.

[84] Flick, K., Scholander, C., Chen, Q., Fernandez, V., Pouvelle, B., Gysin, J., and Wahlgren, M. (2001). Role of nonimmune IgG bound to PfEMP 1 in placental malaria. *Science,* 293, 2098-2100.

[85] Elliot, S.R., Brennan, A.K., Beeson, J.G., Tadesse, E., Molyneux, M.E., Brown, G.V., and Rogerson, S.J. (2005). Placental malaria induces variant-specific antibodies of the cytophilic subtype Immunoglobulin G1 (IgG1) and IgG3 that correlated with adhesion inhibitory activity. *Infect. Immun,* 73, 5903-5907.

[86] Chizzolini, C., Trottein, F., Bernard, F.X., and Kaufmann, M.-H. (1991). Isotypic analysis, antigen specificity and inhibitory function of maternally transmitted *Plasmodium falciparum*-specific antibodies in Gabonese newborns. *Am. J. Trop. Med. Hyg,* 45, 57-64.

[87] Brabin B (1990). An analysis of malaria parasite rates in infants: 40 years after MacDonald. *Trop. Dis. Bull,* 87, R1-R21.

[88] Deloron, P., Dubois, B., Le Hesran, J.Y., Riche, D., Fievet, N., Cornet, M., Ringwald, P., and Cot, M. (1997). Isotypic analysis of maternally transmitted *Plasmodium falciparum*-specific antibodies in Cameroon, and relationship with risk of *P. falciparum* infection. *Clin. Exp. Immunol,* 110, 212-218.

[89] Hogh, B., Marbiah, N.T., Burghaus, P.A., and Andersen, P.K. (1995). Relationship between maternally derived anti-*Plasmodium falciparum* antibodies and risk of infection and disease in infants living in an area of Liberia, West Africa, in which malaria is highly endemic. *Infect. Immun,* 63, 4034-4038.

[90] Branch, O.H., Oloo, A.J., Nahlen, B.L., Kaslow, D., and Lal, A.A. (2000). Anti-merozoite surface protein-1 19-kDa IgG in mother –infant pairs naturally exposed to *Plasmodium falciparum:* subclass analysis with age, exposure to asexual parasitemia,

and protection against malaria. V. The Asembo Bay Cohort Project. *J. Infect. Dis,* 181, 1746-1452.

[91] Achidi, E.A., Salimonu L.S., Perlmann, H., Perlmann, P., Berzins, K., and Williams, A.I.O. (1996). Lack of association between levels of transplacentally acquired *Plasmodium falciparum*-specific antibodies and age of onset of clinical malaria in infants in a malaria endemic area of Nigeria. *Acta Trop,* 61, 315-326.

[92] Phillips, R.E., and Pasvol, G. (1992). Anaemia of *Plasmodium falciparum* malaria. *Bailliere's Clin. Haematol,* 5, 315-330.

[93] Facer, C.A. (1980). Direct Coombs antiglobulin tests in Gambian children with *P. falciparum* malaria II. Specificity of erythrocyte bound IgG. *Clin. Exp. Immunol,* 39, 279.

[94] Facer, C.A. (1980). Direct Coombs antiglobulin tests in Gambian children with *P. falciparum* malaria. III. Expression of IgG subclass determinants and genetic markers and association with anaemia. *Clin. Exp. Immunol,* 41, 81-90.

[95] Rosenberg, E.B., Strickland, G.T., Yang, S.-L., and Whalen, G.E. (1973). IgM antibodies to red cells and autoimmune anemia in patients with malaria. *Am. J. Trop. Med. Hyg,* 22, 146-152.

[96] Fribourg-Blanc, A., Druilhe, P., Brasseur, P., Rhodes-Feuillette, A., Ballet, J.J., and Tharavanij, S. (1985). Immunological evaluation of cell-mediated and humoral immunity in Thai patients with cerebral and non cerebral *Plasmodium falciparum* malaria: II. Evolution of serum levels of immunoglobulins, antimalarial antibodies, complement fractions and alpha interferon. *Southeast Asian J. Trop. Med. Pub. Hlth,* 16, 307-313.

[97] Al-Yaman, F., Genton, B., Reeder, J.C., Mokela, D., Anders, R.F., and Alpers, M.P. (1997). Humoral response to defined *Plasmodium falciparum* antigens in cerebral and uncomplicated malaria and their relationship to parasite genotype. *Am. J. Trop. Med. Hyg,* 56, 430-435.

[98] Carson, J., Helmby, H., Hill, A.V.S., Brewster, D., Greenwood, B.M., and Wahlgren, M. (1990). Human cerebral malaria: association with erythrocyte rosetting and lack of anti-rosetting antibodies. *Lancet,* 336, 1457-1460.

[99] Treutiger, C.J., Hedlund, I., Helmby, H., Carlson, J., Jepson, A., Twumasi, P., Kwiatkowski, D., Greenwood, B.M., and Wahlgren, M. (1992). Rosette formation in *Plasmodium falciparum* isolates and anti-rosette activity of sera from Gambians with cerebral or uncomplicated malaria. *Am. J. Trop. Med. Hyg,* 46, 503-510.

[100] Taylor, T.E., Molyneux, M.E., Wirima, J.J., Borgstein, A., Goldring J.D., and Hommel, M. (1992) Intravenous immunoglobulin in the treatment of paediatric cerebral malaria. *Clin. Exp. Immunol,* 90, 357-362.

[101] Perraut, R., Diatta, B., Marrama, L., Garraud, O., Jambou, R., Longacre, S., Krishnegowda, G., Dieye, A., and Gowda, D. C. (2005). Differential antibody responses to Plasmodium falciparum glycosylphosphatidylinositol anchors in patients with cerebral and mild malaria. *Microbes and Infect,* 7, 682-687.

[102] Spiegelberg, H.L.(1974) Biological activities of immunoglobulins of different classes and subclasses. *Adv. Immunol,* 19, 259.

[103] Morell, A., Skvaril, F., Hitzig, W.H., and Barandun, S. (1972). IgG subclass: Development of the serum concentrations in "normal"infants and children. *J. Pediatrics,* 80, 960-964.

[104] Haddad, D., Liljeqvist, S., Stahl, S., Perlmann, P., Berzins, K., and Ahlborg, N. (1998). Differential induction of immunoglobulin G subclasses by immunization with DNA vectors containing or lacking a signal sequence. *Immunol. Lett,* 61, 201-204.

[105] Jungblut, P.R., Grabher, G., and Stoeffler, G. (1999). Comprehensive detection of immunorelevant *Borrelia garinii* antigens by two-dimensional electrophoresis. *Electrophoresis,* 20, 3611-3622.

[106] Wallis, R.S., Amir-Tahmasseb, M., and Ellner, J.J. (1990). Induction of interleukin 1 and tumor necrosis factor by mycobacterial proteins: The monocyte Western blot. *Proc. Natl. Acad. Sci. USA,* 87, 3348-3352.

In: Progress in Malaria Research
Editor: Lee O. Koning, pp. 127-147

ISBN: 978-1-60021-590-2

Chapter III

A Focus on Malaria Research and Interventions Should Be Based on Accessing the Feasibility, Effectiveness, Safety, Availability, Cost /Affordability and Acceptability of Artemesinin Combination Therapy in Home Management of Malaria in Urban and Rural Communities of Tanzania

Stephen E. D. Nsimba *

Muhimbili University College of Health Sciences (MUCHS),
Department of Clinical Pharmacology, P. O. Box 65010, Dar-Es-Salaam-Tanzania

Abstract

Malaria represents a major health and socio-economic problem in Tanzania (with a total population 35.6 million people) as in all of sub-Saharan Africa. Generally, malaria ranks number one in terms of morbidity and mortality. Malaria case-management has lately been hampered significantly by rapid development and spread of chloroquine parasite resistance in the mainland, like elsewhere, especially for *P. falciparum* malaria to the long-time established first line anti-malarial drug – chloroquine (CQ). The current recommended first and second line antimalarial drugs in the country are sulphadoxine – pyrimethamine (SP) and amodiaquine respectively. However, SP is reported to develop resistance rapidly and has necessitated changing the malaria treatment policy in most subs-Saharan Countries. Tanzania again will be changing first line therapy to artemesinin fixed combination (ACT) therapy by November, 2006.

* Stephen E. D. Nsimba: snsimba@muchs.ac.tz or nsimbastephen@yahoo.co.uk

Early diagnosis and prompt effective treatment represent the fundamental strategy of malaria control. National treatment guidelines are essential tools for health workers to exercise such a control. Following reports of increasing chloroquine (CQ) resistance the government on the Tanzanian mainland changed drug policy from chloroquine to sulphadoxine-pyrimethamine (SP) as first line drug for uncomplicated malaria. For example Zanzibar (Tanzania islands) as well as other countries in the region), the Ministries of Health has embarked directly on more efficacious artemesinin based fixed drug combination therapies a bit earlier than Tanzania mainland because of SP treatment failure mostly in east, central and southern Africa.

Fixed combination therapy (ACT), is a new strategy for malaria treatment, which is based on the hypothesis that two (or more) components of different mechanisms of action protect each other from development of resistance, simultaneously enhancing the efficacy and promoting compliance. Artemisinin as well as its two derivatives, e.g. artemether and artesunate, constitute a family of compounds with several attractive features for such a combination, due mainly to their rapid onset of effective action against multidrug-resistant P. falciparum and their gametocitocidal effect, which potentially reduces transmission of resistant strains. No cross-resistance with other known anti-malarials has been shown both in vivo and *in vitro*.

Introduction

The uncomplicated form of malaria is mainly responsible for febrile illness. Without proper and prompt actions it may progress to severe/complicated forms of malaria with fatal consequences (Snow et al., 1994). Malaria contributes to 10% of infant mortality and 25% of all childhood deaths (Greenwood et al., 1987, Greenwood, 1997). Intervention studies have shown that early treatment of malaria in children (Greenwood et al., 1988, Alonso et al., 1991) and the use of Insecticide Treated Nets (ITNs) (WHO, 1993b) may reduce overall mortality and morbidity. This means that malaria contributes to mortality both directly, and indirectly by its relation to deaths from other causes (Snow and Marsh, 1998, Greenwood, 1999). Thus, an effective malaria control programme must be seen as an integral component of all child health programmes in any malaria endemic country (Greenwood, 1997).

Malaria interferes with productivity and economic well-being. It causes absenteeism from school by pupils and workers alike (Magnussen et al., 2001). It also consumes time from healthy family members who must provide care for the sick. Apart from the consequences of the disease to individuals, households and communities, malaria treatments impose additional economic burdens on most rural populations, hence complicating the fight to alleviate poverty. The situation is made worse by the fact that malaria has become resistant to the more affordable antimalarial drugs. The new drugs recommended to treat malaria in sub-Saharan Africa are expensive and sometimes unavailable (Trigg and Kondrachine, 1998). Thus, malaria and poverty are inter-related. The only parts of Africa free of malaria are the northern and southern regions, which are the richest countries on the continent. The world map of malaria positively corresponds to a world map of poverty. Furthermore, all rich countries are now outside the bounds of malaria risk (Trigg and Kondrachine, 1998, Magnussen et al., 2001) whereas, three hundred years ago it was the main life-threatening disease, for example, in Rome. Areas with severe malaria are poor and continue to have low economic growth. Therefore, the estimated impact of malaria on the economy is very large.

Malaria Control Strategy

The malaria eradication efforts in the 1950s and the 1960s, which were then followed by a re-orientation towards the control of the disease, have been largely unsuccessful, for several reasons including financial, technical and operational constraints. These include the development of resistance to the existing antimalarial drugs and insecticides. The worsening malaria situation in the late 1980s led the World Health Organisation to develop a new Global Malaria Control Strategy (WHO, 1993b) in full partnership with health workers from malaria endemic countries. In 1992, WHO organised a Ministerial Conference on Malaria Control in Amsterdam to endorse the Global Malaria Control Strategy. In contrast to earlier malaria eradication campaigns, the Global Strategy realised that malaria problems varied from country to country, from area to area and even between different groups within the population. Thus, it was agreed that control efforts must be adapted according to the local situations if they are to succeed (WHO, 1993b).

The Global Malaria Control Strategy consisted of four basic elements:

1. To provide early diagnosis and prompt and effective treatment.
2. To plan and implement selective and sustainable preventive measures including vector control.
3. To detect epidemics, as well as containing or preventing them.
4. To strengthen local capacities in basic and applied research to permit and promote the regular assessment of a country's malaria situation, in particular the ecological, social and economic determinants of the disease.

A large proportion of underfives die every year at home without having been able to visit a health facility (Trigg and Kondrachine, 1998, Garg et al., 2001). Access to efficacious drugs is problematic. Moreover, adequate response to malaria epidemics is often delayed and has resulted in high mortality in countries such as Burundi, Ethiopia, Somalia and Kenya (Myers et al., 2000, Hay et al., 2001). Self-treatment, especially in rural areas, is often the rule rather than the exception. In Kilifi, Kenya, 72% of interviewed mothers bought drugs from shops for treating fever in children, mainly chloroquine and antipyretics (Williams et al., 1999). Early treatment of malaria can prevent its progression to a severe disease and death (Koram et al., 1995). However, doses of antimalarials administered in households are often inadequate (Thera et al., 2000). Drug sellers play an important role as the main sources of most antimalarials in many rural communities (Snow et al., 1992, Foster, 1995, McCombie, 1996, WHO, 2000b).

Plasmodium falciparum resistance to CQ, SP and other antimalarials is increasing all the time, mostly in malaria endemic countries. Resistance to CQ in east, central and southern Africa has caused many sub-Saharan countries to change their drug treatment policies by phasing out CQ in the 1990s and replacing it with other first line drugs, such as SP (Bloland et al., 1993). However, until July, 2001 CQ was still the first-line drug for treatment of uncomplicated malaria in Tanzania. Although molecular mechanisms for parasite resistance have been proposed for SP and possibly for CQ (Plowe et al., 1995), the factors influencing the emergence and spread of antimalarial drug resistance within communities are not quite clear. Inadequate dosage regimens have been mentioned as one factor, and are common in self-medication (Carme et al., 1992, Foster, 1995, Mwenesi et al., 1995a). The use of sub-curative doses allows the more resistant part of the parasite population to survive (Hellgren et al., 1994). Presence of sub-curative plasma concentration of an antimalarial drug that will encounter new infections eradicates only the most susceptible strains (Molyneux, 1986).

Roll Back Malaria Initiative (RBM)

The control strategies of 1992 were complemented with an initiative by the Director General of the World Health Organisation, Dr Gro Brundtland, to roll back malaria (RBM) in 1998 based on the belief that malaria deaths can be reduced by half using the available drugs, tools and control measures and by improving health care services and systems (Trigg and Kondrachine, 1998).

Roll Back Malaria is a global partnership founded by governments of malaria-afflicted countries, the World Health Organisation, the UN Development Programme, the UN Children's Fund and the World Bank. Its objective is to reduce by half the burden of malaria for the world's people by the year 2010 by saving lives, reducing poverty, boosting school attendance and making life better for millions of people living in poor countries, especially in Africa. The RBM has the following elements:

1. Evidence-based decisions: (a) surveillance where malaria outbreaks are identified through screening and case detection, (b) health authorities responding to malaria effectively using reliable information, (c) community awareness so that families have the information they need to understand the risks of malaria and take appropriate and timely actions.
2. Rapid diagnosis and treatment: (a) home is the first hospital where a simple packet of effective drugs available to parents can rescue children from malaria, (b) bringing treatment to the people in which prescriptions can be changed to ensure patients are treated with an effective drug by monitoring drug resistance, (c) widely available health services in which rapid diagnostic facilities and effective case management can save people with severe malaria.
3. Multiple prevention: (a) treated bed nets so that people at risk are able to use insecticide-treated nets, (b) mosquito control using the correct mix of control methods for the local situation, (c) safer pregnancies where women are able to take antimalarial drugs and improve the safety of their pregnancy.
4. Focused research: (a) effective actions to roll back malaria are made possible as a result of well-directed research, (b) the industry helping develop effective, safe and inexpensive medicines and insecticides, (c) scientific co-operation accelerating the development of effective vaccines.

5. Well coordinated action: (a) situation analysis where community experience with malaria prevention and treatment are reviewed, (b) a common strategy to roll back malaria is proposed and agreed upon, (c) stronger health systems where public health services, NGOs', private practitioners and local healers implement the strategy in response to peoples' needs, building on effective programmes of child and adult health, (d) governments' health policies allocate sufficient resources to roll back malaria.
6. Dynamic global movement: (a) partnership involving schools, community groups and other organisations join in the synchronised effort to reduce malaria-related illness and death, (b) political support is stimulated through global advocacy efforts, (c) national actions are backed by partnerships with the private sector, foundations and trusts, NGOs', civil society, the media, research and academic institutions, UN agencies and development banks and bilateral development agencies.

RBM is therefore a new global initiative against malaria using interventions that are adapted to local needs and by the reinforcement of the health sector.

Integrated Management of Childhood Illness (IMCI)

One of the most notable strategies to improve child health is through the WHO/UNICEF initiative, Integrated Management of Childhood Illness, IMCI (Gove, 1997, WHO, 1999). From a history of disease-specific programs, IMCI aims to integrate the management of sick children at health facilities (Gove, 1997, WHO, 1999). Children often suffer from more than one condition at the same time, making exact diagnosis difficult as the symptoms of uncomplicated malaria overlap with those of many other acute febrile illnesses (Redd et al., 1992, O'Dempsey et al., 1993). Thus, IMCI's first objective is to train first-level health workers and enable them to use a symptom-based algorithm for assessing, classifying and treating the sick child at health facilities. Under the IMCI algorithm, "malaria" in high-risk settings is defined by the presence of fever or history of fever. Yet, while fever is a rather unspecific symptom (Smith et al., 1995), the scientific community has accepted the gained benefits of treating all fevers as if they were malaria, despite the likelihood of over-treatment. In those cases where fever occurs in conjunction with cough and fast breathing, dual treatment with both antimalarials and antibiotics shall be given to also cover for pneumonia, the next greatest cause of child death after malaria (Gove, 1997, Chandramohan et al., 2002).

The second objective of IMCI is to promote family practices for the prevention of disease, provision of quality home-care and appropriate and early care seeking for sick children (Lambrechts et al., 1999). This component is still not finalised, so far, the focus of IMCI has mainly been on management at health facilities and not on households and the community where the majority of the illness episodes are being treated. However, the IMCI strategy aims at also covering communities/households. More than 70 low- and middle-income countries have now introduced the IMCI strategy and Uganda is one of the leading countries in Africa. In Uganda, health workers have been trained to implement IMCI in

Government and Non-Governmental Organisation (NGO) clinics as part of the RBM effort, but the private sector has not yet been included. In a similar manner in Tanzania, most districts have been covered by the IMCI strategy involving only the public primary health care facilities; the strategy is aiming to reach implementation at a community level soon. However, it has been reported that despite the introduction of the IMCI strategy in holo-endemic areas, malaria management was still problematic as confirmation of diagnosis was not possible (Tarimo et al., 2001a).

Home Based Management of Fever (HBMF)

In an effort to increase proper and timely management of childhood fevers in the community, an integrated community component of IMCI (C-IMCI) was developed since access to health services is limited in sub-Saharan Africa and the majority of African children die at home (Garg et al., 2001). Improving malaria management at health facilities is not enough. The C-IMCI is thus aiming to improve home care; care seeking is now in its early implementation phase. It was recently demonstrated that a 40% underfive mortality reduction (Kidane and Morrow, 2000) and decrease in risk of severe disease (Sirima et al., 2003) could be obtained through presumptive treatment of malaria using community volunteers holding drugs for neighbouring mothers. This means that all services including drugs must be made accessible, available, affordable, safe, efficacious and as close as possible to the people, especially in the rural communities, in order for them to make full utilization of these services.

As vertical strategies, they bring health education and pre-packed antimalarials for fever treatment to the community level (WHO, 2000b, Sirima et al., 2003). Also, the evidence of the mothers' capacity to adequately administer antimalarial treatment to children in the home (Kofoed et al., 2003) has convinced many policy makers and financers to support the undertaking and implementation of this strategy in communities. The Global Fund, RBM, IMCI and HBMF initiatives now support such home management of malaria across sub-Saharan Africa. This implies that "out of health facility management" is also being accepted for malaria, with the use of simple treatments for well-defined symptoms (i.e. fever). The focus is on the mother and local health workers for education of symptoms and management (WHO, 2000b). The community activities of IMCI will also become the vehicle for implementation of other Roll Back Malaria activities. In Uganda, where HBMF is already a national policy, the strategy focuses on early, appropriate home treatment of fever using pre-packaged antimalarial drugs (a combination of chloroquine-Fansidar), as well as the recognition and appropriate care seeking in case of danger signs, such as convulsions (Wendo, 2002).

Combination Therapies and Community Malaria Treatment

Communities in Tanzania, and the African region as a whole, are increasingly practicing home treatment or self-mediactions for malaria and other illnesses before consulting formal health care. While actually it is most desirable for patients to be attended and treated by trained health personnel, but this is not always possible because most of the public health care facilities are compromised in Africa as they either lack trained personnel or essential basic drugs or both. The diagnosis of malaria by mothers and care givers is based on recognition of the symptoms of fever. Households and community level antimalarial drug use represents an important entry point for malaria control programmes in Tanzania and other sub-Saharan countries (Fosters, 1995). It is well known that in Tanzania and other sub-Saharan countries, shops and drug stores are the main sources of antimalarial drugs (Snow et al, 1992; Foster, 1995; Ongore and Nyabola, 1996). However, the course of treatment sold is often sub-optimal (Mwenesi et al, 1995; Nyamongo, 1999; Nsimba et al, 1999). The previous and currently available antimalarial drugs (chloroquine, SP etc) have been cheap, safe and relatively affordable and available to rural communities. It has also been cost effective to treat all fevers or suspected cases of malaria with chloroquine or SP. However, with the increasing cost of the new artemesinin based antimalarials, especially ACTs, a revision of this policy is urgently needed.

Because African countries have plans and some have started using households and communities in fever management as a potential strategy, this necessitates the importance of using antimalarial combination therapies instead of the traditionally well known and used antimalarial monotherapies. Despite the invention of this innovative approach of using artemesinin based fixed combination therapies, there is a need to improve diagnosis and constant monitoring for resistance both at households, communities and in the primary health care facilities while the antimalarial fixed combinations are in use in Tanzania and other sub-Saharan countries. Such strategies for monitoring and improving malaria diagnosis would help these resource poor countries to prevent development of antimalarial resistance and cost of antimalarial treatment that increases every time when the drugs of choice are rendered ineffective and new ones comes in becomes unaffordable for these countries especially those in (sub-Saharan) Africa.

The Burden of Malaria in Tanzania

There are different types of malaria classifications such as mild, moderate and severe. The mild and moderate are considered uncomplicated malaria which are expressed by the following signs and symptoms in underfive children: fever, headache, joint pain, malaise, vomiting or diarrhoea, chest pains, poor appetite and body weakness. Complicated or severe malaria displays symptoms such as extreme weakness, difficulty breathing and convulsions. Thus, the management differs from time to time. Before the policy shift in August, 2001, uncomplicated malaria was managed using CQ, with the first policy shift malaria was managed using SP and paracetamol and soon the second policy shift anytime from

November, 2006, Tanzania will be moving to fixed artemesinin combination therapy. Uncomplicated malaria can develop into complicated/severe malaria if untreated or not properly treated. The objectives of proper treatment of uncomplicated malaria in the country are to provide rapid, long-lasting clinical cures and to reduce morbidity and mortality (Ministry of Health, 2000).

Effective case management is delivered through rapid, accurate diagnosis and prompt access to effective treatment with the aim to prevent progression of the malaria disease to severe forms and death (Trigg and Kondrachine, 1998). Complicated malaria such as cerebral malaria, due to *P. falciparum,* is a medical emergency. The drug of choice for the treatment of severe/complicated falciparum malaria is parenteral quinine, preferably given by intravenous infusion including antipyretics, such as paracetamol (Ministry of Health, 2000).

In Tanzania, malaria severely affects the most vulnerable groups, that is, children under the age of five and pregnant women. It is the leading cause of mortality and morbidity, particularly in underfives. It is estimated that 14-18 million malaria cases occur every year (Ministry of Health, 2000). More than 100,000 malaria-related deaths are reported annually, of which 70,000-80,000 are children under 5 years of age (Ministry of Health, 1999). Malaria is also a major factor in the loss of productivity in the active population (15-55 Years) in Tanzania.

Malaria Control Strategies and Malaria Case Management in Tanzania

The malaria control strategy for Tanzania is in line with the Global Malaria Control Strategy (WHO, 1993b) and the Roll Back Malaria Initiative (1998). The goal is to reduce the morbidity and mortality caused by malaria. Case management, through early diagnosis and prompt treatment with effective drugs, is the basis for malaria control. CQ has been the first line drug for treatment of uncomplicated malaria and has been in use over 40 years in Tanzania. Due to CQ resistance reaching over 42% in the country, the drug was replaced with SP in August 2001 (Kitua et al., 1999, Ministry of Health, 2000). In addition, selective interventions like Insecticide Treated Nets (ITNs) or materials (ITMs) (WHO, 1993b, 2000b), and Intermittent Presumptive Treatment (IPT) are currently being considered as effective preventive measures (Shulman et al., 1999, WHO, 2000b, Schellenberg et al., 2001, WHO, 2002, Schellenberg et al., 2003). Such ITNs, and the newly (recently proposed) introduced Long Lasting Treated Nets (LLTNs) ITMs and IPT interventions are aimed at improving malaria management and is a primary form of prevention in Tanzania and other sub-Saharan countries. Both ITNs and IPT have been reported to reduce malaria morbidity and severe anaemia in children (WHO, 1993b, Shulman et al., 1999, Schellenberg et al., 2001, Schellenberg et al., 2003). A reduction in morbidity and severe anaemia will also decrease the workload of the already compromised public health services and consequently improve their quality. For example, before the change in malaria treatment policy in the country and other malaria endemic countries, chemoprophylactic measures were used, such as taking chloroquine on a weekly basis. The approach had the ability to reduce morbidity and mortality in vulnerable groups, such as children and pregnant women. However, some of these prophylactic options, which were commonly used, are faced with the emergence of (antimalarial and insecticides) resistance which have made these strategies impossible to implement and as a result are no longer used in sub-Saharan countries (WHO, 1993b, 1996).

Irrational use of drugs (taking inadequate dosages / subtherapeutic and / or not completing doses), including antimalarials, is a worldwide problem (Hardon and van der Geest, 1987, Massele et al., 1993b, Mnyika et al., 1995). The main sources of drugs used for self-medication are private drug stores and other drug vendors (Massele et al., 1993b, Mnyika et al., 1995). Self-medication is not always irrational, if properly used it can have large benefits. Apart from irrational use, presence and use of poor quality or expired drugs is another major public health problem in Tanzania and other developing countries especially in sub-Saharan Africa.

Malaria management starts at home where caregivers recognise and respond to a sick child with a fever (Mwenesi et al., 1995a, Tarimo et al., 2000, McCombie, 2002). Whether, when and where to seek treatment of the sick child depends on understanding, perceptions and practices regarding malaria, as well as on the available options in terms of financial, availability, safety, effectiveness of drugs, and geographical access as well as the quality of services. Self-treatment of children with antimalarials is a common practice in homes as a first action (Snow et al., 1992, Foster, 1995, Mnyika et al., 1995, Mwenesi et al., 1995a, McCombie, 1996). It has been regularly shown that children with severe malaria and convulsions often receive treatment from traditional healers, whereas uncomplicated cases seek care from formal facilities (Mwenesi et al., 1995a, Makemba et al., 1996, McCombie, 1996). The majority of antimalarial drugs used for self-treatment in homes are either bought from drug shops (McCombie, 1996), from private and public health care facilities, or taken from remaining stocks from previous malaria episodes (Ongore and Nyabola, 1996). The practice is often accompanied by the use of inadequate doses (Mnyika and Kihamia, 1991, Massele et al., 1993b, Mnyika et al., 1995) and as a result, poor-quality antimalarials have been reported (Kibwage et al., 1992, Murtada and Sesay, 1994). Drug costs may be among the reasons why people buy insufficient drug doses (Foster, 1995, Nyamongo, 1999).

Another important level for malaria management is the primary health care (PHCs) facilities where malaria is often diagnosed presumptively (based on clinical grounds) due to the lack of diagnostic equipment. Mild malaria resembles many other febrile childhood illnesses like ARI/pneumonia, UTI's and measles (WHO, 1992, O'Dempsey et al., 1993, English et al., 1996) making it difficult to diagnose. Most public facilities have little diagnostic aids. Thus, in most rural PHC facilities, adequate malaria case management relies entirely on the clinical skills of the health care providers in assessing and classifying the presenting illness of the patient. Here the competence and performance of the health workers is crucial (Gilson et al., 1993). In Tanzania, most dispensaries and health centres offer both curative and preventive care as described in the paragraph. The IMCI algorithm provides guidelines for the treatment of malaria in children in the country. For example in areas where malaria is endemic, the IMCI strategy recommends that children who present with fever or a recent history of fever should receive antimalarial chemotherapy. It has not been known whether use of laboratory diagnostic aids to confirm if signs are due to malaria would be useful or not. It was recently shown that some diagnostic tests could be potentially useful, however the cost for these tests are not affordable (prohibitive) to many poor rural people (Tarimo et al., 2001a).

This way of seeking care has consequences with mothers not promptly seeking care at health facilities, causing delay of getting prompt treatment. The results highlight the need for educating mothers and other community members on cerebral malaria (convulsions) causes, symptoms and proper treatment. If we are to roll back malaria using both preventive and curative measures and homes must be targeted. For global initiatives, such as Roll Back Malaria (Trigg and Kondrachine, 1998, WHO, 2000a), Integrated Management of Childhood Illnesses (Gove, 1997, Lambrechts et al., 1999) and Home Based Management Fever (Kidane and Morrow, 2000, Sirima et al., 2003) to be effective, it is not enough to provide antimalarials to the communities, but the socio-cultural perceptions and beliefs must be addressed so as to change people's behaviour in this respect. Traditional practitioners need to be included for improved malaria care in the same way as for example they are being involved in HIV/AIDS programmes in sub-Saharan Africa (Green, 2000).

Lack of diagnostic equipments is still a major problem in most public health facilities in Tanzania, as in other sub-Saharan countries. Most diagnostic procedures are usually made presumptively. One could think that care providers over-diagnose and over-prescribed antimalarials. This is supported by the fact that care providers do not use diagnostic equipments because they don't have / are not available, thus, treatment is based on clinical diagnosis and this is likely to result in over-use of antimalarials.

On the other hand due to absence of diagnostic tools, this practice may be considered to be rational in the sense that WHO and IMCI advocate that any child with fever or history of fever should potentially be treated with antimalarials (WHO, 1993b, Trigg and Kondrachine, 1998, Lambrechts et al., 1999). In a study on malaria diagnosis and treatment under the IMCI strategy to assess the relevance of laboratory support, it was noted that though some of the diagnostic tests were attractive and easy to use by relatively inexperienced health workers, unfortunately their costs were prohibitive in poor settings (Tarimo et al., 2001a).

Other researchers, (Redd et al., 1992, Rooth and Bjorkman, 1992, Lubanga et al., 1997, Krause et al., 1998, Font et al., 2001), indicate the challenges in reaching accurate malaria diagnosis in the absence of diagnostic facilities by caregivers. A clinical overlap exists between malaria and pneumonia (English et al., 1996) and this makes it difficult to arrive at correct clinical diagnosis, even for well-trained health workers / clinicians (Redd et al., 1992, Rooth and Bjorkman, 1992, Ray et al., 1995, English et al., 1996).

The roll back malaria initiative advocates diagnostic facilities for effective case management (Trigg and Kondrachine, 1998). The reality is quite different with little or no diagnostic equipment available. This does not however, excuse the striking lack of physical examination of all encounters and too short average consultation times in previous studies (Font et al, 2001; Nsimba et al, 2002). The IMCI strategy of the WHO recommends treating febrile illnesses presumptively with antimalarials, and in that aspect the over-use of drugs. Thus, the prescribing practices observed in these studies may not be irrational if one considers the benefits of preventing the progression of mild to severe form of the disease and therefore reducing both morbidity and mortality. However, efforts have been made to develop guidelines, such as IMCI, to assist the health workers in such settings. According to the IMCI guidelines, one should make a proper assessment to classify the different illnesses for appropriate management (Gove, 1997, WHO, 1999).

Although fever is the characteristic sign of clinical malaria, many *P. falciparum* malaria cases in endemic areas do not present with increased temperature in underfives. In Tanzania it has been reported that 67% of malaria attributable morbidity episodes corresponded to temperatures <37.5°C (Smith et al., 1995). In older children, most of the episodes due to malaria corresponded to increased temperatures. It has further been suggested that febrile temperatures in underfives are frequently a result of other causes, such as respiratory infections, and not necessarily due to malaria, even if the patient is parasitaemic (Smith et al., 1995). Despite these uncertainties in the diagnosis of malaria in endemic areas, it is possible to estimate the proportion of fever cases that may be due to malaria using parasitaemia data. Fever episodes due to malaria may also depend on the season and malaria endemicity (Smith et al., 1998).

Antimalarial Drug Quality in Tanzania and other Sub-Saharan Countries

Failure of a dissolution test of a drug could be a satisfactory indicator of a poor drug bioavailability. Thus, a low dissolution rate accompanied with poor bioavailability of any antimalarial drug would render such a drug ineffective even against sensitive *Plasmodium falciparum* parasites. Effectiveness of any drug depends on the metabolism and absorption after oral administration. Both chloroquine (CQ) and sulfadoxine-pyrimethamine (SP) have good oral bioavailabilities of more than 90% if they are of good quality (Aden-Abdi et al., 1995a). Bioavailability is not only dependent on drug quality, but it may also be affected by specific patient factors, such as mal-absorption syndrome and may be by type of food consumed.

Chloroquine has been popular in the treatment of malaria fevers because it also possesses antipyretic, ant-inflammatory and analgesic actions (Warrell, 1993, McIntosh and Greenwood, 1998). In contrast, SP lacks these properties and is reported to produce slow clinical responses (White, 1999). Lack of such properties can have negative implications on people's acceptance and satisfaction of SP (Tarimo et al., 2001b), especially in rural communities. Low literacy makes it difficult to explain that the effect on fever is not the same as the effect on malaria, and that the effect of the former comes later (Williams et al., 1999, Tarimo et al., 2001b). An advantage of SP is that it has none of the bitter taste often associated with CQ and it is given as single dose treatment. This should make it easier to administer to children and thus attractive even to parents, although the mothers reported that they would like to continue using chloroquine since they believe that chloroquine was still effective by then in treating malaria (Eriksen et al, 2005; Nsimba, 2006). A disadvantage of SP is the occurrence of the rare, but severe, side effect of Stevens Johnson Syndrome (SJS). The true frequency of SJS is not known and under-reporting is probably very common in many developing countries. It has been reported by both mothers, fathers and some health workers that fear of side effects and negative perceptions about using SP was common at that time (Eriksen et al, 2005; Nsimba, 2006). The latter being due to delay in producing clinical response, including effects on reducing fever (Tarimo et al., 2002). Most of the information about SP was reported to come from mass media and health facilities. Thus, there is a need to look for ways and means of how to best inform the public on issues related to drug treatment for any future atimalarial drug policy change in Tanzania.

Table 1. The pharmacokinetic and pharmacodynamic properties of CQ and SP

Drug name	Pharmacokinetics	Pharmacodynamics
CQ	• Can be given orally, IM, IV and rectally • CQ is concentrated in platelets and granulocytes • Half-life has three phases: 3-6 days, 12-14 days and 2 months or more • 90% oral bioavailability • Peak plasma levels are reached within 1-6 hrs after single oral dose of 300 mgs base	• Reduces fever • May cause nausea, vomiting, diarrhoea, dizziness, headache, rashes, itching, abdominal pain, blurred vision, acute cardiovascular effects, tinnitus, reduced hearing, deafness, etc.
SP	• Is given orally • Rapidly absorbed with 90% bioavailability • Half-life of the drugs: Sulfadoxine = 7-9 days and Pyrimethamine = 4 days • Peak plasma concentrations are reached within 2-6 hrs after oral dosing	• Does not reduce fever • May cause nausea, vomiting, skin rashes, haematological reactions, severe cutaneous adverse reactions and Stevens-Johnson's Syndrome affecting people extremely rarely

In many African and Asian countries there have been reports of poor quality of drugs (Mahamood et al., 1994, Ogwal-Okeng et al., 1998, WHO, 2003). This has also been reported in Tanzania (Aden-Abdi et al., 1995b, Rimoy et al., 2002, Risha et al., 2002). The use of poor quality or fake antimalarials may cause therapeutic failures, adverse effects or fatal toxicity and it promotes development of drug resistance (Menkes, 1997, Shakoor et al., 1997, Stenson et al., 1998, Po, 2001). Resistance develops when parasites are exposed to concentrations of the drug not high enough to kill them (Hellgren et al., 1994). Expired drugs have been reported to be used for patients because of economic constraints and lack of adequate drug information (Murtada and Sesay, 1994). Thus, the availability of good quality antimalarial drugs is important for the safe treatment of the disease. A study from South East Asia reported that 38% of the collected samples did not contain the active ingredient (Newton et al., 2001).

The existence of low-quality and fake drugs is considered a problem in many low- and middle-income countries (Roy, 1994, Shakoor et al., 1997, Stenson et al., 1998, Newton et al., 2001, Po, 2001, Taylor et al., 2001). Low-quality drugs have been reported in Tanzania (Aden-Abdi et al., 1995b, Rimoy et al., 2002, Risha et al., 2002, Minzi et al., 2003a). The consequences of using low-quality antimalarials not only produces treatment failures, but also increases the development of resistance and increased mortality (WHO, 2003). Therapeutic failure can occur because of pharmaceutical failure resulting from the poor quality of products, instability of products that leads to the deterioration of their quality before they reach the patient, or the use of counterfeit products. Thus, handling, packaging and transportation of medicines are known to affect the quality of some drugs. For example, it has been reported in several studies that a significant instability of products, such as ergometrine (Hogerzeil et al., 1992, Hogerzeil and Walker, 1996) and other essential drugs, occurs during transportation (Hogerzeil et al., 1991).

Drugs are available in different formulations with differences in quality. In Tanzania, the Pharmacy Board, under the Ministry of Health, is trying to curb the cases of imported and locally manufactured sub-standard drugs and has established a modern drug quality control laboratory as a check for quality control assurance in the country. In most drug stores, drugs are kept in hot climatic conditions, as the rooms have no air-conditioning facilities. Thus, some drugs are liable to decompose due to poor stability while others reach their expiration date Hogerzeil et al, 1992; Kibwage et al, 1992; Hogerzeil and Walker, 1996).

In Tanzania and many other developing countries, the drug regulatory authorities are weak (Kibwage et al., 1992, Murtada and Sesay, 1994, Shakoor et al., 1997). In Lao PDR, enforced regulation via strengthened inspections improved the quality of pharmacy services (Stenson et al., 2001) and drug quality (Syhakhang, 2002).

Future Reflections

Home caregivers play an important role in recognizing and responding to malaria fevers and should be targeted in malaria control programmes. Encouraging findings from an intervention study in Ethiopia by Kidane and Morrow (Kidane and Morrow, 2000) showed that mothers can be taught to recognise and adequately treat fevers in children, resulting in reduction in morbidity and mortality. As it has been reported that convulsions a prominent feature of severe malaria are perceived to be caused by evil spirits and thus are not treated by modern medicine (Comoro et al, 2003). Furthermore, it has been reported that stocking and self-treatment are common (Nsimba et al, 1999; 2002), which is in line with international policies such as RBM, IMCI and HBMF.

If we are to improve malaria case management in children, pregnant women and families, we need to bring health services as close to the people as possible especially in rural communities. At present only artemesinin based combination therapy (artemether-lumefantrine) is available as fixed dose antimalarial drugs in which both of these compounds are co-formulated into a single tablet. However, there are other artemesinin based combination therapies available as individual products that need to be co-administered. Co-packaging of the other combination partner antimalarial drugs in blister forms is highly recommended in order to \make them user friendly and this would increase adherence to complete the prescribed therapies. As a caution to these artemesinin compounds is that they are highly sensitive to moisture, and their shelf life is almost two (2) years and thus, good storage conditions should be available / are essential to be undertaken in order to preserve their shelf-life. This is very important for all sub-Saharan countries.

Furthermore, we need to consider also the other three main actors involved directly or indirectly in malaria case management, namely household members, public health facility workers and private health care providers, such as drug sellers and traditional healers. The focus should be on the households, as we have seen there are deficits in terms of perceptions and various beliefs about severe malaria with convulsions (*degedege)* and SP, as well as decision-making about where and when to seek care taking too long. Furthermore, mothers' lack of adequate knowledge on causes of severe/cerebral malaria (*degedege*) and drug administration for the underfives needs to be addressed. The low quality of care at health facilities in terms of physical examination, consultation time and prescribing antimalarials, proper dispensing of drugs and correct instructions or advise giving to clients must be improved. In general malaria case management in homes and in health facilities should be substantially improved.

Conclusions and Recommendations

There is a belief that convulsions (*degedege*), a prominent feature of severe malaria, are caused by evil spirits. This leads to inappropriate treatments. There is a need to find ways of changing misperceptions and ensure prompt rational malaria case management. Here, decision makers such elders (grandmothers and mothers-in-law) including traditional healers were first contact in management of childhood malaria.

Little home stocking and self-treatment with antimalarials may result in delays in prompt care seeking, as people need to travel to public facilities to get free SP. This may negatively influence malaria morbidity and mortality in underfives. There is a need to find the right balance between improving access/availability and acceptability on one hand, and preserving the effects of SP and any other future first line antimalarial drugs to come such as artemesinin fixed combination therapy in Tanzania.

The performance by health care providers, in terms of consultation time and physical examination, needs to be improved in most public health care facilities in Tanzania as poor performance could lead to inadequate clinical assessment and poor quality of malaria case management. The quality of care should be improved. Any antimalarial policy should take into consideration pharmacological properties of the drug, counselling of patients regarding the course of illness and drug properties as these properties may help to increase acceptability and compliance to a recommended drug (s).

The development and spread of resistance to antimalarial drugs is a major set back to the delivery of prompt, effective, affordable and safe malaria treatment in sub-Saharan countries, as prompt and correct malaria diagnosis and early disease management remain fundamental and indispensable elements of malaria control. Thus, it is in this regard that the World Health Organisation and other Global Initiatives recently reached a decision and made recommendations that all countires faced with the problem of antimalarial drug resistance should adopt strategies of moving towards using combination therapies, particularly those containing artemesinin derivatives.

Any future new antimalarial drug policy to follow in sub-Saharan Africa (SSA) including Tanzania such as the artemesinin based fixed combination should take into consideration of issues of availability/access, affordability/price, safety, effectiveness and acceptability. A deficit in any of the above mentioned properties or criteria can have negative consequences to the consumers as they can lead to poor compliance/poor drug adherence among users.

We need to develop a nation wide multi-sectoral intervention package, targeting home caregivers, health care providers, drug sellers and traditional healers to improve malaria case management in Tanzania and elsewhere in sub-Saharan countries where malaria is endemic.

References

Aden-Abdi, Y., Gustafsson, L. L., Ericsson, Ö. and Hellgren, U. (1995a). *Handbook of drugs for tropical parasitic infections, second edition,* Taylor and Francis Ltd, London, England.

Aden-Abdi, Y., Rimoy, G. H., Ericsson, O., Alm, C. and Massele, A. Y. (1995b). Quality of chloroquine preparations marketed in Dar es Salaam, Tanzania. *Lancet*, 346:1161.

Alonso, P. L., Lindsay, S. W., Armstrong, J. R., Conteh, M., Hill, A. G., David, P. H., Fegan, G., de Francisco, A., Hall, A. J., Shenton, F. C. and et al. (1991). The effect of insecticide-treated bed nets on mortality of Gambian children. *Lancet*, 337:1499-502.

Bloland, P. B., Lackritz, E. M., Kazembe, P. N., Were, J. B., Steketee, R. and Campbell, C. C. (1993). Beyond chloroquine: implications of drug resistance for evaluating malaria therapy efficacy and treatment policy in Africa. *Journal of Infectious Diseases*, 167:932-937.

Carme, B., Koulengana, P., Nzambi, A. and Guillo du Bodan, H. (1992). Current practices for the prevention and treatment of malaria in children and in pregnant women in the Brazzaville Region (Congo). *Annals of Tropical Medicine and Parasitology*, 86:319-322.

Chandramohan, D., Jaffar, S. and Greenwood, B. (2002). Use of clinical algorithms for diagnosing malaria. *Tropical Medicine and International Health*, 7:45-52.

Comoro, C., Nsimba, SED., Massele, AY., Warsame, MY and Tomson, G (2003). Local understanding, perception and reported practices of mothers/care takers and health care providers about childhood malaria in Kibaha district, Coast region, Tanzania. *Acta Tropica*. 87: 305-313.

English, M., Punt, J., Mwangi, I., McHugh, K. and Marsh, K. (1996). Clinical overlap between malaria and severe pneumonia in Africa children in hospital. *Transactions of the Royal Society of Tropical Medicine and Hygiene*, 90:658-662.

Ericksen, J., Nsimba, SED., Minzi, OS., Sanga, AJ., Gustaffson. L., Warsame, M and Tomson, G (2005). Adoption of the new antimalarial drug policy in Tanzania-major changes in treatment practices. *Tropical Medicine and International Health*. 10 (10): 1-9.

Font, F., Alonso Gonzalez, M., Nathan, R., Kimario, J., Lwilla, F., Ascaso, C., Tanner, M., Menendez, C. and Alonso, P. L. (2001). Diagnostic accuracy and case management of clinical malaria in the primary health services of a rural area in south-eastern Tanzania. *Tropical Medicine and International Health*, 6:423-428.

Foster, S. (1995). Treatment of malaria outside the formal health services. *Journal of Tropical Medicine and Hygiene*, 98:29-34.

Garg, R., Omwomo, W., Witte, J. M., Lee, L. A. and Deming, M. S. (2001). Care seeking during fatal childhood illnesses: Siaya District, Kenya, 1998. *American Journal of Public Health*, 91:1611-1613.

Gilson, L., Jaffar, S., Mwankusye, S. and Teuscher, T. (1993). Assessing prescribing practice: a Tanzanian example. *International Journal of Health and Management*, 8:37-58.

Gove, S. (1997). Integrated management of childhood illness by outpatient health workers: technical basis and overview. The WHO Working Group on Guidelines for Integrated Management of the Sick Child. *Bulletin of the World Health Organization*, 75 Suppl 1:7-24.

Green, E. C. (2000). Traditional healers and AIDS in Uganda. *Journal of Alternative and Complementary Medicine*, 6:1-2.

Greenwood, B. (1999). Malaria mortality and morbidity in Africa. *Bulletin of the World Health Organization*, 77:617-618.

Greenwood, B. M. (1997). The epidemiology of malaria. *Annals of Tropical Medicine and Parasitology*, 91:763-769.

Greenwood, B. M., Bradley, A. K., Greenwood, A. M., Byass, P., Jammeh, K., Marsh, K., Tulloch, S., Oldfield, F. S. and Hayes, R. (1987). Mortality and morbidity from malaria among children in a rural area of The Gambia, West Africa. *Transactions of the Royal Society of Tropical Medicine and Hygiene*, 81:478-486.

Greenwood, B. M., Greenwood, A. M., Bradley, A. K., Snow, R. W., Byass, P., Hayes, R. J. and N'Jie, A. B. (1988). Comparison of two strategies for control of malaria within a primary health care programme in the Gambia. *Lancet*, 1:1121-1127.

Hardon, A. P. and van der Geest, S. (1987). Hazards of self-medication. *World Health Forum*, 8:469-471.

Hay, S. I., Rogers, D. J., Shanks, G. D., Myers, M. F. and Snow, R. W. (2001). Malaria early warning in Kenya. *Trends in Parasitology*, 17:95-99.

Hellgren, U., Ericsson, O., Kihamia, C. M. and Rombo, L. (1994). Malaria parasites and chloroquine concentrations in Tanzanian schoolchildren. *Tropical Medicine and Parasitology*, 45:293-297.

Hogerzeil HV, De Goeje MJ and Abu-Reid IO. (1991). Stability of essential drugs in Sudan. *Lancet*, 338: 754-755.

Hogerzeil HV, Battersby A, Srdanovic V and Stjernstrom NE. (1992). Stability of essential drugs during shipment to the tropics. *British Medical Journal*, 304: 210-212.

Hogerzeil HV and Walker GJA. (1996). Instability of (methyl) ergometrine in tropical climates – an overview. *European Journal of Obstretic Gynaecology and Reproductive Biology*, 69: 25-29.

Kibwage, I. O., Ogeto, J. O., Maitai, C. K., Rutere, G., Thuranira, J. and Ochieng, A. (1992). Drug quality control work in Daru: observations during 1983-1986. *East African Medical Journal*, 69:577-580.

Kidane, G. and Morrow, R. H. (2000). Teaching mothers to provide home treatment of malaria in Tigray, Ethiopia: a randomised trial. *Lancet*, 356:550-555.

Kilama, W. L. and Kihamia, C. K. (1991). *Malaria*, Harper Collins Academic, London.

Kitua, A. Y. (1999). Antimalarial drug policy: making systematic change. *Lancet*, 354 Suppl:SIV32.

Kofoed, P. E., Lopez, F., Aaby, P., Hedegaard, K. and Rombo, L. (2003). Can mothers be trusted to give malaria treatment to their children at home? *Acta Tropica*, 86:67-70.

Koram, K. A., Bennett, S., Adiamah, J. H. and Greenwood, B. M. (1995). Socio-economic determinants are not major risk factors for severe malaria in Gambian children. *Transactions of the Royal Society of Tropical Medicine and Hygiene*, 89:151-154.

Krause, G., Schleiermacher, D., Borchert, M., Benzler, J., Heinmuller, R., Ouattara, K., Coulibaly, S., Diasso, I., Ilboudo, A. and Diesfeld, H. J. (1998). Diagnostic quality in rural health centres in Burkina Faso. *Tropical Medicine and International Health*, 3:100-107.

Lambrechts, T., Bryce, J. and Orinda, V. (1999). Integrated management of childhood illness: a summary of first experiences. *Bulletin of the World Health Organization*, 77:582-594.

Lubanga, R. G., Norman, S., Ewbank, D. and Karamagi, C. (1997). Maternal diagnosis and treatment of children's fever in an endemic malaria zone of Uganda: implications for the malaria control programme. *Acta Tropica*, 68:53-64.

Magnussen, P., Ndawi, B., Sheshe, A. K., Byskov, J. and Mbwana, K. (2001). Malaria diagnosis and treatment administered by teachers in primary schools in Tanzania. *Tropical Medicine and International Health*, 6:273-279.

Mahamood, B. M., Ali, H. M., Homeida, M. M. A. and Bennet, J. L. (1994). Bioequivalence of five chloroquine brands marketed in Sudan. *Pharmacy Journal*, 8:164-167.

Makemba, A. M., Winch, P. J., Makame, V. M., Mehl, G. L., Premji, Z., Minjas, J. N. and Shiff, C. J. (1996). Treatment practices for degedege, a locally recognized febrile illness, and implications for strategies to decrease mortality from severe malaria in Bagamoyo District, Tanzania. *Tropical Medicine and International Health*, 1:305-313.

Massele, A. Y., Sayi, J., Nsimba, S. E., Ofori-Adjei, D. and Laing, R. O. (1993b). Knowledge and management of malaria in Dar es Salaam, Tanzania. *East African Medical Journal*, 70:639-642.

McCombie, S. C. (1996). Treatment seeking for malaria: a review of recent research. *Social Science and Medicine*, 43:933-945.

McCombie, S. C. (2002). Self-treatment for malaria: the evidence and methodological issues. *Health Policy and Planning*, 17:333-344.

McIntosh, H. M. and Greenwood, B. M. (1998). Chloroquine or amodiaquine combined with sulfadoxine-pyrimethamine as a treatment for uncomplicated malaria--a systematic review. *Annals of Tropical Medicine and Parasitology*, 92:265-270.

Menkes, D. B. (1997). Hazardous drugs in developing countries. *British Medical Journal*, 315:1557-1558.

Ministry of Health (1991). *Standard Treatment Guidelines and National Essential Drug List for Tanzania*. Dar-es-Salaam, Tanzania

Ministry of Health (2000). *National Guidelines for Malaria*. Dar-es-Salaam, Tanzania

Ministry of Health (2002). Morbidity and mortality statistics. In *Health Statistics Abstract* Health Information and Research Section, Planning and Policy Department, Ministry of Health, Dar-es-Salaam, Tanzania.

Ministry of Health, T. (1999). Morbidity and mortality statistics. In *Health Statistics Abstract* Health Information and Research Section, Planning and Policy Department, Ministry of Health, Dar-es-Salaam, Tanzania.

Minzi, O. M., Moshi, M. J., Hipolite, D., Massele, A. Y., Tomson, G., Ericsson, O. and Gustafsson, L. L. (2003a). Evaluation of the quality of amodiaquine and sulphadoxine/pyrimethamine tablets sold by private wholesale pharmacies in Dar Es Salaam Tanzania. *Journal of Clinical Pharmacy and Therapeutics*, 28:117-122.

Mnyika, K. S. and Kihamia, C. M. (1991). Chloroquine-induced pruritus: its impact on chloroquine utilization in malaria control in Dar es Salaam. *Journal of Tropical Medicine and Hygiene*, 94:27-31.

Mnyika, K. S., Killewo, J. Z. and Kabalimu, T. K. (1995). Self-medication with antimalarial drugs in Dar es Salaam, Tanzania. *Tropical and Geographical Medicine*, 47:32-34.

Molyneux, C. S. (1986). *The epidemiology of drug resistance in malaria: an unfinished conceptual model*. Geneva: WHO

Murtada, M. and Sesay, B. (1994). Expiry dates on pharmaceuticals - Some worrying realities in Sierra leone. *Pharmacy Journal*, 8:202-206.

Mwenesi, H., Harpham, T. and Snow, R. W. (1995a). Child malaria treatment practices among mothers in Kenya. *Social Science and Medicine*, 40:1271-1277.

Mwenesi, H. A., Harpham, T., Marsh, K. and Snow, R. W. (1995b). Perceptions of symptoms of severe childhood malaria among Mijikenda and Luo residents of coastal Kenya. *Journal of Biosocial Science*, 27:235-244.

Myers, M. F., Rogers, D. J., Cox, J., Flahault, A. and Hay, S. I. (2000). Forecasting disease risk for increased epidemic preparedness in public health. *Advances in Parasitology*, 47:309-330.

Newton, P., Proux, S., Green, M., Smithuis, F., Rozendaal, J., Prakongpan, S., Chotivanich, K., Mayxay, M., Looareesuwan, S., Farrar, J., Nosten, F. and White, N. J. (2001). Fake artesunate in southeast Asia. *Lancet*, 357:1948-1950.

Nyamongo, I. K. (1999). Home case management of malaria: an ethnographic study of lay people's classification of drugs in Suneka division, Kenya. *Tropical Medicine and International Health*, 4:736-743.

Nsimba, SED., Massele, AY., Mabatiya, ZA., Warsame, MT., and Tomson, G. (1999). A household survey on sources availability and use of antimalarial drugs in rural area of Tanzania, *Drug Information Journal*. 33:1025-1032.

Nsimba, SED., Massele, AY., Ericksen, J., Gustaffson. L., Tomson, G and Warsame. MY (2002). Case management of malaria in undefives at primary health care facilities in a Tanzanian district. *Tropical Medicine and International Health*. 7: 201-209.

O'Dempsey, T. J., McArdle, T. F., Laurence, B. E., Lamont, A. C., Todd, J. E. and Greenwood, B. M. (1993). Overlap in the clinical features of pneumonia and malaria in African children. *Transactions of the Royal Society of Tropical Medicine and Hygiene*, 87:662-665.

Ogwal-Okeng, J. W., Okello, D. O. and Odyek, O. (1998). Quality of oral and parenteral chloroquine in Kampala. *East African Medical Journal*, 75:692-4.

Ongore, D. and Nyabola, L. (1996). Role of shops and shopkeepers in malaria control. *East African Medical Journal*, 73:390-394.

Plowe, C. V., Djimde, A., Bouare, M., Doumbo, O. and Wellems, T. E. (1995). Pyrimethamine and proguanil resistance-conferring mutations in Plasmodium falciparum dihydrofolate reductase: polymerase chain reaction methods for surveillance in Africa. *American Journal of Tropical Medicine and Hygiene*, 52:565-568.

Po, A. W. (2001). Too much, too little, or none at all: dealing with substandard and fake drugs. *Lancet*, 357:1904.

Redd, S. C., Bloland, P. B., Kazembe, P. N., Patrick, E., Tembenu, R. and Campbell, C. C. (1992). Usefulness of clinical case-definitions in guiding therapy for African children with malaria or pneumonia. *Lancet*, 340:1140-1143.

Rimoy, G. H., Moshi, M. J. and Massele, A. Y. (2002). Comparative bioavailability of oral sugar-coated and plain formulation of chloroquine phosphate marketed in Tanzania. *Tropical Doctor*, 32:15-17.

Risha, P. G., Shewiyo, D., Msami, A., Masuki, G., Vergote, G., Vervaet, C. and Remon, J. P. (2002). In vitro evaluation of the quality of essential drugs on the Tanzanian market. *Tropical Medicine and International Health*, 7:701-707.

Rooth, I. and Bjorkman, A. (1992). Fever episodes in a holoendemic malaria area of Tanzania: parasitological and clinical findings and diagnostic aspects related to malaria. *Transactions of the Royal Society of Tropical Medicine and Hygiene*, 86:479-482.

Roy, J. (1994). The menace of substandard drugs. *World Health Forum*, 15:406-407.

Schellenberg, D., Menendez, C., Kahigwa, E., Aponte, J., Vidal, J., Tanner, M., Mshinda, H. and Alonso, P. (2001). Intermittent treatment for malaria and anaemia control at time of routine vaccinations in Tanzanian infants: a randomised, placebo-controlled trial. *Lancet*, 357:1471-1477.

Schellenberg, J. A., Victora, C. G., Mushi, A., de Savigny, D., Schellenberg, D., Mshinda, H. and Bryce, J. (2003). Inequities among the very poor: health care for children in rural southern Tanzania. *Lancet*, 361:561-566.

Shakoor, O., Taylor, R. B. and Behrens, R. H. (1997). Assessment of the incidence of substandard drugs in developing countries. *Tropical Medicine and International Health*, 2:839-845.

Shulman, C. E., Dorman, E. K., Cutts, F., Kawuondo, K., Bulmer, J. N., Peshu, N. and Marsh, K. (1999). Intermittent sulphadoxine-pyrimethamine to prevent severe anaemia secondary to malaria in pregnancy: a randomised placebo-controlled trial. *Lancet*, 353:632-636.

Sirima, S. B., Konate, A., Tiono, A. B., Convelbo, N., Cousens, S. and Pagnoni, F. (2003). Early treatment of childhood fevers with pre-packaged antimalarial drugs in the home reduces severe malaria morbidity in Burkina Faso. *Tropical Medicine and International Health*, 8:133-139.

Smith, T., Hurt, N., Teuscher, T. and Tanner, M. (1995). Is fever a good sign for clinical malaria in surveys of endemic communities? *American Journal of Tropical Medicine and Hygiene*, 52:306-310.

Snow, R. W., Bastos de Azevedo, I., Lowe, B. S., Kabiru, E. W., Nevill, C. G., Mwankusye, S., Kassiga, G., Marsh, K. and Teuscher, T. (1994). Severe childhood malaria in two areas of markedly different falciparum transmission in east Africa. *Acta Tropica*, 57:289-300.

Snow, R. W. and Marsh, K. (1998). New insights into the epidemiology of malaria relevant to malaria control. *British Medical Bulletin*, 54:293-309.

Snow, R. W., Peshu, N., Forster, D., Mwenesi, H. and Marsh, K. (1992). The role of shops in the treatment and prevention of childhood malaria on the coast of Kenya. *Transactions of the Royal Society of Tropical Medicine and Hygiene*, 86:237-239.

Stenson, B., Lindgren, B. H., Synhakhang, L. and Tomson, G. (1998). The quality of drugs in private pharmacies in the Lao People's Democratic Republic. *International Journal of Risk and Safety in Medicine*, 11:243-249.

Syhakhang, L. (2002). *The quality of private pharmacy services in a province of Lao PGR: perceptions, practices and regulatory enforcements.* Stockholm: Division of International Health (IHCAR), Karolinska Institutet.

Tarimo, D. S. (2002). *Paediatric malaria case management under the strategy of the integrated management of childhood illness and malaria control policy in Tanzania.* Copenhagen: Department of International Health, Institute of Public Health, University of Copenhagen.

Tarimo, D. S., Lwihula, G. K., Minjas, J. N. and Bygbjerg, I. C. (2000). Mothers' perceptions and knowledge on childhood malaria in the holendemic Kibaha district, Tanzania: implications for malaria control and the IMCI strategy. *Tropical Medicine and International Health*, 5:179-184.

Tarimo, D. S., Minjas, J. N. and Bygbjerg, I. C. (2001a). Malaria diagnosis and treatment under the strategy of the integrated management of childhood illness (IMCI): relevance of laboratory support from the rapid immunochromatographic tests of ICT Malaria P.f/P.v and OptiMal. *Annals of Tropical Medicine and Parasitology*, 95:437-444.

Tarimo, D. S., Minjas, J. N. and Bygbjerg, I. C. (2001b). Perception of chloroquine efficacy and alternative treatments for uncomplicated malaria in children in a holoendemic area of Tanzania: implications for the change of treatment policy. *Tropical Medicine and International Health*, 6:992-997.

Tarimo, D. S., Minjas, J. N. and Bygbjerg, I. C. (2002). Sulfadoxine-pyrimethamine monotherapy in Tanzanian children gives rapid parasite clearance but slow fever clearance that is improved by chloroquine in combination therapy. *Tropical Medicine and International Health*, 7:592-598.

Thera, M. A., D'Alessandro, U., Thiero, M., Ouedraogo, A., Packou, J., Souleymane, O. A., Fane, M., Ade, G., Alvez, F. and Doumbo, O. (2000). Child malaria treatment practices among mothers in the district of Yanfolila, Sikasso region, Mali. *Tropical Medicine and International Health*, 5:876-881.

Trigg, P. and Kondrachine, A. (1998). The Global Malaria Control Strategy. *World Health*, 51:4-5.

Warrell, D. A. (1993). Treatment and Prevention of Malaria. In *Bruce-Chwatt's Essential Malariology* (Eds: Gilles, H. M. and Warrell, D. A.) Edward Arnold, London, Boston, Melbourne, pp. 164-193.

Wendo, C. (2002). Uganda leads the way on Africa Malaria Day. *Lancet*, 359:1494.

White, N. J. (1999). Delaying antimalarial drug resistance with combination chemotherapy. *Parasitologia*, 41:301-308.

WHO (1990). *Technical Report Series No. 805. (Practical chemotherapy of malaria: report of a WHO Scientific Group).*

WHO (1993b). *Implementation of the global malaria strategy.* Geneva: WHO.

WHO (1996). *Assessment of Therapeutical Efficacy of Antimalarial Drugs for Uncomplicated Falciparum Malaria in Areas with Intense Transmission.* Geneva: WHO, WHO/MAL/96.1077.

WHO (1999). *Management of childhood illness in developing countries: Rationale for an integrated strategy.* Geneva: WHO, WHO/CHS/CAH/98.1A.

WHO (2000a). Community Action for Malaria Control. *Malaria - Liaison Bulletin of the Malaria Programme WHO/AFRO*, 3:1-4.

WHO (2000b). *Malaria Diagnosis - New Perspectives.* Geneva: WHO, WHO/CDS/RBM/2000.14, WHO/MAL/2000.1091.

WHO (2000c). *The world health report 2000. Health Systems: Improving performance.* Geneva: World Health Organization.

WHO (2002). *Community involvement in rolling back malaria.* Geneva: WHO, WHO/CDS/RBM/2002.42.

WHO (2003). *The quality of antimalarials: a study in selected African countries.* Geneva: WHO, WHO/EDM/PAR/2003.4.

Williams, H. A., Kachur, S. P., Nalwamba, N. C., Hightower, A., Simoonga, C. and Mphande, P. C. (1999). A community perspective on the efficacy of malaria treatment options for children in Lundazi district, Zambia. *Tropical Medicine and International Health*, 4:641-652.

In: Progress in Malaria Research
Editor: Lee O. Koning, pp. 149-169

ISBN: 978-1-60021-590-2

Chapter IV

FDG-PET Imaging in a Primate Model of Severe Human Malaria

Satoru Kawai
Department of Tropical Medicine and Parasitology,
Dokkyo Medical University, Japan

Abstract

The clinical utility of positron emission tomography (PET) is well documented, and high-resolution imaging of ^{18}F-fluorodeoxyglucose (FDG) has been used for many years to study glucose utilization in neoplasms and major organs such as the brain, heart and spleen. However, little attention was directed to the use of FDG-PET for parasitic diseases including malaria. Recently, to elucidate the clinical features of severe malaria, we performed whole-body FDG-PET of *Plasmodium coatneyi*-infected acute phase Japanese macaques (*Macaca fuscata*). Our previous studies demonstrated that the Japanese macaque is highly susceptible to *P. coatneyi* infection and that pathologic findings in infected monkeys are similar to those observed in human falciparum malaria. The *P. coatneyi*-infected Japanese macaque thus appears to be a useful model for pathological and pathophysiological studies of severe falciparum malaria. We present here direct evidence concerning glucose uptake by FDG-PET scanning in *P. coatneyi*-infected macaques, and demonstrate the relationship of such uptake to histopathological changes observed in the tissue.

We focused on the cerebral metabolic changes induced by severe malaria. We observed diffuse and heterogeneous reduction of metabolism in the cerebral cortex in the acute phase of malaria infection. Histopathological examination revealed preferential sequestration of parasitized red blood cells (PRBCs) in the cerebral microvasculature. However, neither hemorrhagic change nor necrosis was observed in HE- and Nissl-stained brain tissues. This suggests that reduction of cerebral metabolism occurs before parenchymal changes appear in the brain. This may be one reason why more than half of cerebral malaria patients have no neurological sequelae after recovery.

The current study revealed also distinct elevation of FDG up-take in the spleen of infected monkeys. The infected monkeys clearly exhibited increase in splenic FDG uptake indicating marked enhancement of glucose metabolism. The Standardized Uptake

Values (SUVs) of the spleen in the infected monkeys were significantly higher than those in the uninfected monkey. At autopsy, splenomegaly was clearly present in all infected monkeys, and histopathologic findings included hyperplasia of lymphoid follicles in white pulp, a large number of activated macrophage, and congestion of PRBCs and malaria pigments in red pulp. Increase in splenic glucose uptake may thus be closely related to activation of splenic clearance system against blood-stage malarial parasites.

These findings will improve understanding of physiological alterations of the host in serious malarial infection. We believe that whole-body FDG-PET may be useful for evaluating and monitoring pathophysiological processes involved in severe malaria.

Introduction

The major clinical features of malaria are paroxysms of high fever, hemolytic anemia, and splenomegaly. In addition, falciparum malaria often causes serious or fatal complications such as cerebral malaria, hypoglycaemia, renal failure, hepatic dysfunction, and adult respiratory distress syndrome [1]. Several clinical indicators are associated with increased risk of fatal outcome of falciparum malaria, but the actual causes of death and mechanisms contributing to it are not well established. To elucidate the clinical features of severe malaria, we performed whole-body positron emission tomography (PET) scanning with ^{18}F-fluorodeoxyglucose (FDG) of *P. coatneyi*-infected Japanese macaques [2, 3]. We present here direct evidence concerning glucose uptake by FDG-PET scanning in *P. coatneyi*-infected acute phase Japanese macaques, and demonstrate the relationship of such uptake to histopathological changes observed in tissue.

What Is FDG-PET?

PET is a molecular imaging technique that provides images of physiologic processes. PET was developed in the early 1970s soon after x-ray computed tomography (CT) and at about the same time as magnetic resonance (MR) imaging [4]. The initial uses of PET were to help characterize disorders of the brain and heart by quantitatively imaging biologically important molecules labeled with short-lived positron emitting radionuclides [5]. The radiopharmaceutical that has had the most impact on clinical PET imaging is FDG, which was first described in the late 1970s [5, 6]. Over the last decade its applications in clinical neurology, cardiology and especially in clinical oncology have increased considerably, paralleled by an increasing availability of PET cameras [5-8].

The mechanism of cellular uptake of FDG in tumor cells has been described in detail [5]. FDG, an analogue of glucose, is metabolized similarly to glucose in that FDG is transported across cell membranes by glucose transporter proteins and is enzymatically phosphorylated. Phosphorylated glucose enters the glycolytic pathway for energy production. Phosphorylated FDG, however, is not further metabolized and remains trapped in the cell. FDG thus accumulated within cells in proportion to the cellular rate of glycolysis. The primary exception to the metabolic trapping is in the liver, where the large concentration of phosphatase enzymes results in dephosphorylation of the FDG-6-phosphate and clearance of FDG from the liver [5].

FDG has been shown to accumulate in a diverse spectrum of malignant tumors because of their increased glucose metabolism [9]. Recently FDG has been used extensively with PET for differentiating malignant from benign tumor staging, and for evaluating treatment efficacy in cancer patients [10]. On the other hand, it has also been demonstrated that elevated accumulation of FDG is associated with inflammatory and infectious diseases [11-14]. Sugawara and others evaluated the feasibility of use of FDG-PET in patients with a variety of infections, and concluded that FDG-PET appears to be a promising modality for rapid imaging of active human infections [14]. In these previous studies using PET, however, little attention was directed to the use of FDG-PET for parasitic diseases including malaria [11].

Nonhuman Primate Model of Severe Human Mararia

In some studies of the pathological mechanisms of falciparum malaria, nonhuman primate models have been used. They include rhesus monkey (*Macaca mulatta*) infected with *P. coatneyi* or *P. fragile*, Japanese macaque (*M. fuscata*) infected with *P. coatneyi* and squirrel monkey (*Saimiri sciureus*) infected with *P. falciparum* [15-18]. Aikawa and others demonstrated that these infected monkeys produced parasitized red blood cell (PRBC) sequestration in the microvessels that was similar to that in human falciparum malaria [15-18]. Therefore, nonhuman primate models have been considered promising candidates for the assessment of severe human malaria with cerebral involvement.

We have been studying the pathophysiological mechanisms of sever malaria using the Japanese macaque experimentally infected with *P. coatneyi* (CDC strain) [2, 3, 17, 19-22]. The monkey infected with *P. coatneyi* develop a fulminating acute infection with pronounced parasitemia and became moribund with severe manifestations such as tremors, vomiting, dyspnea, anemia, and hemoglobinuria. Histopathological examinations of tissues from the infected monkey have revealed sequestration events and cytoadherence associated with knobs on PRBCs to endothelial cells in cerebral microvessels and capillaries of major organs [17]. Moreover, rosette formation associated with *P. coatneyi*-infected erythrocytes *in vitro* has been identified [22, 23]. Therefore, sequestration events and rosette formation with *P. coatneyi*-infected erythrocytes have been considered major factors in the pathogenesis of severe manifestations with cerebral involvement in infected monkeys as in severe human malaria.

Pathophysiology of Cerebral Malaria

Cerebral malaria (CM) is a severe complication of falciparum malaria that occurs in approximately 2% of patients infected by *P. falciparum*. Cerebral dysfunction is detectable as a variety of symptoms, including extreme lethargy and stupor, and can proceed to coma and eventual death if the disease is not controlled [24]. Several hypotheses have been proposed to explain the development of the neurological complications. The central histopathologic features in most patients with CM include sequestration of PRBCs within the cerebral microvasculature, mainly cortical and perforating arteries, with perivascular ring hemorrhages and white matter necrosis [25]. The presence of PRBC sequestration in cerebral microvessels has been reported a major factor in the pathogenesis of human CM when the rate of PRBC sequestration in cerebral microvessels was compared between cerebral and noncerebral falciparum malaria cases. MacPherson and others reported earlier that over three times as many vessels contained PRBCs in CM patients than in the noncerebral malaria patients [26]. Thus, the pathogenesis of CM is clearly related to blockade of cerebral microvessels by sequestration of PRBCs.

On the other hand, some authors have tried to explain the pathophysiology of CM by proposing that cytokines or other soluble mediators could cause the symptoms of coma directly, independently of sequestration [27, 28]. Cytokines such as tumour necrosis factor (TNF)-α, interleukin (IL)-1, and IL-10, or neuro-active mediators such as nitric oxide (NO) can be toxic to the central nervous system when overproduced. Therefore, current several investigators assume that multiple factors determine why some acute *P. falciparum* infections exhibit cerebral symptoms whereas others with equal or even higher blood parasitemia do not.

Cerebral Metabolic Rate of Glucose (CMRglc) in Acute Phase of Severe Malaria

Although CM is the most important fatal complication in severe malaria with a mortality rate between 25% and 50%, the great majority (90%) of patients who survive CM do so without suffering from residual neurological sequelae [24]. Currently, there are several theories on recovery system from CM [28]. However, detailed mechanism and cerebral metabolic alterations in the patients surviving complicated CM remains unclear.

To further elucidate the clinical features of CM, we focused on the cerebral metabolic changes induced by severe malaria, and we performed whole-body FDG-PET scanning of the infected macaques. In this study, two monkeys, J31 (male) and J32 (female) were examined. Both monkeys were bred and grown in animal facilities in Japan. The investigators adhered to the Guidelines for the Use of Experimental Animals authorized by the Japanese Association for Laboratory Animal Science. Healthy monkeys were examined by FDG-PET as control studies, and artificial infection was performed for the same monkeys by injecting about 1×10^9 frozen *P. coatneyi*-infected erythrocytes intravenously as previously reported [17].

The PET scans of monkeys were performed twice, before (first PET scan) and after (second PET scan) malarial infection. On administration for FDG and during FDG-PET scans, both monkeys were initially anesthetized with intramascular injection of Ketamine-HCl (15 mg/kg), and maintained with inhalation of 1.0-2.0% isoflurane in air (4 L/min). The FDG-PET images were obtained after administration of approximately 74-144 MBq (2-4 mCi) of FDG intravenously. To obtain an accurate input function, which was used for evaluating the cerebral metabolic rate of glucose (CMRglc) from the PET images, intermittent arterial blood samplings were performed through a small catheter placed in the femoral artery just after FDG injection.

After inoculation of *P. coatneyi*, the monkeys developed a fulminating acute infection. Monkey J31 initially tolerated malarial infection without any behavioral change. Subsequent clinical signs of the monkey ranged from partial anorexia to severe manifestations, such as complete anorexia, restlessness, and depression, correlated with the rapid increase in parasitemia, whereas J32, which had a low level of parasitemia, exhibited no severe manifestations other than mild anorexia. Parasitemias of monkeys J31 and J32 were 17.9% (Day 13) and 1.8% (Day 12), respectively, on second PET scans.

Figure 1 shows axial CMRglc images for J31 before and after malarial infection. Diffuse and heterogeneous metabolic reduction occurred in the frontal and temporal lobes, and no differences were found between the right and left hemisphere. Figure 2 shows sagital images of J31 and J32 before and after malarial infection. In both cases, regional CMRglc decreased in the cerebral cortex, but was almost unchanged in the basal ganglia. However, shown in figures 2b and 2d, CMRglc images of J31 with a high parasitemia exhibited a more heterogeneously reduced pattern than those of monkey J32 with a low parasitemia. Table 1 shows serial changes in regional CMRglc of monkeys J31 and J32 evaluated by regions of interest (ROI) analysis. Because FDG had been injected under anesthesia, regional CMRglc values were small and metabolic activity in gray matter was suppressed to the same level as in white matter. Although there was a strong biasing effect of anesthesia, regional CMRglc in the frontal and temporal lobes decreased by 10–20 % with malarial infection, as shown in table 1. Furthermore, CMRglc reduction in the cerebellum was not as significant as in the frontal and temporal lobes in both monkeys. The ROI analysis showed slightly increased regional CMRglc in the basal ganglia.

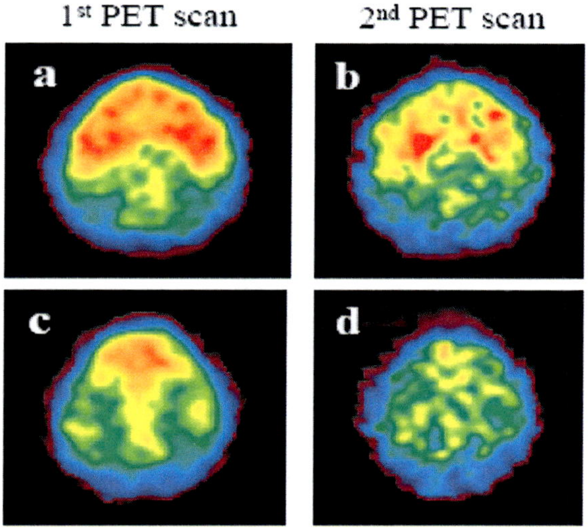

Figure 1. Axial images CMRglc before and after malarial infection for Japanese macaque J31. (a), (c) cross-section of heads of the caudate and frontal and temporal lobes. (b),(d) cross-section of frontal and parietal lobes above limbic structures. Diffuse and heterogeneous reduction of metabolism occurred in the frontal and temporal lobes in the phase of malarial infection. (a), (b) uninfected J31 (1st PET scan), and(c), (d) infected J31, with parasitemiaof 17.7% (2nd PET scan).

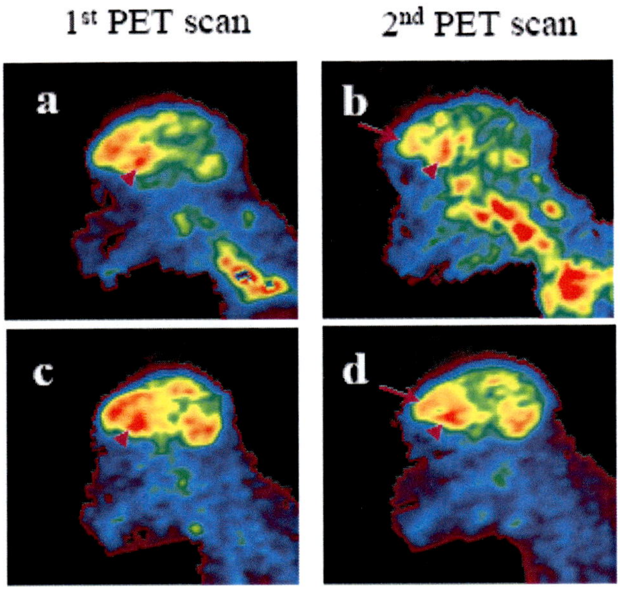

Figure 2. Sagittal images of CMRglc before and after malarial infection for two macaques J31 and J32. These four images are cross-section of the left basal ganglia indicated as arrowheads. In both cases, regional CMRglcdecreased in the frontal lobes (arrow), but was almost unchanged in basal ganglia (arrow head). (a) uninfected J31, and (b) infected J31, with parasitemiaof 17.7%. (c) uninfected J32, and (d) infected J32, with parasitemiaof 1.8%.

Table 1. Serial changes in the regional cerebral metabolic rateof glucose (CMRglc) associated with malarial infection*

	J31			J32		
	1st scan (micromol/ g/min)	2nd scan (micromol/ g/min)	change %	1st scan (micromol/ g/min)	2nd scan (micromol/ g/min)	change %
Prefrontal	2.52	2.18	-13.5	2.83	2.30	-18.7
Lateral frontal	2.22	1.75	-21.2	2.46	2.16	-12.2
Temporal	2.57	2.23	-14.3	2.97	2.41	-19.0
Parietal	1.78	1.67	- 5.9	2.17	2.01	-7.4
Basal ganglia	2.77	2.78	+0.4	2.72	2.75	+1.1
Cerebellum	1.94	1.87	- 3.6	2.58	2.40	-7.0

* Metabolic change (%) is defined as [100 x (regional CMRglc in second scan-regional CMRglc in first scan) / regional CMRglc in first scan]. Regional CMRglc values of each portion used for calculating serial metabolic changes are averaged values over the right and left hemispheres.

Although monkey J31 had a higher parasitemia than monkey J32 and exhibited severe clinical manifestations, there was little difference between monkey J31 and J32 in cerebral metabolic reduction pattern, as shown in table 1. Therefore, this reduction in cerebral metabolic activity may develop before neurologic symptoms are clearly observed in severe malaria.

Warrell and others [29] previously reported that cerebral blood flow (CBF) in patients with CM was within normal range, and that cerebral oxygen consumption and cerebral arteriovenous oxygen content difference were subnormal. Furthermore, Newton and others [30] reported that CBF velocity increases by 30% in children with CM. Recently, Clavier and others [31] also reported normal-range jugular bulb venous oxygen saturation. These findings are consistent with the reduction in cerebral metabolic activity we directly observed for the first time. Conversely, Kampfl and others [32] performed single photon emission computed tomography examination of distributional changes in CBF in a *Plasmodium falciparum*-infected human CM patient, and found that focal right hemispheric hypoperfusion and decreased oxygen saturation correlated with precision with the right hemispheric localizing signs of the patient. Local cerebral hypoperfusion should induce metabolic changes in the same region. We believe that the cerebral metabolic reduction observed in this study may protect against local hypoperfusion.

Correlation of Findings of Cerebral FDG-PET Imaging with Pathological Changes

Our previous studies showed that *P. coatneyi*-infected Japanese macaques produced PRBC sequestration in the cerebral microvessels that was similar to that in human CM patient [17]. In the current study, by using this primate model, we investigated the relationship between the findings of cerebral FDG-PET imaging and histopatholocal changes of the brain tissue. After the second FDG-PET scans, the monkeys were exsanguinated under anesthesia. They were then autopsied and their major organs including the brain were weighed and processed for histopathological examination.

Histopathological examination, as shown in figure 3, showed preferential sequestration of PRBCs in the cerebral capillaries, as observed in human CM patients. In both monkeys, the degree of sequestration in the frontal and temporal lobes did not clearly differ from that in the parietal lobe and cerebellum. The degree of sequestration in monkey J31 appeared to be slightly higher than that in monkey J32. Hemorrhagic change or neuronal necrosis was not found in HE- and Nissl-stained tissues of monkeys J31 and J32.

This suggests that the reduction in cerebral metabolic activity observed by FDG-PET occurs before parenchymal changes appear in the brain of CM patients, and that initial reduction of metabolism is reversible. We believe that reduction in cerebral metabolic activity is a hypoxic adaptation to impaired microcirculation in brain tissue, which may be induced by nitric oxide or other cytokines. We have observed increase in plasma levels of tumor necrosis factor-α and interferon-γin *P. coatneyi*-infected Japanese macaques (Kawai S and others, unpublished data). Moreover, plasma levels of soluble intrercellular adhesion molecule-1 and soluble vascular cell molecule-1 are significantly increased in the severe phase of malaria infection in this animal model [21]. Increase in plasma levels of some cytokines or other molecules are thought to be a critical step in the pathogenesis of severe malaria *in vivo*. White suggested that coma in CM is a neuroprotective reaction. Such a reduction in metabolism is considered suitable for decreasing energy consumption and minimizing brain damage with pathological changes [33]. This may be one of the reasons why most CM patients have no neurological sequelae after recovery, and why recovered CM patients exhibit reversible coma. Follow-up examinations of a human patient who recovered from CM showed regular cerebral perfusion and oxygenation patterns [32].

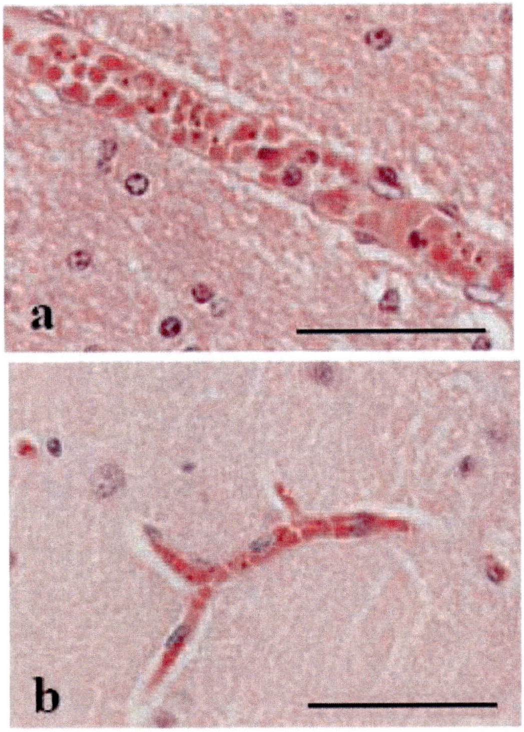

Figure 3. HE-stained (a) frontal lobe and (b) cerebellum of J31, autopsied just after the 2nd PET scan. Although sequestration of parasitized red blood cells has noted in the cerebral microvessels, neither hemorrhagic change nor neuronal necrosis was found in parenchymal regions. Bar = 50μm.

Enhancement of Splenic Glucose Metabolism During Acute Malarial Infection

The pathophysiology of the spleen's involvement in malaria is poorly understood, although it clearly plays a major role in clearance of the infection [34]. Our current study revealed also distinct elevation of FDG uptake in the spleen of *P. coatneyi*-infected acute-phase Japanese macaques. High FDG accumulation in the spleen has been recognized in patients with malignant lymphoma and sarcoidosis [35, 36], but has not been reported in infectious diseases including malaria. Our study is the first to report marked increase in splenic glucose uptake due to serious malarial infection.

In this study, four monkeys, J30 (female), J32 (male), J31 (female) and J33 (female) were examined (table 2).

Table 2. Hematological and splenic data in the experimental animals

	Before infection						After infection				
animal No. age (year) /sex	J-30 3/F	J-31 3/M	J-32 3/F	J-33 3/F	mean	SD	J-31	J-32	J-33	mean	SD
HCT (%)	40.3	36.6	38.0	44.9	40.0	3.2	20.7	26.7	27.5	25.0 *	3.0
HGB (g/dl)	12.2	11.4	11.7	13.6	12.2	0.8	6.5	8.0	8.0	7.5 *	0.7
MCV (fl)	88.2	89.3	80.9	83.5	85.5	3.4	90.8	80.7	87.6	86.4	4.2
MCH (pg)	26.7	27.8	24.9	25.3	26.2	1.2	28.5	24.2	25.5	26.0	1.8
MCHC (%)	30.3	31.1	30.8	30.3	30.6	0.3	31.4	30.0	29.1	30.2	1.0
blood glu. (mg/dl)	85	108	87	137	104.3	20.9	79	63	60	67.3 *	8.3
paraitemia (%)	-	-	-	-	-	-	17.9	1.6	37.0		
SUV in spleen	1.8	0.7	2.3	ND	1.6	0.7	5.1	5.9	4.4	5.1 *	0.6
spleen weight at autopsy (g)	5.5						17.3	11.9	13.2	14.1	2.3
mean percentage of white pulp (%)	28						41*	42*	39*	40.7	1.2

F= female; M= male; HCT= hematocrit; HGB= hemoglobin; MCV= mean corpuscular volume; MCH= mean corpuscular hemoglobin; MCHC= mean corpuscular hemoglobin concentration; blood glu.= blood glucose level; SUV= standard uptake value; ND= no data

*$P < 0.05$, Student's *t* test.

Of the macaques, J30 was used as an uninfected control, and the other three macaques (J31, J32, J33) for the infected group. PET scans of J31 and J32 were performed twice, before and after infection. J30 and J33 were scanned once, without infection and only after infection, respectively (table 2). PET scan after infection was obtained on Day 13 (J31 and J33) or Day 12 (J32). Using attenuation-correlated images, injected doses of FDG, body weights and cross-calibration factors between PET and dose calibrator, functional images of standardized uptake values (SUVs) were produced. SUV was defined as follows:

SUV = radioactive concentration in tissue (MBq/g) /
(injected dose (MBq) / monkey body weight (g)).

We manually placed one round region of interest (ROI) on the area corresponding to the center of the spleen on the SUV image of each animal. Mean SUV value of the ROI was considered a quantitative index of tissue uptake of FDG.

Parasitemias of J31, J32, and J33 were 17.9%, 1.6%, and 37.0%, respectively, on second FDG-PET scans (table 2). HCT (25.0±3.0%) and HBG (7.5±0.7g/dl) at the second PET scan were significantly decreased in all infected monkeys (P <0.05), but MCV, MCH, and MCHC did not differ significantly from the first PET scan (P >0.05). The mean blood glucose level at first PET scan was 104.3±20.9mg/dl. At the second PET scan, blood glucose level was significantly lower in all infected monkeys (67.3±8.3mg/dl, P <0.05), but no correlation was found between peripheral parasite count and blood glucose level in the infected monkeys.

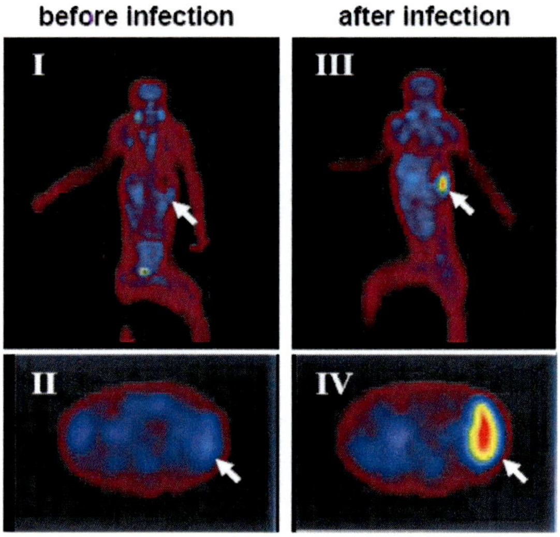

Figure 4. Sagittal and transverse FDG-PET images in a monkey at the level of the spleen before and after *P. coatneyi*-infection. I: Sagittal image in J31 before infection. II: Transverse image in J31 before infection. III: Sagittal image in infected monkey J31 with high parasitemia. IV: Transverse image in infected monkey J31 with high parasitemia. Markedly increased FDG uptake was recognized in this monkey after infection. Arrow indicates position of the spleen.

Whole-body FDG-PET scanning in the uninfected control monkey revealed no remarkable activation of FDG uptake in any organ (figure 4-I and II). On the other hand, the infected monkeys clearly exhibited increase in splenic FDG uptake, indicating marked enhancement of glucose metabolism (figure 4-III, arrow). The increase in FDG uptake in infected monkeys was diffuse throughout the entire spleen, and focal activation was noted in no particular region of the organ (figure 4-IV, arrow).

Table 2 summarizes the SUV levels of spleen in the four macaques including the uninfected control monkey J-30. The mean level of SUV in uninfected monkeys was 1.6±0.7, while the infected monkeys had significantly higher mean SUV levels (5.1±0.6, $P<0.05$).

Histopathological Changes in the Spleen During Acute Phase of Severe Malaria

All animals were exsanguinated under anesthesia after second PET scan. At autopsy, splenomegaly was clearly present in all infected monkeys. The spleen of the infected monkeys was significantly heavier than that of the uninfected control monkey ($P<0.05$, table 2). Dark red color and fragile parenchyma were observed on the cut surface of the spleen in the infected monkeys.

On light-microscopic examination of HE-stained sections, the organization of white pulp in the infected monkeys was more clearly than that in the uninfected control monkey (figures 5-A and B). Appearance of and remarkable increase in size of germinal centers were observed in infected monkey spleen. The percentage of white pulp in splenic tissue from the infected monkeys was significantly higher than that in the uninfected control tissue, and the percentage of area occupied by germinal centers in white pulp was also increased and contributed to the increasing white pulp ($P<0.05$, table 1).

In the infected monkeys J31 and J33 with high parasitemia, there was massive congestion of PRBCs, which contained early-to-middle trophozoites, uninfected erythrocytes, and numerous malarial pigments in the venous sinuses and splenic cords of red pulp (figures 5-C and D). In addition, macrophages containing malarial pigment were frequently recognized in the red pulp at high magnification (figure 5-E and F, arrow). On the other hand, infected monkey J32 with low parasitemia exhibited scattered pigment in the red pulp (data not shown).

On HLA-DP, DQ, DR immunostaining of white pulp, in the uninfected control tissue, positive reaction was predominantly found in the coronas around germinal centers, and weakly positive reaction was recognized throughout entire germinal center (figure 6-A). In the infected monkeys, however, strongly HLA-DP, DQ, DR positive reaction was recognized throughout the entire germinal center, and a large number of positive cells were scattered over the corona and the marginal zone (figure 6-B).

In an attempt to examine the activity of B lymphocytes in white pulp, immunostaining with anti-IgG antibody was employed. In the uninfected control tissue, distinct IgG-positive cells were observed as a prominent ring around the germinal center, which continued along the marginal zone (figure 6-C), whereas strongly IgG-positive reaction was recognized over the entire germinal center in infected monkey tissues (figure 6-D).

On CD68 immunostaining, the splenic macrophages in the infected monkeys were found to be larger than those in the uninfected control tissue (figures 6-E and F). The mean sizes with standard deviations of CD68-positive area of each macrophage excluding the nucleus are shown in figure 7. The mean sizes of CD68-positive area in uninfected control monkey J30, infected monkey J32 with low parasitemia, and those with high parasitemia (J33) were $34.0\pm17.4\mu m^2$, $60.4\pm31.9\mu m^2$, and $78.4\pm26.1\mu m^2$, respectively (figure 7). Differences among the three groups were significant ($P<0.05$)

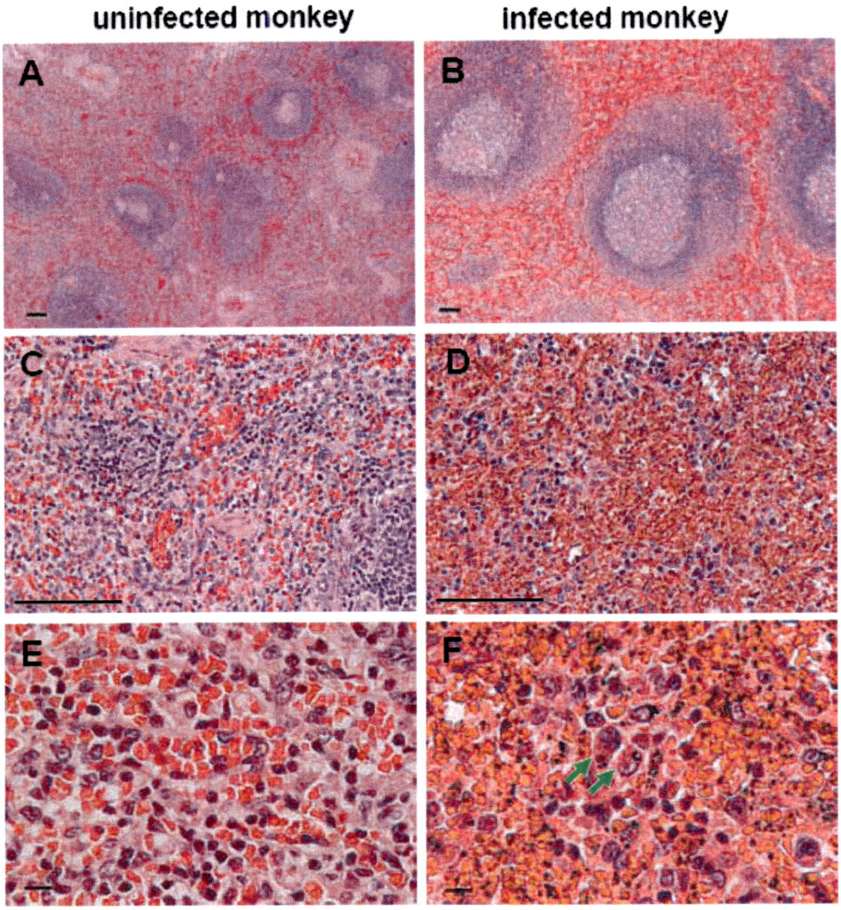

Figure 5. HE-stained sections of spleen of uninfected monkey J30 (left column: A, C, E) and J31 infected with *P. coatneyi* (right column: B, D, F). A and B: The remarkable increase in size of germinal centers contributed significantly to the increase in white pulp in infected monkey tissue. (original magnification x40, Bar = 100μm). C and D: There was massive congestion of PRBCs, uninfected erythrocytes, and numerous malarial pigments were massively congested in the venous sinuses and splenic cords (original magnification x100, Bar = 100μm). E and F: Macrophages containing malarial pigment were frequently recognized in the red pulp at high magnification (arrows) (original magnification x400, Bar = 10μm).

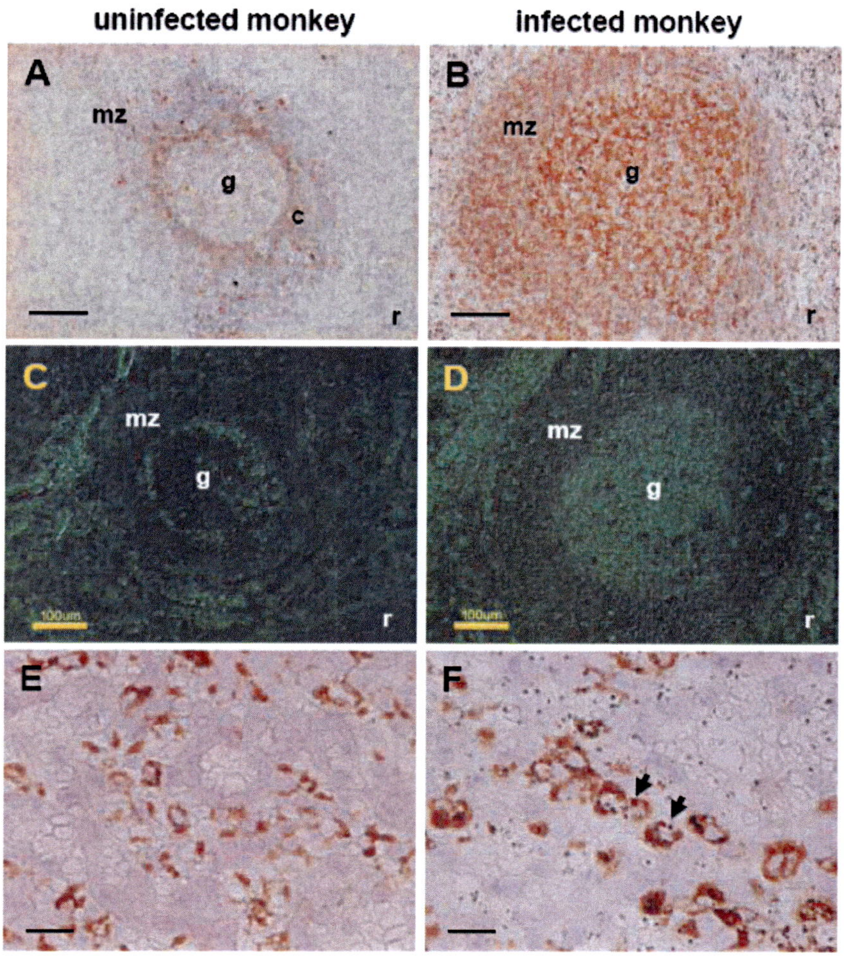

Figure 6. Immunohistochemically-stained sections of spleen of uninfected monkey J30 (left column: A, C, E) and J31 infected with *P. coatneyi* (right column: B, D, F). A and B: white pulp stained with anti-HLA-DP, DQ, DR antibody. g = germinal center, c = corona, mz = marginal zone, r = red pulp (original magnification x100, Bar =100μm). C and D: immunofluorescencestaining of white pulp using anti-monkey IgG antibody (original magnification x100, Bar=100μm). E and F: macrophages in red pulp stained with anti-CD68 antibody. Arrows = malarial pigment (original magnification x400, Bar = 10μm).

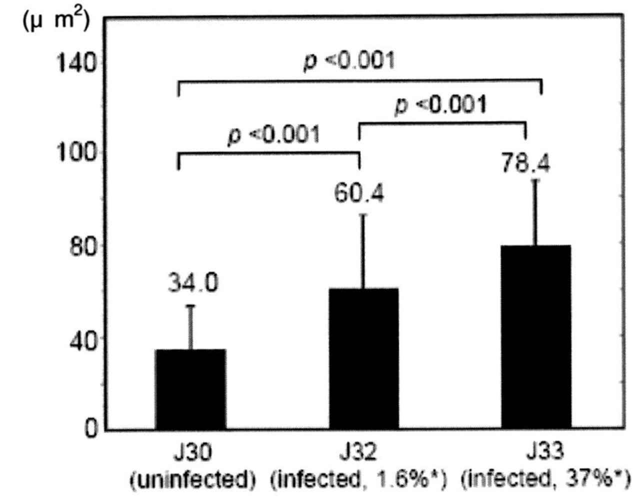

Figure 7. Size of macrophages immunopositive for CD68 in splenic tissues from uninfected monkey J30, *P. coatneyi*-infected monkey J32 with low parasitemia and infected monkey J33 with high parasitemia. (mean ±SD). * : parasitemia at autopsy.

Correlation of Findings of Splenic FDG-PET Imaging with Pathological Changes

In malarial infection, the spleen plays a critical role in clearance of PRBCs and immunity against blood-stage parasites [37]. It is the major site of elimination of PRBCs via erythrophagocytosis, elaboration of protective immune mechanisms, and hypersensitivity reaction manifesting as splenic enlargement. In the current study, we found characteristic features of malaria in the spleen of infected monkeys. Splenomegaly was clearly detected in all infected monkeys, and histopathologic findings included hyperplasia of lymphoid follicles in white pulp, a large number of activated macrophages, and congestion of PRBCs and malaria pigments in red pulp. Similar histopathological changes in spleen have been observed in patients with acute falciparum malaria and in laboratory experiments using rodent models [34, 38]. Furthermore, in the current study, *P. coatneyi*-infected monkeys exhibited increase in splenic FDG uptake indicating marked enhancement of glucose metabolism. Increase in splenic glucose uptake may thus be closely related to activation of splenic clearance systems against blood-stage malarial parasites.

As is well known, the germinal centers in splenic white pulp are sites of active production of B lymphocytes during antigenic stimulation [39]. Proliferation of B lymphocytes in the germinal centers is associated with phenotypic changes and differentiation into plasma cells and memory B lymphocytes. In addition, dendritic cells and macrophages are present in germinal centers, where they present antigens to T lymphocytes [40]. Histopathological examination of spleen in the current study revealed enlargement of the germinal centers in infected monkey tissue, which could be discriminated by immunostaining with anti-IgG antibody as well as by specific staining for MHC class II molecules. Although we did not specify the cell type that was positive, it is apparent that the majority of cells in germinal centers were activated B lymphocytes following proliferation, since activated B lymphocytes exhibit positive reaction for both MHC class II molecules and IgG. Scharko and others have studied FDG distribution in activated lymphoid tissues of rhesus macaques after simian immunodeficiency virus infection and showed higher uptake in B cells compared with those in CD4+ and CD8+ T cells [41]. Similar observations are found in recent studies on accumulation of FDG in inflammatory tissue [42, 43]. Therefore, we suggest that one of possible reasons for the increase in splenic FDG uptake of *P. coatneyi*-infected monkeys may reflect the activation of B lymphocytes in the white pulp.

Kawabe and others observed high FDG uptake by the tonsils and follicular hyperplasia with proliferation of lymphocytes in the germinal centers in chronic tonsillitis, and concluded that increased glucose metabolism in active inflammation involving lymphocyte proliferation was a cause of high FDG uptake by tonsils [44]. Kato and others also described massive lymphocytic infiltration and lymph follicles at sites of high FDG accumulation in the pancreas [45]. The mechanism of cellular FDG uptake in active inflammation involving lymphocyte proliferation is currently not fully understood, but is probably related to the fact that lymphocytes use glucose as an energy source during their metabolic activity. We infer from these studies that levels of splenic glucose utilization during acute malaria appear to be affected by lymphocyte proliferation and activation in lymphoid follicles.

A characteristic feature of malaria is the development of splenomegaly associated with splenic macrophage hyperplasia. In a previous study on the mechanism of splenic macrophage hyperplasia, the number of splenic macrophages in *P. berghei*-infected mice dramatically increased within 4 days after infection [46]. On the basis of this study, Wyler and Gallin found that most of the increase in splenic macrophages during acute phase do not appear to derive from local proliferation and suggested that splenic macrophages presumably increase as a result of "trapping" of blood monocytes [46]. In the current study, we found a large number of activated macrophages in the enlarged spleen of infected monkeys. In addition, we observed marked increase in splenic FDG uptake, which was diffuse throughout the entire spleen. These findings suggest that both high density and functional activity of splenic macrophages may contribute to high FDG accumulation.

Some studies have investigated FDG uptake and distribution in inflammatory tissue that was induced experimentally in animal models. For instance, Yamada and others demonstrated that subcutaneous injection of turpentine oil could produce inflammation in rats, and high FDG uptake in the inflammatory site was observed [47]. In this paper, moreover, they pointed out that grain counting on micro-autoradiography showed a high density was found in neutrophils and macrophages. Ogawa and others reported that macrophages are mainly responsible for the accumulation of FDG in atherosclerotic lesions in experimental animals [48], as atherosclerotic plaque is rich in macrophages and there is a strong correlation between accumulation of FDG and density of macrophages. These findings are direct evidence about increase of activated cellular FDG uptake by inflammatory cells such as macrophage. Therefore, hyperplasia and activation of splenic macrophages in malaria appears to be a cause of high FDG accumulation, and it is thought that splenic macrophages use glucose as an energy source for chemotaxis and phagocytosis.

Another possible reason for the increase in splenic FDG uptake is glucose consumption by the malarial parasite itself. It is known that host glucose is the main energy source for asexual stages of *P. falciparum*, and that the more mature form of the parasite consumes up to 70 to 80 times the amount of glucose required by uninfected erythrocytes *in vitro* [49, 50]. Interestingly, in the current study, blood glucose level was significantly lower at second PET scan, whereas splenic FDG level was markedly increase in all infected monkeys. Histopathological examination of infected tissue revealed massive congestion by numerous PRBCs in the red pulp. These findings suggest that the increased accumulation of FDG in the spleen of the infected monkeys may have been due to PRBC congestion itself. The parasites appear to consume enormous amounts of glucose as an energy source for development or survival after being trapped in the spleen. The mechanisms of survival of PRBC in the spleen are not yet clearly understood, but might depend upon local alterations of splenic conditions such as pH, glucose concentration, and oxygen partial pressure that influence disruption of PRBCs [51].

Our findings demonstrated drastic changes in the tissue of the spleen due to acute *P. coatneyi* infection, including hyperplasia of splenic lymphoid follicles and macrophages indicating activation of these cells in response to antigenic stimulation. However, several investigators have reported that both activation and suppression of the splenic immune system are observed in primate malaria, rodent malaria, and patients with human malaria [52-55]. For instance, Kakinuma and others reported that splenic lymphoid follicles from macaques infected with *P. knowlesi* were small and indistinct, indicating immuno-suppresive reaction [52], whereas Abildgaad and others reported that they were large and hyperplastic [53]. In addition, Maegraith stated that hyperplasia of lymphocytes was evident in the splenic white pulp during the recovery period and after treatment for human patient with malaria [54]. It seems likely that the changes in the splenic immune system are associated with dynamic alterations exhibited by hyperplastic or atrophic cell reactions during different phases of disease. In the current study, we obtained direct evidence for the correlation between glucose uptake and pathologic characteristics of the spleen in the acute phase of malaria. It is possible that level of glucose uptake in the spleen varies depending on disease status during the course of infection. Thus, further studies are needed to characterize the relationships between splenic FDG uptake and disease status of malaria, such as the chronic phase and recovery phase after treatment.

Conclusion

Several authors have demonstrated that many events take place in the brain and the spleen during severe malaria, including changes in histological, immunological, and physiological characteristics. Although some techniques have been proposed for noninvasive evaluation of alterations, it is difficult to accurately evaluate physiological conditions during the course of malaria infection. PET is one example of such a technique, and has the potential to yield the physiological information necessary not only for diagnosis of cancers or site of inflammation based on altered tissue metabolism, but also for monitoring of the effects of treatment on tissue metabolism. In this study, to elucidate the clinical features of severe malaria, we performed whole-body PET scanning with FDG of *P. coatneyi*-infected Japanese macaques. We observed diffuse and heterogeneous reduction of metabolism in cerebral cortex in acute phase of malaria infection. Furthermore, we determined correlations of splenic glucose uptake and histopathological changes in the primate model. These findings will improve understanding of physiological alterations of the host in serious malarial infection. We believe that whole-body FDG-PET may be useful for evaluating and monitoring pathophysiological processes involved in severe malaria.

Acknowledgments

I am grateful to many colleagues in Gunma University Graduate School of Medicine for their help in the experiment. Particular thanks to Dr. Munehiro Sugiyama, Dr. Eiji Ikeda and Prof. Mamoru Suzuki for manuscript review. Preparation of this review was supported by a Grant-in-Aid Ministry of Education, Culture, Sports, Science and Technology of Japan (1859040) and a Grant-in-Aid of Ministry of Health, Labor and Welfare (H17-Shinkou-ippan-019).

References

[1] Molyneux, M. E. (2000). Impact of malaria on the brain and its prevention. Lancet, 335, 671-672.

[2] Sugiyama, M., Ikeda, E., Kawai, S., Higuchi, T., Zhang, H., Khan, N., Tomiyoshi, K., Inoue, T., Yamaguchi, H., Katakura, K., Endo, K. and Suzuki, M. (2004). Cerebral metabolic reduction in severe malaria: Fluorodeoxyglucose-positoron emission tomography imaging in a primate model of severe human malaria with cerebral involvement. *Am. J. Trop. Med. Hyg*, 71, 542-545.

[3] Kawai, S., Ikeda, E., Sugiyama, M., Matsumoto, J., Higuchi, T., Zhang, H., Khan, N., Tomiyoshi, K., Inoue, T., Yamaguchi, H., Katakura, K., Endo, K., Matsuda, H. and Suzuki, M. (2006). Enhancement of splenic glucose metabolism during acute malarial infection: correlation of findings of FDG-PET imaging with pathological changes in a primate model of severe human malaria. *Am. J. Trop. Med. Hyg*, 74, 353-360.

[4] Phelps, M. E., Hoffman, E. J., Mullani, N. A. and Ter-Pogossian, M. M. (1975) Application of annihilation coincidence detection to transocial reconstruction tomography. *J. Nuc.l Med*, 16, 210-214.

[5] Rohren, E.M., Turkington, T.G. and Coleman, R.E. (2004). Clinical applications of PET in oncology. *Radiology*, *231*, 305-332.

[6] Gallagher, B. M., Fowler, J. S., Gutterson, N. I., MacGregor, R. R., Wan, C. N. and Wolf, A. P. (1978). Metabolic trapping as a principle of radiopharmaceutical design: some factors resposible for the biodistribution of [^{18}F] 2-deoxy-2-fluoro-D-glucose. *J. Nucl. Med*, *19*, 1154-1161.

[7] Kumar, A., Braum, A., Schapiro, M., Grady, C., Carson, R. and Herscovitch, P. (1992). Cerebral glucose metabolic rates after 30 and 45 minutes acquisitions: a comparative study. *J. Nucl. Med*, *33*, 2103-2105.

[8] Schwaiger, M. and Hicks, R. (1991). The clinical role of metabolic imaging of the heart by positron emission tomography. *J. Nucl. Med*, *32*, 565-578.

[9] Warburg, O., Wind, F. and Niglers, E. (1930). On the metabolism of tumors in the body. In O. Warburg (Ed.). *Metabolism of Tumors*: (pp.164-170). London, England: Constable.

[10] Wahl, R. L. (1994). Positron emission tomography: application in oncology. In I. P. C. Murray and H. W. Strauss (Eds.). *Nuclear Medicine in Clinical Diagnosis and Treatment*: (pp. 801-820). London, England: Churchill Livingston.

[11] Winter, F. D., Vogelaers, D., Gemmel, F. and Dierckx, R. A. (2002). Promising role of 18-F-fluoro-D-deoxyglucose positron emission tomography in clinical infectious disease. *Eur. J. Clin. Microbiol. Infect. Dis*, *21*, 247-257.

[12] Kawabe, J., Okamura, T., Shakudo, M., Koyama, K., Wanibuchi, H., Sakamoto, H., Matsuda, M., Kishimoto, K., Ochi, H. and Yamada, R. (1999). Two cases of chronic tonsillitis studied by FDG-PET. *Ann. Nucl. Med*, *13*, 277-279.

[13] Bakheet, S. M., Powe, J., Kandil, A., Ezzat, A., Rostom, A. and Amartey, J. (2000). F-18 FDG uptake in breast infection and inflammation. *Clin. Nucl. Med*, *25*, 100-103.

[14] Sugawara, Y., Broun, D. K., Kison, P. V., Russo, J. E., Zasadny, K. R. and Wahl, R. L. (1998). Rapid detection of human infections with fluorine-18 fluorodeoxyglucose and positron emission tomography: preliminary results. *Eur. J. Nucl. Med*, *25*, 1238-1243.

[15] Aikawa, M., Brown, A., Smith, C. D., Tegoshi, T., Howard, R. J., Hasler, T. H., Ito, Y., Perry, G., Collins, W. E. and Webster, K. (1992). A primate model for human cerebral malaria: *Plasmodium coatneyi*-infected rhesus monkeys. *Am. J. Trop. Med. Hyg*, *46*, 391-397.

[16] Fujioka, H., Millet, P., Maeno, Y., Nakazawa, S., Ito, Y., Howard, R. J., Collins, W. E. and Aikawa, M. (1994). A nonhuman primate model for human cerebral malaria: Rhesus monkeys experimentally infected with *Plasmodium fragile*. *Exp. Parasitol*, *78*, 371-376.

[17] Kawai, S., Aikawa, M., Kano, S. and Suzuki, M. (1993). A primate model for severe human malaria with cerebral involvement: *Plasmodium coatneyi*-infected *Macaca fuscata*. *Am. J. Trop. Med. Hyg*, *48*, 630-636.

[18] Gysin, J., Aikawa, M., Tourneur, N. and Tegoshi, T. (1992). Experimental *Plasmodim falciparum* cerebral malaria in the sequirrel monkey *Saimiri sciureus*. *Exp. Parasitol*, *75*, 390-398.

[19] Matsumoto, J., Kawai, S., Terao, K., Kirinoki, M., Yasutomi, Y., Aikawa, M. and Matsuda, H. (2000). Malaria infection induces rapid elevation of the soluble Fas ligand level in serum and subsequent T lymphocytopenia : possible factors responsible for the differences in susceptibility of two species of *Macaca* monkeys to *Plasmodium coatneyi* infection. *Infect. Immun*, *68*, 1183-1188.

[20] Kawai, S., Yoshino, M., Matsumoto, J., Kirinoki, M., Aikawa, M. and Matsuda, H. (2003). *Plasmodium coatneyi*-infected erythrocytes bind to C32 amelanotic melanoma cells under static and flow conditions. *J. Vet. Med. Sci*, *6*, 375-380.

[21] Kawai, S., Matsumoto, J., Aikawa, M. and Matsuda, H. (2003). Increased plasma levels of soluble intracellular adhesion molecule-1 (sICAM-1) and soluble vascular cell molecule-1 (sVCAM-1) associated with disease severity in a primate model for severe human malaria: *Plasmodium coatneyi*- infected Japanese macaques (*Macaca fuscata*). *J. Vet. Med. Sci*, *65*, 629-631.

[22] Kawai, S., Kano, S. and Suzuki, M. (1995). Rosette formation by *Plasmodium coatneyi*-infected erythrocytes of the Japanese macaque (*Macaca fuscata*). *Am. J. Trop. Med. Hyg*, *53*, 295-299.

[23] Tegoshi, T., Udomsangpetch, R., Brown, A., Nakazawa, S., Webster, H. K. and Aikawa, M. (1993). Ultrastructure of rosette formation by *Plasmodium coatneyi*-infected erythrocytes of rhesus. *Parasitol. Res*, *79*, 611-613.

[24] Marsh, K. (1999). The Clinical Features of Cerebral Malaria. In M. Wahlgren and P. Perlmann (eds.), *Malaria: Molecular and Clinical Aspects* (pp.91-98). Amsterdam: Harwood Academic Publishers.

[25] Aikawa, M., Iseki, M., Branwell, J. W., Taylor, D., Oo, M. M. and Howard R. J. (1990). The pathology of human cerebral malaria. *Am. J. Trop. Med. Hyg*, *43*, Suppl., 30-37.

[26] MacPherson, G. G., Warrell, D. A., White, N. J., Looareesuwan, S. and Warrell, D. A. (1985). Human cerebral malaria. A quantitative ultrastructural analysis of parasitized erythrocyte sequestration. *Am. J. Pathol*, *119*, 385-401.

[27] Clark, I. A., Yaman, F. M. and Jacobson, L. S. (1997). The biological basis of malarial disease. *Int. J. Parasitol*, *27*, 1237-1249.

[28] Adams, S., Brown H. and Turner G. (2002). Breaking down the blood-brain barrier: signaling a path to cerebral malaria? *TRENDS in Parasitol*, *18*, 360-366.

[29] Warrell, D. A., White, N. J., Veall, N., Looareesuwan, S., Chanthavanich, P., Phillips, R. E., Karbwang, J., Pongpaew, P. and Krishna, S. (1988). Cerebral anaerobic glycolysis and reduced cerebral oxygen transport in human cerebral malaria. *Lancet*, *2*, 534-538.

[30] Newton, C. R., Marsh, K., Peshu, N. and Kirkham, F. J. (1996). Perturbations of cerebral hemodynamics in Kenyans with cerebral malaria. *Pediatr. Neurol*, *15*, 41-49.

[31] Clavier, N., Rahimy, C., Falanga, P., Ayivi, B. and Payen, D. (1999). No evidence for cerebral hypo- perfusion during cerebral malaria. *Crit. Care Med*, *27*, 628-632.

[32] Kampfl, A., Pfausler, B., Haring, H. P., Denchev, D., Donnemiller, E. and Schmutzhard, E. (1997). Impaired microcirculation and tissue oxygenation in human cerebral malaria: a single photon emission computed tomography and near-infrared spectroscopy study. *Am. J. Trop. Med. Hyg*, *56*, 585-587.

[33] White, N. J. (1999). Cerebral perfusion in cerebral malaria. *Crit. Care Med* , *27*, 478-479.

[34] Warrell, D. A., Turner, G. D. and Francis, N. (2002). Pathology and pathophysiology of human malaria. In D. A. Warrell, and H. M. Gilles (Eds.), *Essential Malariology*: (Fourth edition, pp. 236-251). New York: Edward Arnold.

[35] Moog, F., Bangerter, M., Diederichs, C. G., Guhlmann, A., Merkle, E., Frickhofen, N. and Reske, S. N. (1998). Extranodal malignant lymphoma: detection with FDG PET versus CT. *Radiology*, *206*, 475-481.

[36] Lewis, P. J. and Salama, A. (1994). Uptake of fluorine-18 fluorodeoxyglucose in sarcoidosis. *J. Nucl. Med*, *35*, 1647-1649.

[37] Engwerda, C. R., Beattie, L. and Amante, F. H. (2005). The importance of the spleen in malaria. *TRENDS in Parasitol*, *2*, 75-80.

[38] Stevenson, M. M. and Kraal, G. (1989). Histological changes in the spleen and liver of C57BL/6 and A/J mice during *Plasmodium chabaudi* AS infection. *Exp. Mol. Pathol*, *51*, 80-95.

[39] Gartner, L. P. and Hiatt, J. L. (2000). Spleen. *Color Atlas of Histology*: (Third edition, pp. 190-191). Philadelphia: Lippincott Williams and Wilkins.

[40] Abbas, A. K., Lichtman, A. H. and Pober, J. S. (2003). The major histocompatibility complex. *Cellular and Molecular Immunology*: (Fifth edition, pp.65-80). Philadelphia, Pennsylvania: Saunders.

[41] Scharko, A. M., Perlman, S. B., Hinds II, P. W., Hanson, J. M., Uno, H. and Pauza, C. D. (1996). Whole body positron emission tomography imaging of simian immunodeficiency virus-infected rhesus macaques. *Proc. Natl. Acad. Sci. USA*, *9*, 6425-6430.

[42] Ishimori, T., Saga, T., Mamede, M., Kobayashi, H., Higashi, T., Nakamoto, Y., Sato, N. and Konishi, J. (2002). Increased ^{18}F-FDG uptake in a model of inflammation: concanavalin A-mediated lymphocyte activation. *J. Nucl. Med*, *43*, 658-663.

[43] Shozushima, M., Tsutsumi, R., Terasaki, K., Sato, S., Nakamura, R. and Sakamaki, K. (2003). Augmentation effects of lymphocyte activation by antigen- presenting macrophages on FDG uptake. *Ann. Nucl. Med*, *17*, 555-560.

[44] Kawabe, J., Okamura, T., Shakudo, M., Koyama, K., Wanibuchi, H., Sakamoto, H., Matsuda, M., Kishimoto, K., Ochi, H. and Yamada, R. (1999). Two cases of chronic tonsillitis studied by FDG-PET. *Ann. Nucl. Med*, *13*, 277-279.

[45] Kato, T., Fukatsu, H., Ito, K., Tadokoro, M., Ota, T., Ikeda, M., Isomura, T., Ito, S., Nishino, M. and Ishigaki, T. (1995). Fluorodeoxyglucose positron emission tomography in pancreatic cancer: an unresolved problem. *Eur. J. Nucl. Med*, *22*, 32-39.

[46] Wyler, D. and Gallin, J. (1977). Spleen-derived mononuclear cell chemotactic factor in malaria infections: A possible mechanism for splenic macrophage accumulation. *J. Immunol*, *118*, 478-484.

[47] Yamada, S., Kubota, K., Kubota, R., Ido, T. and Tamahashi, N. (1995). High accumulation of fluorine-18-fluorodeoxyglucose in turpentine-induced inflammatory tissue. *J. Nucl. Med*, *36*, 1301-1306.

[48] Ogawa, M., Ishino, S., Mukai, T., Asano, D., Teramoto, N., Watabe, H., Kudomi, N., Shiomi, M., Magata, Y., Iida, H. and Saji, H. (2004). ^{18}F-FDG accumulation in atherosclerotic plaques: Immunohistochemical and PET imaging study. *J. Nucl. Med*, *45*, 1245-1250.

[49] Zolg, J. W., MacLeod, A. J. and Scaife, J. G. (1984). The accumulation of lactic acid and its influence on the growth of *Plasmodium falciparum* in synchronized cultures. *In Vitro*, *20*, 205-215.

[50] Sherman, I. W. (1988). Mechanisms of molecular trafficking in malaria. *Parasitol*, *96*, S57-S81.

[51] Goodman, J., Newman, M. I. and Chapman, W. C. (2003). Splenic function. In J. P. Greer, J. Foerster, J. N. Lukens, G. M. Rodgers, F. Paraskevas, B. Glader, (Eds.), *Wintrobe's clinical hematology* (Eleventh edition, Vol 2, pp. 190-191). Philadelphia: Lippincott Williams and Wilkins.

[52] Kakinuma, C., Futamura, Y., Kaga, N. and Shibutani, Y. (1999). Plasma cytokine concentrations and splenic changes in cynomolgus monkeys (*Macaca fascicularis*) with malaria. *Lab. Anim. Sci*, *49*, 101-104.

[53] Abildgaad, C., Harrison, S. and Denardo, S. (1975). Simian *Plasmodium knowlesi* malaria: studies of coagulation and pathology. *Am. J. Trop. Med. Hyg*, *24*, 764-768.

[54] Maegraith, B. G. (1973). Malaria. In H. Spencer (ed.), *Tropical pathology*: (pp.319-349). New York: Springer-Verlag.

[55] Zingman, B. S. and Viner, B. L. (1993). Splenic complications in malaria: Case report and review. *Clin. Infect. Dis*, *16*, 223-232.

In: Progress in Malaria Research
Editor: Lee O. Koning, pp. 171-192

ISBN: 978-1-60021-590-2

Chapter V

The Oral Transmission of Malaria

Filiberto Malagon**, *Jose Luis Tapia*, *Judith Vazquez*, *Francisco del Toro and Lilia Robert
Laboratorio de Malariologia; Departamento de Microbiologia y Parasitologia,
Facultad de Medicina; Universidad Nacional Autonoma de Mexico

Abstract

Transmission of malaria through the oral route is analyzed looking at the evolutionary origin of Apicomplexa, Coccidia, Haemosporidia, and *Plasmodium* parasites. Discussion is done on the two ways of oral transmission proposed: by ingesting the meat of an infected animal, or by ingestion of the infective form of a coccidian. This discussion is linked to experimental observations to sustain a theory that consider that the original coccidian from which *Plasmodium* evolved is an *Isospora* that did not disappear in the process of speciation and, it is still with us forming part of the cycle of a parasite that behave like plasmodium and/or coccidian, depending on the host they infect. The stage of the parasite that make connection between *Plasmodium* and coccidian, may be the sporozoite, although merozoites may be involved in infections transferred by blood forms.

Key words: Malaria, oral transmission, apicomplexa, Haemosporidia, *Plasmodium,* Coccidia, *Isospora*, evolution.

* Address: Laboratorio de Malariologia, Departamento de Microbiologia y Parasitologia; Facultad de Medicina, UNAM; Ciudad universitaria, Mexico 04510, D.F. Mexico; e mail: malagon@servidor.unam.mx

Introduction

Transmission is a process through which a pathogen is transferred from a host to another, and biologically is a means for the dispersion of a parasite species. In malaria in 1894, transmission of malaria parasites was quite unknown, however, spread by air or water were the most favored. It is well known that Manson had propounded a theory that mosquitoes transmitted malaria, theory that was the motive of the studies of Ross (1926) who at the very end of the XIX century, together with Grassi discovered that malaria was transmitted from person to person, by *Anopheles* mosquito bites. Grassi himself described a detailed account of the parasite development in the mosquito presented at the Lincei Academy (Capanna, 2006) leaving to posterity a master piece of work still very much estimated. Since then, all discussion about natural transmission of malaria means to talk about infected mosquito bites, if speaking about horizontal transmission and, of congenital transfer of the parasite when thinking in vertical transmission. However, other demonstrated forms of transmission are not usually considered. Although, transmission of human malaria by other routes has never been demonstrated, it does not mean that they do not exist. Some experiments on malaria transmission in other animal species, done through the time, indicate that *Homo sapiens* may perhaps behave in a similar way. There are several old experimental observations on monkey and bird malarias being transmitted by the oral route. Among these experiences, Shortt and Menon (1940) reported infection of *Macaca radiata* and *M. mulatta* after oral inoculation of blood infected by *P. knowlesi*, and of chickens fed with blood infected by *P. gallinaceum*; Beltrán and Larenas (1941) infected chickens after oral inoculation with blood infected also with *Plasmodium gallinaceum* and, Young (1941) observed infection of pigeons inoculated by the oral route with blood infected by *P. relictum*. Several other experimental ways for transmitting malaria in birds were performed by Sergent (1937). More recently, the author (Malagon, et al. 1994) reported the infection of mice fed with blood infected by *P. yoelii*. To discuss on the possibility that oral infection of malaria is taking place now, many biological aspects of the problem have to be analyzed, and that is the purpose of the present work.

Preamble

What Malaria Is?

In recent years the application of molecular tools to the phylogeny and evolution of parasites, and particularly in malaria, has produced a conflict of identity on the haemosporidian that have to be named "malaria parasites" (Perez-Tris, 2005). As malaria is the central subject of this work, it seems necessary to make clear the position under which this discussion is written. Perez-Tris and co-workers, seem to be confused on what a symptom is.

It is well known that malaria is the name the Romans coined in the middle of the XVIII century, to refer to a malady they thought was born from the bad air (mal aria) coming from the marshes in the vicinity of Rome, which also was called the "roman fever" (Bruce-Chwatt, 1980). Malaria is a term to name an intermittent febrile illness associated to the unhealthy atmosphere caused by the exhalations of marshes, as defined on those times, before the microorganisms that caused it were discovered. It is clear that in its origin malaria was a name with no taxonomical connotation, but was just the name of a disease. When parasites causing the illness called malaria were discovered, soon they were called malaria parasites, to refer to all parasites causing the disease. In the beginning those parasites to be referred as malaria parasites could be from the *Oscillaria, Haemamoeba, Plasmodium, Laverania, Haematozoon* and *Haemomonas* genera (Belding, 1965), however as time passed, genus *Plasmodium* was the only one to design the human parasites causing malaria, the term malaria parasites was later extended to all parasites of the genus *Plasmodium* infecting other mammals, birds and reptiles, most of them without producing visible clinical signs of a picture of human malaria-like disease, in their own hosts. In those animal species in which *Plasmodium* parasites cause disease, is difficult to say that they are those animal species in which *Plasmodium* parasites cause disease, is difficult to say that they are suffering from malaria, because no a clinical frame exists to define when an animal is clinically expressing a malaria picture, nor either the way to recognize in animals, others than monkeys and apes, many of the symptoms observed in human malaria. Strictly speaking, malaria parasites have to be used just in reference to those parasites producing malaria in humans independently of its taxonomic position, and perhaps extended to those parasites that produce a malaria-like disease in other animals, just defining the symptoms to be found to call it malaria or malaria-like. However, tradition is stronger than reason.

Phylogenetic studies, already have and, will undoubtedly have an enormous influence in taxonomy, however, the taxonomic reconstruction of the tree of life have to take into consideration the emerging phylogenetic views, together with traditional taxonomic knowledge.

By the force of tradition, in the present work the term malaria parasites is used, and introduce in some instances the name *Plasmodium* parasites, instead.

Evolution of the Apicomplexa

Life is, fundamentally, the expression of two kinds of living organisms, bacteria and eukaryotes. Eukaryotes probably evolved from a Gram-negative eubacterium (actinobacteria), 850 million years ago (Mya) (Cavalier-Smith 2002), and from those original eukaryotes diverged all extant eukaryote organisms with all their structural complexity, among them the Apicomplexa and the malaria parasites.

Chatton associated the Haemosporidia parasites in their most ancient forms to Dinoflagellate, since 1937 he argued that the specialized argyrofilic apparatus, characteristic of flagellates still persists on the cuticle of many Sporozoa, and later in 1953 Grassi suggested the flagellate ancestry of Coccidiomorpha and Gregarinomorpha (cited by Garnham, 1966). Many years had to pass, to find out that Chatton and Grassi suggestions were true. Gutteridge (1971) when working with the DNA of the monkey malaria parasite *Plasmodium knowlesi*, found a law density satellite DNA using centrifugation with CsCl densities, and later Kilejian (1975) working with Mitochondrial DNA of the bird malaria *P. lophurae*, found the same element with similar procedures, but he also observed specimens in electron microscope to find out that this DNA was conformed in circles of about 10μm in length, and suggested to characterize the satellite DNAs observed at CsCl densities of 1.677 and 1.679 g/ml found in rodent and primate malaria parasites. Both authors thought that this DNA was coming from mitochondrial DNA of their respective parasites. However, Wilson (1994, 1996,1997) working on *Plasmdium falciparum* found that the 35 kb circled DNA was the residual genome of a secondarily acquired plastid, gained by endosymbiotic interaction of a progenitor of the phylum Apicomplexa with an alga in ancient times and, suggested that the ancestor from which the Apicomplexa evolved was an alveolate or a dinoplagellate that phagocytosed an alga containing a cyanobacterium as an endosymbiont. In a next step Kohler (1997), doing a nice ultra-structural study, found that the 35 kb genome, also called apicoplast, was contained in a 4 layered membranous sac laying into the cytoplasm and proximal to the nucleus, he described it like a true plastid with no photosynthetic functions. In opinion of Fast (2001), Apicomplexa and Dinoflagellate plastids appear to be the result of a single endosymbiotic event which occurred early in eukaryotic evolution, thus the ancestral state of apicomplexan parasites was photosynthetic, condition that was lost through evolution. McFaden, (2000) stated that dinoflagellate and apicomplexan diverged from those ancestral photosynthetic protozoa 400 million years ago (Mya), apicomplexan lost their photosynthetic character and became intracellular parasites, while some dinoflagellate conserved it. Taking into consideration the possible bias of the molecular predictions, at this time, available evidences support the idea that Apicomplexa evolved from a dinoflagellate or both diverged from the same ancestor, in any case, a partial or totally true prediction was made by Chatton 70 years ago!!.

Cocccidial Origin of Haemosporidia

Although *Coccidium oviform*, a common parasite of the rabbit was recognized in the middle of the nineteenth century, Remak was the first to establish the intracellular nature of the parasite and Eimer in describing the development of the parasites in the epithelial cells of the mouse intestine (Foster, 1965). Later, several workers described the life cycle of coccidian with its alternation of sexual and asexual generation. In 1847 Kauffmann described sporulation inside the oocyst, which was completed with more detail in 1865 by Stieda in the rabbit coccidian. Schuberg described the life cycle of *Eimeria falciformis* in the mouse, in 1895, confirming Eimer's work. In the 1890's a great deal of work was done on coccidian, because they were thought to be a cause of cancer.

More than 30 years of experience in the study of coccidian parasites had passed, when malaria parasites were discovered by Laveran in 1880, and nearly 50 after their discovery, when in 1899 Mesnil and Schaudinn drew attention to the similarity of the life cycles of coccidian and haemosporidian parasites, although only a fragment of the cycle of haemosporidian was known at that time. However, one year later the description of the sporogonic cycle of the malaria parasites by Grassi, confirmed this view (cited by Garnham, 1966). In opinion of Coatney (1973) most workers agreed that malaria parasites descended from a coccidian ancestor. However, two possibilities arose, first that the coccidian that evolved into *Plasmodium* were living in the vertebrate host and second that they were living in the vector. That haemosporidian commenced evolution from a coccidia in the invertebrate host make no sense to Garnham (1966), because "it would be necessary to assume that the sporozoites (within resistant oocyst) were ingested by the insects, in whose mid-gut gametogony would ensue. If such development had formed part of Haemosporidia evolution, some coccidian parasites of dipteroid insects might have been expected to have survive until today, but they have never been found, and coccidians are poorly represented even in other orders of insects". To Coatney (1973), the greatest weight of available evidence seem to support the position that a tissue invading parasite of vertebrate intestine, in a reptile, found its way into the blood of the animal and eventually into blood sucking diptera. Bats seem to Killick-Kendrick to be the most likely animals in which mammalian Plasmodium parasites first became established (Scholtisheck 1977), because they are old mammals, modern bats are hosts of many haemosporidids, their migratory habits could have resulted in a dispersal of ancestral forms of *Plasmodium* to both Asia and Africa, probably before the continental drift, cavernicolous habits of some bats put them in close contact with specialized cave dwelling-mosquitoes.

Today, reptiles are the oldest animals in evolution being infected by *Plasmodium* parasites, and they are very common hosts of several genus and many species of coccidia. Among those genus, *Eimeria, Isospora, Caryospora, Cyclospora, Cryptosporidium, Sarcocystis* and *Besnoitia*, are included, together with many other genera less known. It is reasonable to think that ancient reptiles were also common hosts of Coccidia. According to Muller and Reisz (2006) reptiles started their history in the late carboniferous, 305 Mya thus, possibly that was the time for the beginning of the coccidia-haemosporidia evolution history too. If the Plasmodium parasites emerged at about that time, transmission had to be done by other means different to the bite of haematophagous dipterans, because no one of the extant dipteran malaria vectors existed. Perhaps it is not casual that one of the oldest haematophagous dipterans, the sand flies (Diptera: Psychodidae), are the only known vectors of reptilian malaria parasites (Klein 1987) today. Sandflies are one of the oldest haematophagous dipterans which according to Filho and Brasil (2003) had a common phlebotomine ancestor present in the Triassic before separation of the continents (240 Mya). However, the oldest fossil record recently discover in a Burmese amber, (Poinar G and Poinar R., 2004), showed that a sandfly (*Palaeomyia burmitis*) of the early Cretaceous trapped into amber (144 My) was infected by a leishmanial trypasomatid and probably was transmitting the infection to Cretaceous dinosaurs. Today, this finding probably documents the oldest date of sand flies infection with a protozoan parasite, and opens the possibility that sandflies were infected with *Plasmodium* parasites and transmitting the infection among reptiles at that time. Considering that the reptiles emerged 305 Mya when speciation of *Plasmodium* could start, and the oldest fossil record of the Phlebotomine of 144 Mya, the time distance between both events leave a gap of about 150 My (million years), lapse of time during which Plasmodium parasites evolved but no haematophagous dipterans existed to carry out transmission.

A Plasmodium parasite flowing in the blood of reptiles, in absence of its insect vector, had at least three possibilities of transmission among individuals of the same host species: the parasites harbored by the reptile mother could be transmitted to their offspring by trans-ovarian infection (although it is not observed in today Plasmodium life cycle), parasites could pass from one to another reptile by cannibalism, and also transmission could be done by the oocysts of the original coccidian, if this had not disappeared . In the frame of evolution, however, *Plasmodium* parasites or the sensibility to be infected by them could be inherited to all birds and mammals evolved from the reptiles, and still in absence of *Plasmodium* vectors, the parasites could be transferred to predators of reptiles.

When vectors appeared, horizontal transmission would occur from reptiles to reptiles and from reptiles to other animal species that were sharing their environ and, the vectors living with them. Once the original reptilian plasmodium parasite got establish in other animals, co-evolution (Lambrechts et al. 2006) started between the parasite and its hosts and speciation occurred.

Vertebrate coccidia develop its life cycle in the intestinal epithelium, comprehending development of schizogony, gametogony and sporogony (see figure 1). In addition, some genera develop extra-intestinal tissue stages, in the same host or in another, like *Toxoplasma*, *Sarcocystis*, *Besnoitia* and *Isospora*. Those coccidian that speciate into *Plasmodium* had to have that extra-intestinal invasive behavior, so it invaded liver and then blood. During development of intestinal coccidia stages, just two forms of the parasite are invasive, the merozoites and the sporozoites. Any of these two forms could reach peripheral blood from intestine to establish in liver and blood cells, to include later a hematophagous insect into its development, to conform its life cycle like now it is known.

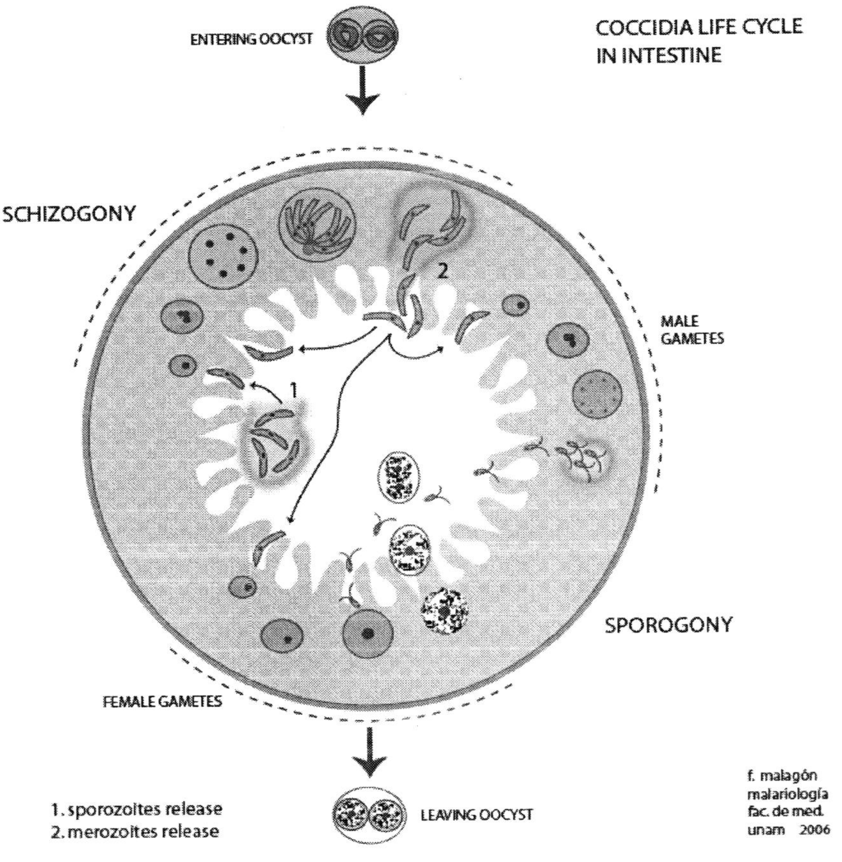

Figure 1. The coccidial stages of development.

According with fossil records, mosquitoes of the subfamily Culicine diverged in the Eocene 60 Mya (Rai and Black, 1999), to give rise to the *Anopheles*, while early fossils of modern mammals range from 50 to 70 Mya (Benton, 1999), bats among them, which probable indicate that mammals and the vectors of their *Plasmodium* parasites came to life at about the same time, so that, adaptation of mammals *Plasmodium* to *Anopheles* mosquitoes probably occurred in a relatively short time.

Usually, it is assumed that whatever the way a coccidia of reptiles evolved into *Plasmodium*, the coccidia proto-plasmodium disappear in the process of speciation, millions of years ago. Perhaps it is just one of the possibilities, because not necessarily speciation convey disappearance of the individuals from which speciation took place, it is to be consider that speciation is a process that happen to occur in an individual and not in a population as a whole, even if at last the new individual or individuals form another population, the original population not necessarily fades away (Mahner and Bunge, 1997). In first and extreme scenery, all proto-plasmodium coccidian became *Plasmodium* and only *Plasmodium* parasites were left (very improbable). In second scenery, some coccidia evolved to *Plasmodium* and both, coccidian and *Plasmodium*, remained until *Plasmodium* could produce sporogonic development in invertebrate hosts, then the intestinal coccidia disappeared. Third scenery, coccidian learn to become *Plasmodium* without leaving to be coccidium, both types of individuals remain, and according to circumstances, they develop as a true coccidian and in others it is both coccidian and *Plasmodium* and, in still other, they are just *Plasmodium* without loosing their possibility to return to coccidian life (see figure 2). Since the evolutionary point of view, the third possibility is the best to guarantee the parasite survival.

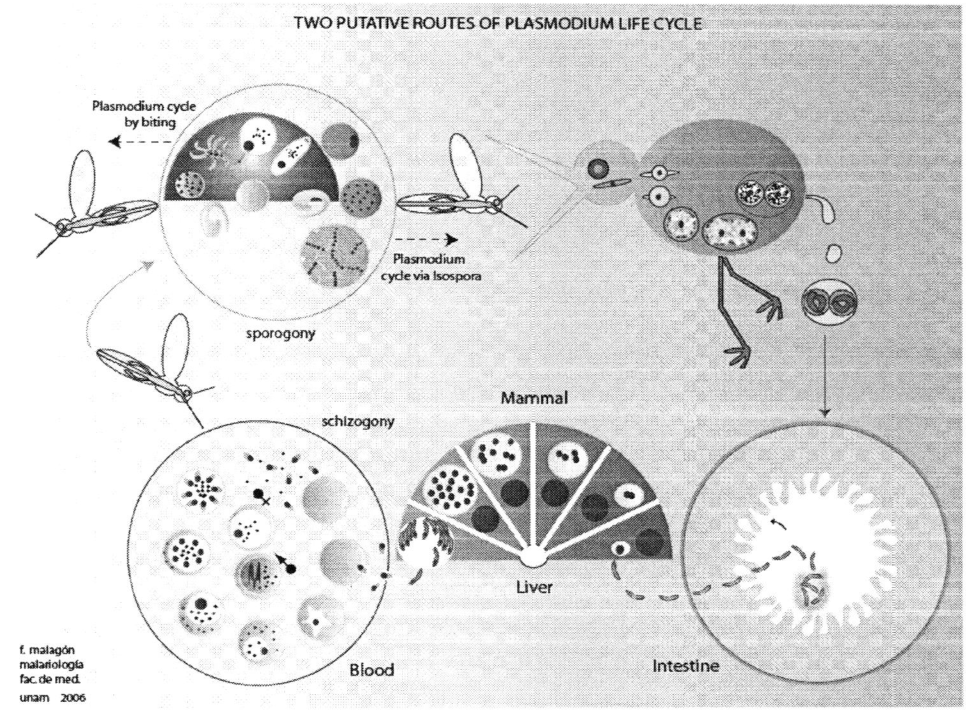

Figure 2. Theoretical view of malaria parasites life cycle.

Experimental Insights

Axenic Forms of Plasmodium to Coccidia

Working on cultivation of blood forms of *Plasmodium berghei* parasites in axenic media, eventually, a new type of cell appeared, which did not reproduce by schizogony, properly speaking, but in a fashion like a multiple budding, just the smallest forms would be recognized as a sort of merozoites, they grew constantly and were maintained by sub-cultivation. These forms were mostly non infecting to the mouse and did not produce an immune state against the blood forms of the same parasites, by the contrary, animals inoculated with the axenic forms were more susceptible to the infection and developed fatal infection in a shorter time. Electron microscopy was performed on axenic forms to see if some apicomplexan organelles could be detected. No organelles proper to apicomplexan parasites were observed, however, one of those forms showed some elongated elements inside, which were very difficult to associate with malaria parasites growing in the blood. Several days of analysis were necessary to find out that for the disposition and form of those intracellular elements, that image could well represent a small coccidian sporocyst containing four sporozoites-like bodies inside (see figure 3).

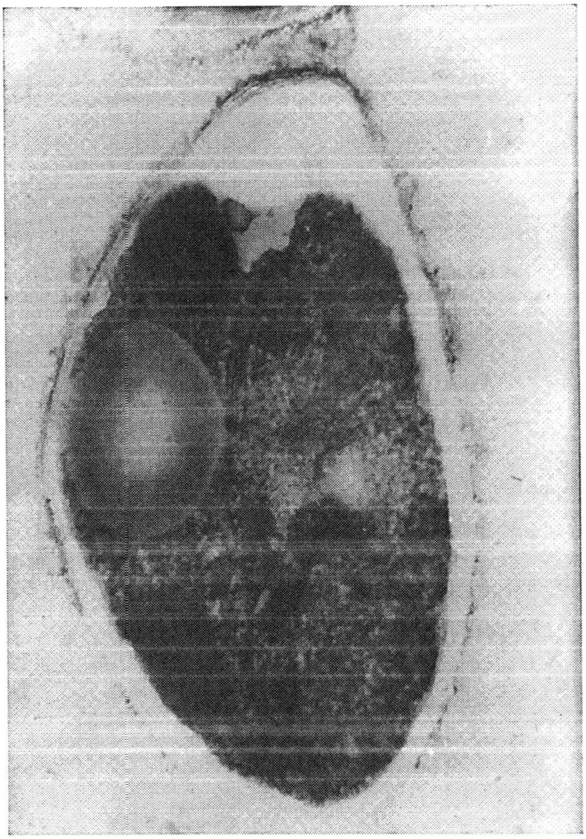

Figure 3. Sporocyst-like body found in axenic culture of *Plasmodium vivax*. Electron microscopy X5000.

It was thought that if the cultures were really producing coccidial forms, it would be possible to produce an intestinal infection with them. According with this line of thought, cats were selected to attempt an infection with axenic forms. Small cats obtained just few days after weaning were isolated and submitted to a regimen of water, milk and meat previously sterilized, and to Sheather coproparasitoscopic studies for three weeks to discard coccidial infection (in no one of the kittens coccidian infection was detected). Experimental cats received doses of axenic forms grown for a week, and suspended in their own culture, while control cats received sterile culture media, both by the oral route. Daily Sheather coproparasitoscopic examination was performed on all cats for one month or until detection of coccidial infection. No one of the control cats shed oocysts, while all experimental cats shed oocyst. Most cats shed very few oocysts but one shed abundant oocysts. This last animal was sacrificed and mucosal smears from the small intestine were done and stained with Giemsa. All shed oocysts were *Isospora* sp of at least two forms one elongated and one oval in form, with immature sporocysts from 10 to 14 µm in maximum length. The mucosa smears exhibited several coccidial forms, intracellular and extracellular trofozoites, intracellular schizonts, gametocytes, and very young oocysts (Malagon and Tapia, 1985 A).

These experiments, however, allowed some conclusions to be advanced: first, that malaria parasites submitted to cultivation and growth in axenic media, produce adapted cells that can (at least some of them) differentiate into coccidian forms, second, that those axenic forms cannot be defined as *Plasmodium* parasites, nor either Coccidia, but they seem to be something like intermedial forms that eventually can develop as *Plasmodium* blood forms and others as intestinal Coccidia. Finally, it was assumed that what can happen in a culture medium, can happen in nature when conditions are present.

Mosquito Bird Experience

During a monographic course on malaria, when analyzing malaria transmission and development of oocysts and sporozoites, a discussion with the students was done about an old statement of Missiroli (1934), that sporozoites are not sporozoites, but they are sporocysts. At the end of the discussion, an experiment was proposed to discard the Missirolis' ideas, assuming that if sporozoites were sporocysts, they would probably develop into a true oocyst and develop an infection in the intestine of insectivorous animals that eat mosquitoes infected by sporozoites. Thirty four mosquitoes *Anopheles albimanus* infected by feeding them on a *Plasmodium vivax* infected patient were the remnants of the course. These mosquitoes had been kept under refrigeration for about three weeks. Looking for an experimental model adjusted to what could happened in nature, any insectivorous animal would be proper, like bats, frogs, lizards or birds among others, from this animals the birds were chosen, because chickens could be easily obtained, and in principle, if well manage, chickens are sterile when hatching from the egg. Just hatched Rhode Island Red chickens were used in the experiment. They were isolated and only sterile water with minerals was provided for the first 24hours. For feeding it was reproduce what would be the normal feeding of home poultry in Mexican towns, broken maize, which was sterilized, and water with added salts also sterilized to feed chickens. Although the chickens are borne sterile, and no predictable chance existed in the laboratory environ to get infected by a coccidian, daily coproparasitocopic (Sheater, 1923) examinations were done for 10 days to monitor any eventual infection of the chickens, before they were fed with the mosquitoes. As the amount of infected mosquitoes was small it was decided to feed only two chickens thus, experimental chickens would be offered with 14 infected mosquitoes each. Two other control chickens were fed with also 14 refrigerated non-infected *Anopheles albimanus* mosquitoes each. Six of the 34 infected mosquitoes were dissected to look after sporozoites or their remnants. It was assumed that if sporozoites had any connection with coccidian stages of development, they would be forms resistant to adverse conditions of the environment, so they would be alive in spite of refrigeration. In three of them something like modified sporozoites were observed.

The day previous to infection all chickens were fasted. Next day, mosquito's bodies were mixed with a small amount of broken maize and offered to each chicken, it was repeated one by one until each ate all its mosquitoes. Daily direct and Sheater coproparasitoscopic examinations were performed to all chickens.

By the fifth day after mosquito feeding, the experimental chickens shed coccidial oocysts, while control chickens remain negative up to three weeks later, when fecal examination was discontinued. No more oocysts were shed after the fifth day. Feces from the fifth and sixth day were preserved in 0.5% potassium dichromate in water according to Ryley (1973). Two days later the feces were washed and concentrated, few oocyst were recovered and many were damaged, oocysts empty or broken, or complete but with no sporocysts just with some granular material inside.

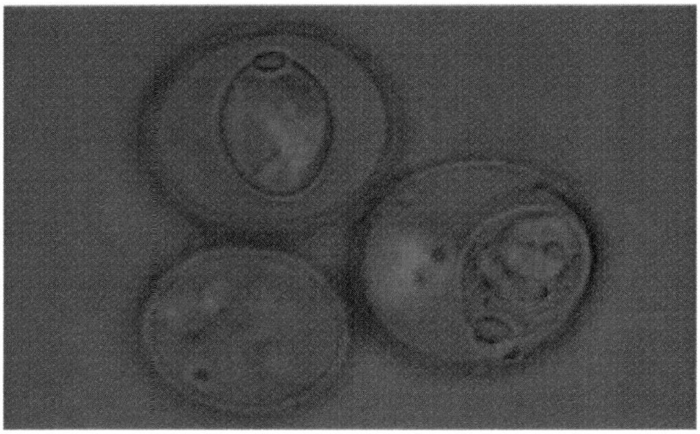

Figure 4. Isosporan oocysts shed by chickens fed with *P. vivax* infected mosquitoes. Light microscopy, X100.

Oocysts freshly observed, the same day they were shed, were spherical, some of them with a discrete micropile, containing two oval or elongated sporocysts whit a prominent Stieda body, some showing four sporozoites completed formed by sporocyst (see figure 4). Most oocysts measured from 26 to 28 μm in diameter, some others were smaller from 16 to 20μm degenerated in appearance, with no sporocysts nor sporozoites but just granular particles of different sizes. Chickens fed with *Anopheles albimanus* mosquitoes infected with *P. vivax* shed coccidia of the genus *Isospora*. In no moment the chickens became ill. Finally the chickens were sacrificed and samples of blood and intestinal mucosa (small and large intestine) were prepared and stained with Giemsa. *Plasmodium* parasites were not observed in blood nor either coccidian forms in intestine (Malagon et al. 1988).

Isosporan oocysts shed by the chickens do not seemed to be the result of an intestinal infection. Chickens do not looked ill at any moment; they grew quite well, with no diarrhea. No stages of coccidial development were detected in the intestine mucosa. The amount of shedded oocyst was small. Everything pointed to just an intestinal transport of oocysts ingested from an outsource. However, under the conditions of the experiment, a coccidial oocyts outsource (different to the mosquitoes ingested) seem impossible: chicken cages were knew and thoroughly washed and dried before use; food and water dispensers were sterilized, maize in bags and water in bottles were sterilized and kept closed until use; food and water was changed every day; no insects or ticks or arthropods of any kind were in the room, nor either on the chickens. Literature on the subject point out this facts: home poultry infections by coccidian parasites are usually produced by genus *Eimeria*, and in few instances by *Isospora* (McDougald, 1998), however, when *Isospora* infection is present, it does not produce disease, and it is so uncommon that Lindsay and Blagburn, (1994) suggested that a diagnoses of isosporan oocyst in poultry, probably correspond to pseudo infections produced by water or food contaminated with wild bird feces, no wild birds or home birds of any kind were around in the lab. Moreover, the control chickens eating uninfected mosquitoes did not shed oocysts. Transovarian transmission is another consideration to be done, in which the chicken would be born already infected by its mother by transovarian transmission. In this case, however, parasites growing in the intestinal epithelium could cause perhaps some grade of illness, and isolation of parasites from that epithelium could be expected. Although study in chickens by Jacobs and Melton (1966) reported to have found one egg infected by the tissue coccidia *T. gondii* out of 327 coming from chickens with chronic toxoplasmosis, however, since then, not many studies on the matter have been reported, probably because it is very uncommon and results are negative (Biancifiori et al. 1986, de Camargo et al., 1995). The transovarian infection of pathogens in chickens is mostly due to species of Salmonella (Indar et al. 1998). Apparently no transovarian infection by chicken *Isospora* is documented in the literature, perhaps because Isospora does not infect them. The other and last possibility of a source of coccidians for the chickens, apart from malaria parasites, are the mosquitoes themselves, i.e. that mosquitoes the chicken ate were infected by an *Isospora*. However, mosquitoes were reared in an insectary and do not came from the wild, also, and most important, no one has ever seen a coccidial oocyst developed into a mosquito. In conclusion, the chickens fed with *A. albimanus* infected by *P. vivax* shed diplosporocystic tetrazoic isosporan oocyts. By the arguments exposed, the *Isospora* shed by the chickens most probably came from the mosquitoes they ate, and those mosquitoes were infected by *Plasmodium vivax*, a Haemoporidia evolved from coccidia, probably an *Isospora*. If the shed *Isospora* does not emerged from *P. vivax*, there is not a reasonable argument to demonstrate where the *Isospora* came from.

When Plasmodium parasites develop in the vertebrate, schizogony and gametogony is present in their blood. Male and female gametes develop while infecting erythrocytes, but they do not continue maturation, until drawn by the Anopheles mosquito. Once in the stomach of the mosquito, asexual forms of the parasite are lysed and digested, and sexual forms mature through different stages to reach the sporozoite infective form (see figure 5). In the invertebrate host, all stages previous to sporozoites are transient, and at last only sporozoites remain, and are present during all the mosquito's life. Perhaps the only *Plasmodium* parasite stage, from which the *Isospora* could emerge, was the sporozoite. Was Missiroli right, After all?.

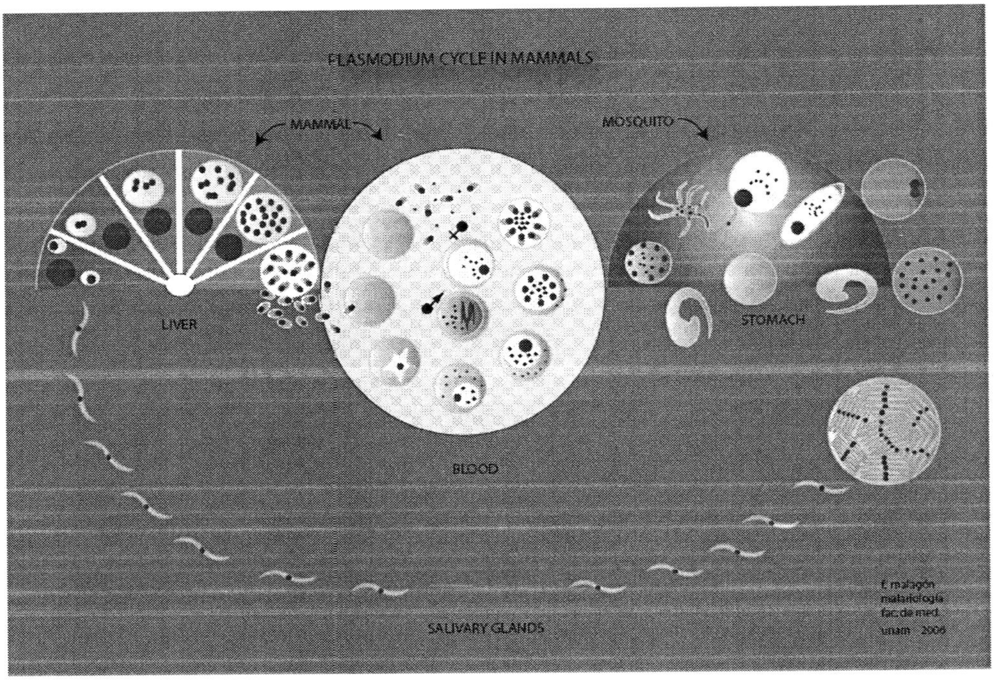

Figure 5. Mammalian malaria parasites life cycle.

The Oral Transmission

According to those previous experiences there were strong possibilities that malaria were being transmitted by the oral route (Malagon, 1992). During an indicative small experiment in which a potential antimalaric was put to test, 4 mice were infected with *P. yoelii,* two received the antimalaric, and the other two non, a single animal was added which received just the antimalaric but no parasites. All the five animals were left in the same cage. The results were contrary to the expected, animals treated died in a shorter time than the not treated, at last all died except the one that received only the "antimalaric". A blood smear was done to the surviving mouse before it was discarded. Surprisingly, the mouse had plasmodium parasites in its blood. Retrospective analysis was done to detect mistakes in the experiment, nothing was found to explain why an animal non-inoculated with parasites resulted infected just for being in contact with infected mice, with no mosquitoes around. It was realized that the only way this animal could acquired the infection was by mouth, this idea gain credibility because it had been observed that when a mouse tail is bled for sampling parasitemia, and the mouse returned to its cage, some of the other mice in the cage lick the remnants of the tails blood. To see if this assumption was correct a series of experiments were done on a total of 116 mice at 72 H post-weaning. Experimental mice were inoculated by mouth with 0.2ml of citrated mouse blood infected with *Plasmodium berghei yoelii*, while control mice were inoculated with non-infected blood, by the same route and doses. Results confirmed what previously was suspected, malaria was transmitted by the oral route, and about 30% of experimental mice acquired the infection against no infection in the control mice. When writing the experience it was surprising to find out that such observation was already done in birds and monkeys (Malagón et al. 1993).

Infections obtained after feeding mice with citrated infected blood collected by cardiac puncture gave the feeling of doing a very artificial experiment that in no way occur in nature. Thus to experiment with a model which resemble more the natural transmission, new experiments were conducted to transmit the malaria parasites through cannibalism. In these assays, mice were infected with *P. berghei yoelii*, and four days later sacrificed and the fresh corps offered to each of the one day starved experimental mice. Control mice were offered with fresh corps of non-infected mice. From all experimental mice, 35% were infected and none of the control mice. Infection through oral route by cannibalism was somewhat more efficient than by drinking blood. Some of the more evident conclusions were: transmission can take place among individuals of the same species by cannibalism. Although, Plasmodium parasites are selective on the species of hosts it infects, when transmission is by mosquito or blood transfer, it is not know if that restriction of host species is also present when parasites enter by the digestive tract. By extension, this mode of transmission probably is not confined to a laboratory but it may be occurring in nature, with other species of Plasmodium and other hosts (Malagon etal.1994), and that transmission of malaria parasites not necessarily require the mosquito to get dispersed.

Considering that parasites of the genus *Babesia* have many biologic similitude with *Plasmodium* parasites (Malagon and Tapia, 1985 B), transmission of babesial infections through the oral route by blood feeding and by cannibalism had to be tested. Hundred and thirty five mice were inoculated by mouth with doses of 20, 50 and 100 μL of *Babesia microti* infected blood, infection occurred in 5, while through cannibalism, 12 mouse out of 79 resulted infected. Again Cannibalism was the best way to infect animals by oral route. Based on the non specific host selection of *Babesia*, (Denning, 1962, 1973) it was then concluded that transmission by the oral route make possible the human infection by carnivorism and, introduces *Babesia* parasites into a flux of dispersion through the food chains in nature (Malagon and Tapia, 1994).

The Evolutionary Records of Malaria Parasites

To calculate the time, at which evolutionary changes on coccidia occurred to give rise to *Plasmodium*, is for its own nature speculative. First, because it was usually thought that malaria parasites did not leave fossil records, which give the most reliable estimates for dating past life, and second, because the use of modern molecular based-evolutionary time scale is at the moment in conflict with the time estimates from fossil records, for calculating very substantially longer times of divergence than the obtained by the paleontologists, when dating life evolution. Benton (1999) is of the opinion that calculated molecular dates are wrong because the molecular clock does not tick regularly through geological times, apart of different methodological handicaps of molecular time estimates in the opinion of others (Rodriguez-Trelles et al 2002; Labandeira, 2005; Elhaik et al. 2006). However, the fossil record studies in the panorama of malaria seem to have a new perspective. The most recent findings (Poinar, 2005) showed that malaria parasites can be detected in mosquitoes in a state of enough conservation as to be able to approximate a diagnoses of species, as occurred with *Plasmodium dominicana* n. sp. (Plasmodidae: Haemospororida), an extinct *Plasmodium* infecting *Culex* mosquitoes living in the mid-Tertiary (25 to 30 Mya), relative of *P. juxtanucleare* of birds. This mosquito found in Republica Dominicana opens the old discussion on the origin of new world *Plasmodium* of primates, very interesting but out of the scope of the present work. Five years ago, also for the first time, it was possible to detect, with the help of molecular tools the presence of *Plasmodium falciparum* DNA in the fossil of babies found in the nearby of Rome (Lugano, Umbria), buried in the V century (Abbot, 2001), which open the possibility of looking for DNA traces of *Plasmodium* in many vertebrate animal fossils and haematophagous dipterans in the future.

The Theory

With the frame given above it seem to be reasonable to assume that malaria parasites started speciation from a coccidian parasite (perhaps an *Isospora*) living in the intestine of a reptile.

Isospora parasite was first described by Labbè in 1893 in the feces of a passerine bird and was called *Diplospora lacaseii*. This coccidium has been subjected to much discussion and controversy, because by its endogenous growth it was compared to haemogregarines, and by its morphology to *Toxoplasma*. Moved by this confusion, professor Garnham (1950) created a new genus: *Atoxoplasma*, for haemosporidian parasites growing asexually in blood monocytes. Later, it was discover that *Atoxoplasma* was in fact an *Isospora*, which, unlike other Coccidia, the first part of its life cycle takes place in mononuclear phagocytes, producing five asexual generations in them and then two additional asexual generations and the sexual stages taking place in the intestinal epithelium, as described by Box (1977) in *Isospora serini* infecting canaries, and others (Upton et al. 2001). Several genera of Coccidia, which develop isosporic oocysts in their life cycle, show the ability to invade and growth in extra-intestinal tissues like *Toxoplasma, Sarcocystis, Besnoitia* and *Isospora* among others.

The extant isosporic coccidia are distributed among fishes (Belova and Krylov, 2000), amphibians (Modry et al. 2001A), reptiles (Bovee, 1962), birds (Dolnik, 2006) and mammals (de Otazu et al, 2004).

Genus *Isospora* is widely spread in today reptile hosts from vast geographical territories on the earth. They are found infecting Skinks, from Egypt (El-Toukhv et al. 1996), and New Caledonian (Modry and Jirku, 2006) lizards from Dominican Republic (Cisper et al., 1995), Israel and Australia (Paperna and Finkelman, 1998), Brasil (Lainson, 2003) Saudi Arabia (al Yousif and al-Shawa, 1998) and Malaysia (Maupin et al. 1998); geckoes, from Mauritius (Leinwand et al., 2005) and New Caledonian (Modry et al., 2004); chameleons from Madagascar (Modry, et al., 2001B); snakes, from Ecuador (Asmundsson et al., 2001); turtles from North America (McAllister et al., 1994); and caimans from Paraguay (Aquino-Shuster and Duszynski, 1989), just to give an example, among other reptile groups and territories. This wide distribution of isosporan infections in reptiles may well represent the richness of *Isospora* in reptile hosts at the time when eventually *Plasmodium* species evolved from an *Isospora* living in their intestine.

Therefore, considering that extra-intestinal invasion behavior and a similar distribution of *Isospora* was present in ancient times, this coccidium could be present in reptiles and even in their ancestors, so that, reptiles could inherit the isosporids and/or the susceptibility to be infected by them. In opinion of the author, the best coccidian candidate to be the Plasmodium ancestor, and eventually the versatile coccidian-*Plasmodium* parasite described below is the *Isospora*.

The *Isospora* living in the reptile gut that evolved into Plasmodium behaved as an extraintestinal tissue coccidia, to grow in the liver and blood of their hosts, and in the lack of an haemathophagous insect, for that *Plasmodium* to survive, it had to keep its coccidia cycle running, apart of the possibility of spreading through cannibalism and predation, and later to be followed by the first haematophagous insect *Plasmodium* transmitter, the Phlebothomine.

The Chicken Experiment

Interpretation of the chickens' experiment above described can be, that stages of the malaria parasites contained in the mosquito were stimulated by the chickens' digestive canal to differentiate into coccidian.

For the analysis already done, the sporozoite, or a modification of it, would be the candidate stage to differentiate into Coccidia. Birds, or at least chickens, probably acts as a host that only enable the parasite to grow and differentiate into coccidial oocysts without properly infecting them, in some way just allowing them to reach maturity from an stage that can direct its growth and differentiation into probably different directions, depending on the composition of the environ they enter. Therefore if the environ is conformed by the secretions of the gastrointestinal duct of a chicken, the sporozoite directs its differentiation to develop into an isosporan oocyst. Chickens pass the oocyst in feces to the environ where they can be collected by a new host. The *Isospora* parasite release the sporozoites when entering a new suitable host and several ways of development could probably be expected, depending on the species of host invaded: 1. Parasites cross the epithelial cells of the intestine without staging in them, enter blood vessels and infect liver first and erythrocytes later; 2. Invade intestinal epithelial cells and reproduce asexually, and then the new brood invade the liver, and then the erythrocyte, 3. Invade intestinal epithelial cells and accomplish a typical coccidial growth, only, 4. Invade intestinal epithelial cells and accomplish a typical coccidial growth, apart of extraintestinal tissue invasion, so Plasmodium and coccidial development coexist.

In this example, taken from the experiment above described, the process of differentiation from *Plasmodium* to Coccidia, has taken place in the gut of the chicken, however, this conversion probably would take place in other insectivorous animal, like bats, birds, frogs and reptiles like lizards and geckoes, among others. Whether the *Plasmodium* sporozoites present in the mosquitoes infect the epithelial cells of those animals` intestine, or just differentiate into a coccidian with no infection, the result in any case, would be the elimination in feces of coccidial oocysts to the environ, from which the new host introduce them by mouth. Oocysts in intestine would behave like the original coccidia mother crossing the intestinal barrier and invading liver and blood, to be taken again for a mosquito, which in turn it can transmit the infection to a vertebrate host in the way now recognized or, can be eaten by an insectivorous animal in whose intestine the coccidial form develops following the routes illustrated in figure 2.

The theory proposes the existence of a parasite, just one parasite, with a large versatility for survival, that could thrive on intestine and/or extra-intestinal tissues (liver and blood) of their vertebrate hosts with development of schizogony in intestine, liver, blood cells and epithelial blood vessels, depending on their hosts species, and sporogony in *Anopheles* or *Culex* mosquitoes and phlebothomines, depending on the *Plasmodium* species involved and, whose transmission could be done by infected mosquitoes or phlebothomines bites and, coccidial oocysts present in the soil, and entering by oral route. In fact a parasites, just one and the same parasite, that fuses the properties and characteristics of Plasmodium and coccidum parasites in one.

Apart from this, transmission in nature of *Plasmodium* parasites by the oral route can also be done by eating the flesh of infected animals by other animals susceptible to be infected by that Plasmodium species, by cannibalism or depredation.

Epidemiological Facts

There are in malaria many instances in which acquisition of the parasites by the human host is inexplicable. This phenomenon is more visible in countries in which malaria has been eradicated. Most of the malaria incidence in these countries comes from their citizens going abroad for business or holydays, to malaria endemic areas. However, certain number of cases occurs in individuals with no history of international travels, blood transfusion, organ transplantation or parenteral injections. Two, now famous, cases of *Plasmodium falciparum* malaria in England occurred in 1983 (Withfield et al. 1984), which after epidemiological study they were found to be acquired locally, at 31 years of the last indigenous case of malaria reported, but through an inexplicable way of transmission. Cases were living at 10 and 15 km of Gatwick airport. Case one was the owner of a pub frequented by airport crew, case two happen to travel near the pub when probably she got infected. Epidemiologists thought that infection was due to the bite of an infected Anopheles mosquito coming from the tropics by aircraft, and drive by a vehicle from the airport to the site of transmission. It was a case of "airport malaria", like many others registered in European countries, in which also imported African *Anopheles* vectors are thought to be involved in transmission of local malaria at the neighborhood of the airports, (Lusina, et al. 2000; Baixench, 1998), however, Currently, there is no proof that tropical *Anopheles* are imported into Europe (Mouchet, 2000). There are also reports of autochthonous malaria in areas far away from airports in which *Anopheles* mosquitoes are also incriminated, although, the probable source of infection for mosquitoes is not confirmed. In some of these cases tropical mosquitoes traveling in the luggage has been incriminated (Dawson, 1996).

Another case occurred in 2003, in a girl 14 years old from Maryland, who acquired *P. falciparum* infection just by sharing the room in a hospital, for less than 24 hours, with a 9 years old boy being treated for *P. falciparum* infection acquired in Gambia, in this case, an interpretation on how transmission was occurred, was not attempted (Eliades, 2005).

Another story of malaria without mosquitoes. An invitation arrived to participate in a clinical session for the presentation of a malaria case attended in a hospital, in Mexico City. Israel as this baby was named, was borne in that hospital; his mother was a woman in her twenties. Mother and baby left the hospital 2 days after delivery, in good health conditions. One week later Israel returned at the hospital once again with fever and diarrhea, after clinical study the diagnoses was, bacterial enteritis, and was sent home with antibiotic treatment. He was better for a couple of days and then the fever return, and the baby was admitted again in the hospital, this second clinical study arrived to the diagnoses of appendicitis. The surgeon, however, was not sure of this diagnoses and return the baby for laboratory studies. Casually, malaria parasites were observed when blood biometry was performed. Infection by *Plasmodium vivax* with severe parasitemia and important anemia was the diagnoses. The treatment consisted in administration of chloroquine, and blood transfusion.

The main question was how Israel acquired the malaria infection?

Israel's home was located in a poor area of the southeast Mexico City. Last cases of autochthonous malaria in Mexico city were reported in the 1940s`, nowadays Mexico city is not considered an area of malaria transmission, his mother has no antecedents of malaria in her life, nor she had moved or visited the malaric areas in the last 5 years, she has never received blood transfusion, nor either organ transplantation. Israel has not received blood transfusion before diagnoses was done. Entomological work was done in Israel's home and neighborhood houses; however, no mosquitoes of any kind were collected. Ocular inspection did not detected mosquito breeding places around, in fact, no tap water was available at his home, it has to be collected and transported from several blocks apart. Her mother used to bring Israel with her to collect the water, where a merchant man lived who used to travel to malaria endemic areas to get his merchandises, only a brief contact of Israel with this man his mother recorded. However, the general hygiene of Israel home surroundings was very poor, his family was formed by a small sister, his two grand parents, and his mother, all of them living in two rooms 3X4 m very unclean, two pigs at three meters of his door were being reared by his mother. His grand mother and his small four years old sister attended Israel while his mother was at work. As no mosquitoes were found, there was no way to know how Israel acquired malaria, however, it was clear that transmission through mosquito bite was not possible, nor either by trans-placental transmission. At last, there is no way to know how malaria transmission took place.

In Brasil and countries of the Amazon region *Anopheles* mosquitoes may be found infected in nature in rates of more than 8% (da Silva-Vasconcelos, et al. 2002). However, in hypo and meso-endemic malarious areas of Mexico, and other countries of Central and South America is common to observe outbreaks of malaria in which no infected mosquitoes are detected, (although they are not published). In some instances perhaps the amount of mosquitoes infected is so low that when malaria control teams arrive is too late to find the mosquitoes involved in transmission, exactly as described by the Australians in the outbreak of North Queensland (Hanna et al., 2004), although, it happen to occur not in a surprising and unexpected outbreak but in endemic areas where outbreaks are expected events.

It is time to think in other ways of malaria transmission to understand what is going on with malaria, instead of forcing interpretations for every inexplicable malaria transmission event to fit it into the mosquito transmission concept.

References

Abbot, A. (2001). Earliest malaria DNA found in Roman baby graveyard. *Nature*. 412:847.

Al Yousif, M. S. and al-shawa, Y. R. (1998). A new coccidian parasite (Apicomplexa: Eimeriidae) from the legless lizard *Diplometopon zarudnyi* (Amphisbaenia: Trogonophidae) in Saudi Arabia. *J. Egypt Soc. Parasitol.* 28:257-261.

Aquino-Shuster, A.L. and Duszynski, D. W. (1989). Coccidian parasites (Apicomplexa: Eimeriidae) from two species of caimans, *Caiman yacare* daudin and *Caiman latirostris* daudin (Alligatoridae), from Paraguay. *J. Parasitol.* 75:348-352.

Asmunsson, I. M., Upton, S. J. and Freed, P. S. (2001). Five new species of Coccidia (Apicomplexa: Eimeriidae) from colubrid snakes of Ecuador. *J. Parasitol.* 87:1077-1081.

Baixench MT, Suzzoni-Blatger J, Magnaval JF, Lareng MB, Larrouy G. 1998. Two cases of inexplicable autochthonous malaria in Toulouse, France. *Med. Trop.* (Mars) 58:62-4.

Belding, D. L. (1965). Textbook of Parasitology. Third edition, pp. 246-248. New York, Appleton-Century-Crofts.

Belova, L. M. and Krylov, M. V. (2000). Distribution of coccidians (Sporozoa: Coccidiida) in various systematic groups of Fishes. *Parazitologiia.* 34:522-533.

Beltrán, E. and Larenas, R. (1941). Producción de malaria aviar con *Plasmodium gallinaeum* por via oral. *Rev. Inst. Salubr. Enferm. Trop. México.* 2:87-94.

Benton, M. J. (1999). Early origins of modern birds and mammals: molecules vs. Morphology. *BioEssays.* 21:1043–1051.

Biancifiori, F., Rondini, C., Grelloni, V., Frescura, T. (1986). Avian toxoplasmosis: experimental infection of chicken and pigeon. *Comp. Immunol. Microbiol. Infect. Dis.* 9:337-246.

Bovee, E. C. (1962). *Isospora crotali* in the Florida diamond-back rattlesnake. *J. Protozool.* 9:459-466.

Box, E.D. (1977). Life cycles of two *Isopora* species in the canary, *Serinus canaries* Linnaeus. *J. Protozool.* 24(1):57-67.

Bruce-Chwatt, L. J. (1980). Essential Malariology. London, William Heinemann Medical Books Ltd.

Capanna, E. (2006). Grassi versus Ross: Who solved the riddle of malaria? *Internatl. Microbiol.* 9:69-74.

Cavalier-Smith, T. (2002). The phagotropic origin of eukariotes and phylogenetic classification of Protozoa. *Intl. J. Syst. Evol. Microbiol.* 52:297-354.

Cisper. G. L., Huntington, C., Smith, D. D., Powell, R., Parmerlee, J. S. Jr. and Lathrop, A. (1995). Four new coccidian (Apicomplexa: Eimeriidae) from anoles (Lacertilia:Polychrotidae) in the Dominican Republic. *J. Parasitol.* 81: 252-255.

Coatney, G.R., Collins, W.E., Warren, M. and Contacos, P.G. (1977). The Primates malaria. Whashington D.C. U.S. Government Printing Office.

da Silva-Vasconcelos, A., YukioNeves, K. M., Neves, M. E., Lessa de Souza, R. T., da Luz Lacerda, R. N., Sibajev, A., Tsouris, P., Povoa, M. M., Momen, H., Rosa-Freitas M. G.. (2002). Biting indices, host-seeking activity and natural infection rates of Anopheleine species in Boa Vista, Roraima, Brasil from 1996 to 1998. *Mem. Inst.* Oswaldo Cruz, Rio de Janeiro. 97:151-161.

de Camargo, M.C., Antunes, C. M., Chiari, C. de A. (1995). Epidemiology of *Toxoplasma gondii* infection in the municipality of Ribeirao das Neves, MG. I. Importance of domestic animals as sources of *T. gondii* infection in humans. *Rev. Soc. Bras. Med. Trop.* 28:211-214.

Dawson, M., Johnson,P.T., Feldman, F., Glover, R., Koehler, J., Blake, P. and Toomey, K.E. (1997). Probable Locally Acquired Mosquito-Transmitted *Plasmodium vivax* Infection -- Georgia, 1996. *CDC MMWR* Weekly. 46:264-267

Denning, H. K. (1962). Experimentelle Ubertragung von *Babesia bovis, B. bigemina, B. equi, B, Caballi,* und *B. trautmani* auf saugende Mause. Z. Tropenmed. Parasitol. 13:472-479.

Denning, H. K. (1973). *Babesia galagolata* n. sp., eine babesienart des Galagos (*Galago crassicaudatus*). Z. Parasitenkd. 41:282-290.

De Otazu, R.D., Garcia-Nieto, L., Izaguirre-Gondra, E., Mayayo, E., Ciani, S. and Nogales, F.F. (2004). Endometrial coccidiosis. *J. Clin. Pathol.* 57:1104-1105.

Dolnik, O. (2006). The relative stability of chronic *Isospora sylvianthina* (Protozoa: Apicomplexa) infection in blackcaps (*Sylvia atricapilla*) : evaluation of a simplified method of estimating isosporan infection intensity in passerine birds. *Parasitol. Res.* Accepted on 28th July.

Elhaik, E., Sabath, N., and Graur, D. (2006). The ''Inverse Relationship Between Evolutionary Rate and Age of Mammalian Genes'' is an artifact of increased genetic distance with rate of evolution and time of divergence. *Mol. Biol. Evol.* 23(1):1–3

Eliades, M.J., Shah, S., Nguyen-Dinh, P., Newman, R.D., Barber, A.M., Roberts, J.M., Mali, S., Monica E. Parise, M.E., Richard Steketee, R. (2005). Malaria Surveillance --- United States, 2003. CDC MMWR Surveillance Summaries. 54:25-39.

El-Toukhv, A. A., Abdel Aziz, A. and Abdel Gawad, M. A. (1996). Light and electron microscopy studies of *Isospora chalchidis* (Amoudi, 1989) infecting *Chalcides ocellatus* in Egypt. *J. Egypt Soc. Parasitol.* 26:79-91.

Fast, N.M., Kissinger, J.C., Roos, D.S., Keeling, P.J. (2001). Nuclear-encoded, plastid-targeted genes suggest a single common origin for Apicomplexan and Dinoflagellate plastids. *Mol. Bio. Evol.* 18:418-426

Filho, J.D. and Brasil, R.P. (2003). Relationships of new world phlebotomine sand flies (Diptera: Psychodidae) based on fossil evidence. *Mem. Inst. Oswaldo Cruz. 98* suppl 1:145-149.

Foster, W.D. (1965). A history of parasitology. Chapter XI. *The parasitic protozoa.* Edimburgh and London. E. and S. Livingstone Ltd.

Garnham, P.C.C. (1950). Blood parasites of eastern vertebrates with a brief description of exoerythrocytic schizogony in *Plasmodium pitmani. Parasitol.* 40:328-337.

Garnham, P.C.C. (1966). Malaria parasites and other Haemosporidia. Oxford. Blackwell Scientific Publications.

Gutteridge, W. E., Trigg, P. I. and Williamson. D. H. (1971). Properties of DNA from some malarial parasites. Parasitol. 62:209–219.

Indar, L., Baccus-Taylor, G., Commissiong, E., Prabhakar, P. and Reid, H. (1998). Salmonellosis in Trinidad: evidence for transovarian transmission of *Salmonella* in farm eggs. *West Indian Med. J.* 47:50-53.

Hanna, J.N., Scott A Ritchie, S.A., Eisen, D. P., Cooper, R.D., Brookes D.L. and Montgomery, B.L. (2004). An outbreak of *Plasmodium vivax* malaria in Far North Queensland. M.J.A.180: 24-28.

Jacobs, L. and Melton, M. L. (1966). Toxoplasmosis in chickens. J. Parasitol. 52:1158-1162.

Kilejian, A. (1975). Circular mithocondrial DNA from the avian malarial parasite *Plasmodium lophurae*. *Bioch. Bioph. Acta.* 390:276-284.

Klein, T.A., Young, D.G., Telford S.R. Jr. and Kimsey, R. (1987). Experimental transmission of *Plasmodium mexicanum* by bites of infected Lutzomyia vexator (Diptera:Psychodidae). *J. Am. Mosq. Control Assoc.* 3:154-164.

Kohler, S., Delwiche, Ch.F., Denny, P.W., Tilney, L.G., Webster, P., Wilson, R.J.M., Palmer, J.D., Ross, D.S. (1997). A plastid of probable green algal origin in apicomplexan parasites. *Science.* 275:1485-1489.

Labandeira, C. C. (2005). Invasion of the continents: Cyanobacterial crusts to tree-inhabiting arthropods. *Trends in Ecology and Evolution.* 20:253-262.

Lainson, R. (2003). Some coccidial parasites of the lizard *Amphisbaena alba* (Reptilia:Amphisbaenia: Amphisbaenidae). *Mem. Inst.* Oswaldo Cruz, Rio de Janeiro, 98:927-936.

Lambrechts, L., Fellous, S. and Koella, J.C. (2006). Coevolutionary interactions between host and parasite genotypes. *Trends in Parasitology.* 22:12-16.

Leinwand, I., Kilpatrick , A. M., Cole, N., Jones, C. G. and Daszak, P. (2005). Patterns of Coccidial prevalence in lizards of Mauritius. *J. Parasitol.* 91:1103-1108.

Levine, N.D. (1973). Introduction , History and Taxonomy. Chapter I, in: Hamond and Long, editors, The coccidian. Pp.4, Baltimore ,University Park Press.

Lindsay, D.S. and Blagburn, B. L (1994). Biology of mammalian *Isospora. Parasitol. Today.* 10:214-220.

Lusina, D., Legros, F., Esteve, V., Klerlein, M. and Giacomini, T. (2000). Airport malaria: four new cases in suburban Paris during summer 1999. *Eurosurveillance.* 5:76-80.

Mahner, M. and Bunge, M. (1997). Foundations of Biophilosophy. Berlin, Springer Verlag.

Malagon, F. and Tapia, J. L. (1985) A. La naturaleza coccidial de los plasmodia. In: Quiroz and Garcia (editors), Parasitologia. Volumen conmemorativo XXV aniversario de la Sociedad Mexicana de Parasitologia, A.C. pp 38-53. Mexico, D.F. Facultad de Medicina Veterinaria y Zootecnia, UNAM.

Malagon, F. and Tapia, J. L. (1985) B. Babaesiosis humana y malaria. Revista Mexicana de Patologia Clinica. 32:116-119.

Malagon, F., Del Toro, F., Tapia, J. L., Vazquez, J. (1988). Eliminacion de ooquistes de Isospora por pollos alimentados con mosquitos infectados por *Plasmodium vivax*. Rev. Mex. Parasitol. 1:32-33.

Malagon, F. (1992). On the current existence of a coccidial line of development in the malaria parasites: a theory. *Mem. Inst.* Oswaldo Cruz, Rio de Janeiro, 87 suppl. III:151-153.

Malagon, F., Castillo, L. and Tapia, J. L. (1993). Experimental transmission of murine malaria by the oral route. *Parasitol. Res.* 79:527-528.

Malagon, F., Castillo, L. and Tapia, J.L . (1994). Experimental transmission of murine malaria by cannibalism on mice infected by Plasmodium berghei yoelii. *Acta Protozoologica,* 33:191-193.

Maupin, R. S., Diong, C. H. and McQuistion, T. E. (1998). Two new coccidian parasites from the grand anglehead lizard, *Gonocephalus grandis* from Peninsular Malaysia. *J. Parasitol.* 84:1210-1212.

McAllister, C.T. Upton, S.J. and Trauth, S.E. (1994). New host and geographic records for coccidia (Apicomplexa: Eimeriidae) from North American turtles. *J. Parasitol.* 80:1045-9.

McDougald, L. R. (1998). Intestinal protozoa important to poultry. Poult. Sci. 77:1156-1158.

McFaden, G.I. (2000). Mergers and acquisitions: malaria and the great chloroplast heist. *Gen. Biol.* 1:1026.1-1026.4

Missiroli, A. (1934) Sullo sviluppo dei parassiti malarici. *Riv. Malar.* 13:539-552.

Modry, D., Slapeta, J. R., Jirku, M., Obornik, M., Lukes, J. and Koudela, B. (2001) A. Phylogenetic position of a renal coccidium of the European green frogs, *Isospora lieberkuehni* Labbe,1894 (Apicomplexa: Sarcocystidae) and its taxonomic implications. *Int. J. Syst. Evol. Microbiol.* 51:767-772.

Modry D, Daszak P, Volf J, Veseley M, Ball SJ and Koudela B. (2001) B. Five new species of coccidia (Apicomplexa: Eimeriidae) from Madagascan chameleons (Sauria: Chamaeleonidae). *Syst. Parasitol.* 48:117-123.

Modry, D., Jirku, M. and Vesely, M. (2004). Two new species of *Isospora* (Apicomplexa: Eimeriidae) from geckoes of the genus *Rhacodactylus* (Sauria: Gekkonidae) endemic to New Caledonia. *Folia Parasitol.* (Praha), 51:283-286.

Modry, D. and Jirku, M.(2006). Three new species of coccidian (Apicomplexa: Eimeriorina) from the Marble-throated skink, *Marmorosphax tricolor* Bavay, 1869 (Reptilia: Scincidae), endemic to New Caledonian with a taxonomic revision of Eimeria spp. From scincid hosts. *Parasitol. Res.* 99:419-428.

Mouchet, J. (2000). Airport malaria: a rare disease still poorly understood. *Eurosurveillance.* 5:75-76.

Müller, J. and Reisz, R.R. (2006). The Phylogeny of Early Eureptiles: Comparing Parsimony and Bayesian Approaches in the Investigation of a Basal Fossil Clade. *Syst. Biol.* 55: 503 – 511.

Paperna, I. and Finkelman, S. (1998). The fine structure of reptilian *Isospora* species with intranuclear endogenous development. *Parassitologia.* 40:283-296

Pérez-Tris. J., Hasselquist. D., Hellgren, O., Krizanauskiene, A., Waldenstrom, J. and Bensch. (2005). What are malaria parasites? *Trends in Parasitology.* 21:209-211.

Poinar, G. Jr. and Poinar, R. (2004). Evidence of vector-borne disease of Early Cretaceous reptiles. *Vector Borne Zoonotic Dis.* 4:281-484.

Poinar, Jr. G. (2005) *Plasmodium dominicana* n. sp. (Plasmodidae: Haemospororida) from Tertiay Dominican amber. *Syst. Parasitol.* 61:47-52.

Potgieter, F. T. and Els, H. J. (1977), Light and electron microscopic observation on the development of *Babesia bigemina* in larvae, nymphae and non-replete females of *Boophilus decoloratus*. *Onderstepoort J. Vet. Res.* 44:213-231.

Rai, K.S. and Black, W.C. (1999). Mosquito genomes: structure, organization, and evolution. *Adv. Genet.* 41:1-33.

Rodrıguez-Trelles, F., Tarrio, R. And Ayala, F. (2002) A methodological bias toward overestimation of molecular evolutionary time scales. *Proc. Natl. Acad. Sci. U. S. A.* 99: 8112–8115.

Ross, R. (1926). Studies on malaria. London ,John Murray.

Ryley, J. F. (1973). Oocysts isolation techniques. In: Hammond and Long (Ed) The Coccidia. (Pp. 425-427) Baltimore, University Park Press.

Sergent, E. (1937). Transmission de *Plasmodium relictum* selon de modes non habituels. *Arch. Inst. Pasteur Alger.* 15:11-17.

Sheater, A. L. (1923). The detection of intestinal protozoa and mange parasites by a floatation technique. *J. Comp. Path. Ther.* 36:266-275.

Shotisheck, E. and Chobotar B. (1977). Taxonomy, cytology and evolution of the sporozoa sensu lato. Hunter H. (Editor). Proceedings of the Fifth Interntional Congress of Protozoology. pp. 29-41.

Shortt, H.E. and Menon, K.P. (1940). Experimental production of monkey and avian malaria by an unusual route of infection, *J. Malar. Inst. India.* 3:195-198.

Upton, S.J., Wilson, S.C., Norton, T.M. and Greiner, E.C. (2001). A new species of *Isospora* Schneider, 1881 (Apicomplexa: Eimeriidae) from the Bali (Rothschild's) mynah *Leucopsar rothschildi* (Passeriformes: Saturnidae), and comments concerning the genera *Atoxoplasma* Garnham, 1950 and *Isospora*. *Syst. Parasitol.* 48: 47–53.

Williamson, D. H., Gardner, M. J., Preiser, P., Moore,D. J., Rangachari, K. and Wilson, R. J. M. (1994). The evolutionary origin of the malaria parasite's 35 kb circular DNA; new evidence supports a possible rhodophyte ancestry. *Mol. Gen. Genet.* 243:249–252.

Wilson, R. J. M., Williamson, D.H. and Preiser, P. (1994). Malaria and other apicomplexans: the "plant" connection. *Infect. Agents Dis. 3*:29–37.

Wilson, R.J.M., Denny, P.W., Preiser, P.R., Rangachari, K., Roberts, K., Roy, A., Whyte, A., Strath, M., Moore, D.J., Moore, P.W. and Williamson, D.H. (1996). Complete gene map of the plastid-like DNA of the malaria parasite *Plasmodium falciparum*. *J. Mol. Biol.* 261:155-172.

Wilson, R.J.M. and Williamson, D.H. (1997). Extrachromosomal DNA in the Apicomplexa. *Microbiol. Mol. Biol. Reviews.* 61:1-16.

Whitfield, D., Curtis, C.F., White, G.B., Targett G.A.T., Warhurst, D.C. and Bradley D.J. (1984). Two cases of falciparum malaria acquired in britain. *Brit. Med. J.* 289:1607-1609.

Young, M.D. (1941). The oral transmission of *Plasmodium relictum* in the pigeon. *Public Health Rep.* 56:1430-1440.

In: Progress in Malaria Research
Editor: Lee O. Koning, pp. 193-204
ISBN: 978-1-60021-590-2

Chapter VI

Artemisinin-Based Combination Therapy in an Area of Seasonal Unstable Malaria Transmission in Central Sudan, Africa

***Abdelrahim Osman Mohamed**[*1] **and Elfatih M. Malik**[2]*
Faculty of Medicine, University of El Imam El Mahdi[1] P.O. Box 209 Kosti, Sudan and National Malaria Control Program[2] Federal Ministry of Health, Khartoum, Sudan.

Abstract

Background

Malaria has remained the major killer in Africa as a million children die of the disease every year. This problem is compounded by the emergence of resistance to the commonly used anti-malarial treatments. However, the collective action of the international community led to the establishment of the global fund which made more resources available for malaria control. WHO on view of an increasing resistance to chloroquine, recommended the use of artemisinin- based combination therapies for treatment of malaria. Every country or region in the same country has chosen its first and second lines of treatment. Northern Sudan has chosen artesunate/sulphadoxine-pyremethamine (AS/SP) and artemether/lumefantrine (ART/LUM) respectively as a first and second line treatment while southern Sudan has selected artesunate/amodiaquine (AS/AQ) as the first line of treatment. Central Sudan represents an area of seasonal unstable transmission of malaria where we have run two clinics to test the efficacies of these chosen lines of treatment for two consecutive years. Here we present the results of the second year.

* Address: Abdelrahim O. Mohamed, University Of El Imam El Mahdi, P. O. Box 209 Kosti, Sudan. Email: Abdelrahim_Osman@yahoo.com

Patients and Methods

Sixty two patients with uncomplicated *P. falciparum* malaria were treated with AS/SP and 29 patients with ART/LUM in two different health centers. The patients were of all ages and did not have another cause of fever.

Results

All patients responded adequately to the first and the second lines of treatment without adverse side effects.

Conclusions

AS/SP and ART/LUM are efficacious for the treatment of malaria in an area of seasonal unstable transmission.

Introduction

Malaria has continued to be the major killer in Africa and in Sudan. There are 300 to 500 million attacks of malaria every year with 90% in sub-Saharan Africa. More than one million die every year in Africa most of them are children under 5 years of age. The increasing mortality and morbidity from malaria is due to the failure of the first line treatment which has complicated the management of *P. falciparum* malaria in the world [1].

Chloroquine Resistance: Chloroquine came into use during world war two and continued for decades. Until recently chloroquine; a 4-aminoquinoline has been the first line of treatment of malaria in Africa and hence in the Sudan. It has been inexpensive, safe and widely available. *Plasmodium falciparum* resistance to chloroquine has challenged malaria control efforts. The resistance to chloroquine has been located to a mutant *P. falciparum* chloroquine resistance transporter protein (*pf*CRT) and a multidrug resistance protein (pfMDR1) [2,3]. Chloroquine resistance is strongly linked to a point mutation of pfCRT by substitution of threonine for lysine at amino acid position 76 (K76T) as all resistant isolates in many studies have shown this mutation [2,4]. The studies could not equally correlate resistance with pfMDR1 and concluded that mutations of pfMDR1 and other mutations play secondary roles in the parasite resistance to chloroquine [4]. The transporters work by different mechanisms preventing accumulation of the drug in the food vacuole of the parasite and rescuing the parasite and its gametocytes leading to propagation of the resistance [3]. Chloroquine resistance in the Sudan has been reported since 1978 [5] and in eastern Sudan 1986 [6]. Recently reports have estimated the resistance to chloroquine to mount to 80% in New Halfa eastern Sudan [7], 75.9% and 32.1% in another report from Gadaref eastern Sudan and an area in the capital respectively[8]. In this latter study all resistant parasites curry the mutant allele of *Pfcrt K76T*. There was also a report of chloroquine resistance in Southern Sudan mounting to 17% in children younger than 5 years of age in the Upper Nile [9] and > 90% in Kajo Kaje of Western Equatoria [10]. Recently it has been argued that mutant parasites may not be as fit as the wild forms and hence will not be responsible for the deadly malaria in the Sudan [11,12]. Failure of chloroquine has been also reported in most of African countries including Uganda where resistance reaches 80% [13,14], East Africa 50-80% [13], Zambia 54% [15], in Chad up to 33% [16] and even in West African countries [17]. This resistance to chloroquine rendered the drug useless for malaria treatment.

Sulfadoxine/pyrimethamine (SP) has been used as a second line treatment in the Sudan and in fact some African countries have moved to SP as the first line of treatment after the failure of chloroquine like in Malawi, Kenya and Tanzania [4]. SP is a fixed combination therapy of two antifolate drugs, pyrimethamine working on dihydrofolate reductase (DHFR) and sulphadoxine working on dihydropteroate synthase (DHPS) [18]. This SP combination deprives the parasite from *de novo* folic acid synthesis and hence stops its growth. Multiple mutations on DHFR and DHPS genes produce resistance to SP. SP also has a long half life with suboptimal concentrations making researchers anticipate short therapeutic life of SP [19]. It is already not functional in south East Asia and resistance has appeared in Africa. Resistance to SP has been reported in Sudan in Sennar area as early as 1991 [20] but remained low ranging between 2-7% in the Northern Sudan. In the Southern Sudan a report by Stivanello and co-workers has shown that the failure rate was 60-78% (95% CI) in a 28 days follow-up study in Western Equatoria State [10] and hence they recommended that SP could not be part of the forthcoming combination therapy. Many African countries also reported varying ranges of resistance to SP, in Uganda, East and West Africa. Experience in Southeast Asia and South America has shown that the useful therapeutic life of SP as monotherapy is very short and does not exceed 5 years [19] therefore to lengthen its life span combination with other therapy is recommended. Other mono-therapies used in Africa included mefloquine which is out of use in Thailand and Southeast Asia linked to increased copies of pfMDR1[21]; amodiaquine a 4-aminoquinoline with reasonable cost but suffers concerns about hepatotoxicity and cross resistance with chloroquine [13] and others all suffering resistance. Amodiaquine has been used in combination with SP which showed efficacy superior to either drugs alone and has been recommended as an interim inexpensive regimen before the adoption of artemisinin-based combination therapies (ACTs) [22].

Artimesinin based combination therapy: Combination chemotherapy is well established in the treatment of cancer, tuberculosis and HIV. If drug resistance develops by spontaneous point mutation the probability of resistance to two structurally distinct drugs with different modes of action is a product of two mutation frequencies which are very low in malaria parasite. For antimalarial drug combination to be effective, the pharmacokinetics of the two or three components must be well matched or otherwise the parasite biomass must be reduced sufficiently by one of the drugs so that the chance of mutation to other slowly eliminated one is reduced [23]. Artemisinin derivatives are yet the most active available antimalarial. When given for three days they reduce the parasite biomass to a level that can be handled by the other component drug. It has been reported that adding artemisinin to a standard drug like SP, mefloquine, amodiaquie and chloroquine will increase efficacy without increasing toxicity [24,25]. Meta analysis of 16 randomized studies all over the world and investigating 6000 patients have proved that addition of 3 days of artesunate to standard antimalerial treatments reduces treatment failure, recrudescence and gametocyte carriage [26]. Artemisinins exhibit a quick onset of action and are effective with high efficacy against the blood stages of

Plasmodium and has been shown to reduce the number of gametocytes in the blood [27]. Artemisinins have been also reported to reduce transmission rates in areas of low transmission. Metabolism of artemisinins in the liver microsomes of humans is by cytochrome P450, primarily by CYP 2B6. Artemisinins have very short half-life of < 10 min and their mode of action is by interference with plasmodial sarcoplasmic/endoplasmic ATPase (SERCA) [27]. Several ACTs have been developed including the combination of ART/LUM (Coartem) and the combination of artesunate with amodiaquine (AQ), mefloquine (MQ) or sulfadoxine-pyrimethamine[27]. ART/LUM is the first fixed dose combination therapy developed in China and has been used in the adult oral dose of 80/480 initially at 0, 8, 24, and 48 hours. The drug is not for use with pregnant women and children < 10 kg of weight. Lumefantrine absorption is improved by simultaneously taking fatty food with the drug [28]. The 4-dose regimen in Thailand gave cure rate of only 83% and gave cure rates in Africa of 93% in Gambia and only 86% in Zambia [28]. The dose then was lengthened following evidence that 6-dose cure rates were more than 96% in Southeast Asia, 99% when assessed at day 14 in Burundi, 97.7%/98% with supervised/unsupervised respectively of extensive randomized 28 day end point study in Uganda [28]. The dosage for non-immune patients was adjusted to be given at 0, 8, 24, 36, 48 and 60 hours [23]. WHO has recommended all countries in sub-Saharan Africa to shift to the use of ACTs following the accumulating evidence that they are the best treatment for uncomplicated malaria [29].

The high prevalence of chloroquine resistance (ranging between 30-80%) and the relatively low level of SP failure (ranging between 2 -7%) has prompted the national malaria control programme to adopt a combination therapy based on artemisinin, AS/SP as a first line of treatment of uncomplicated *P. falciparum* malaria in northern Sudan. The government of southern Sudan following the experience in neighbouring countries and previous studies by *Medicines Sans Frontiers* has chosen AS/AQ as the first line treatment. AS/SP is provided in tablet form as SP and artesunate in separate compartments of the same blister strip (co-blister). However, in this study AS was provided in separate blister strip and SP in a tin from different manufacturers. Coartem has been chosen as the second line for treatment of uncomplicated malaria. Coartem is provided as fixed combination of 1:6 artemether and lumefantrine tablets produced by Norvatis.

Base-line information about the efficacy of treatment is needed in different parts of the country and hence the objective of this study was to evaluate the efficacy of AS/SP and ART/LUM (coartem) in a seasonal unstable transmission area.

Materials and Methods

Study Area

Sudan is the largest country in Africa with an area of 2.6 M sq kilometres extending from 4° north to 22° north. There are different rain regions in the country ranging from 9 month in the south to dry desert in the far north hence the flora and malaria transmission vary accordingly. The figure shows the map of the Sudan with depicted malaria endemicity. Kosti town with 300,000 population in the White Nile State is 300 Km south of Khartoum on the

White Nile. The rainfall in Kosti area is seasonal from May to September and therefore malaria transmission is seasonal and unstable. In the year 2005 the rainfall was average with the total of 357.4 mm with the peak in august (166.9 mm) and malaria transmission was low with peak transmission September-October. Two health centres were chosen for the study, Quarter 28 health centre (Clinic A) with a large catchments area with many primary schools in the region. The other health centre is Sika Hadid health centre (Clinic B) serving a small area near the river and the railway station. Most of the patients in clinic B have health insurance, as they are mostly employees.

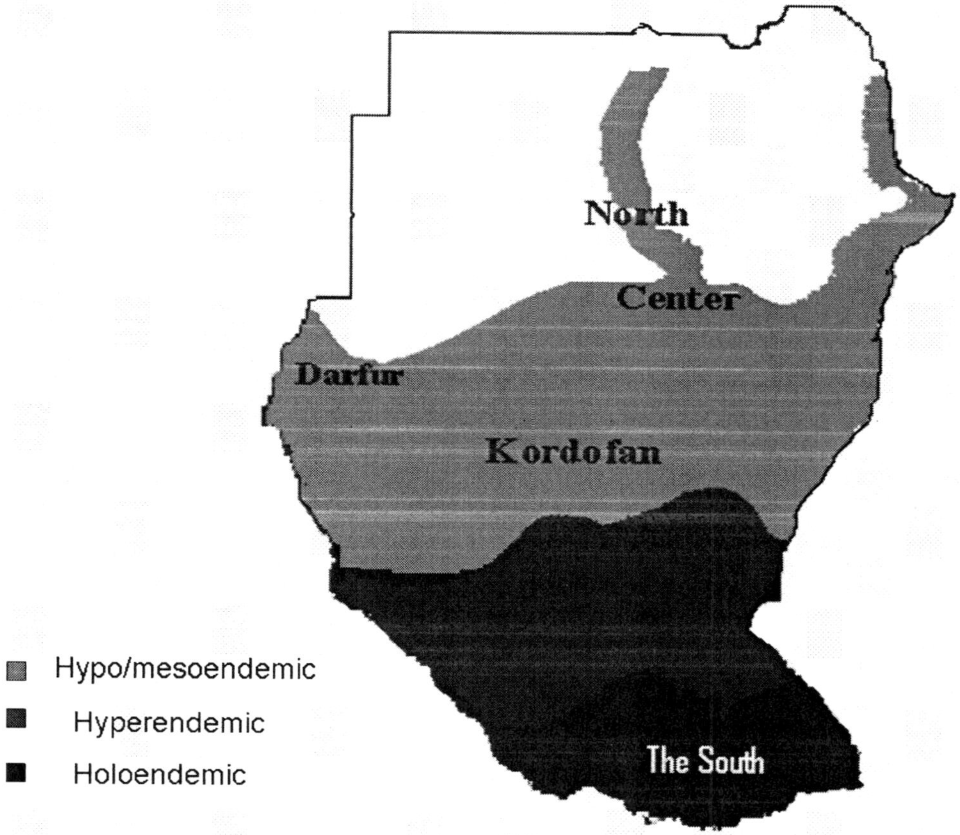

Figure 1. Malaria endemicity in the Sudan; Adapted from [34].

Study Design

This study is a one arm prospective study for the evaluation of the clinical and parasitological response to directly observed treatment with AS/SP in Clinic A and Coartem (Novartis Pharma Ltd, Beijing, China) in Clinic B for uncomplicated malaria. The study followed the minimum requirements for efficacy studies as determined by the WHO task force [30]. The target group has been all ages. Inclusion criteria included parasite counts between 1,000 and 100,000 asexual parasites/μL of blood with absence of other infections causing febrile illness. The history of antimalarial intake did not imply exclusion from the study. The sample size was predetermined following the WHO protocol and would be 50 to 70 patients with a calculated treatment failure of 5% [30]. Patients fulfilling the criteria had been included for each group after informed consent from the patient or guardian. The patients were recruited during the period sixth October to 29th October 2005 in clinic A and follow up continued for 28 days for each patient. In clinic B the recruitment period was from October 5, to October 29, 2005 and the patients were followed up for 28 days each. Patient sheets were designed to record personal data, physical examination findings, parasitological examination and counts, treatment and follow up results. Patients were followed up for clinical data, side effects and assessment for treatment failure which were recorded on days 1, 2, 3, 7, 14, 21 and 28. End-points were expressed as adequate clinical and parasitological response (ACPR) or failure of treatment. Treatment failure was expressed as early treatment failure (ETF) when there was development of danger signs or severe malaria on the first 3 days of treatment in the presence of parasitaemia, parasitaemia on day 2 higher than day 0, parasitaemia on day 3 with the presence of fever or parasitaemia on day 3 $\geq$ 25% of day 0. Late clinical failure (LCF) is reported when there were danger signs or severe malaria after day 3 with the presence of parasitaemia or presence of parasitaemai and fever on any day from day 4 to 28. Late parasitological failure is indicated by the presence of parasitaemia with axillary temperature $<$ 37.5 from day 7 to day 28[30]. Rescue treatment was provided for eventually failing treatment which was coartem for AS/SP and quinine for coartem. Thick and thin blood films were taken and examined on days 0, 2, 3, 7, 14, 21 and 28. Parasitaemia was measured by counting the number of asexual parasites in the thick blood film against an average of 200 leucocytes using hand tally-counters based on a mean count of 8000 leucocytes/μl blood [30]. All positive and negative slide smears were reconfirmed by an experienced microscopist at the national malaria referral laboratory and consistency was obtained in almost all samples. Blood was collected on filter paper on day 0 and any other day with positive blood smear for PCR. However, none of the samples was positive on subsequent visits and so PCR was not performed. Treatment was given according to the weight of the patient as indicated by the national protocol (SP, 1.25 mg pyrimethamine/Kg body weight and AS 4 mg/Kg body weight). Coartem was given as indicated by the national protocol at 0, 8, 24, 36, 48, 60 hours which comprises 24 tablets for adults. Children receive doses according to their weights, 5-<15kg body weight receives one tablet for each dose, 15-<25 kg, 2 tablets are given for each dose, 25-< 35 kg receive 3 tablets each dose to total of 18 tablets. Whenever the patient vomited within 30 minutes would receive another full dose of treatment.

Ethical clearance: Ethical clearance for the study was obtained from the Federal Ministry of Health. All patients were included in the study after informed consent from the patient or accompanying guardian.

Statistical Methods: Data were entered into computer database and double-checked. Analysis was done using SPSS software package.

Results

In Clinic A, 277 patients were seen with 118 (42.6%) having positive blood films for *P. falciparum* malaria. Sixty two patients fulfilled criteria for inclusion and 59 patients completed treatment with (AS/SP) and follow up (table 1), their ages ranged between 1 and 60 years with mean age of 16.2 years. The other patients chose not to participate or were not from the study area and hence could not come for follow up. In clinic B, 645 patients were examined and 100 (15.5%) had positive blood films for *P. falciparum* malaria. Twenty nine patients were treated with the second line treatment coartem with 26 patients completing 28 days follow-up (table 1). Their ages ranged between 3 and 50 years with mean age of 21.3 years (table 2). Unfortunately the predetermined protocol rejected the results of the second line as the number of the patients was below the acceptable number in the protocol. During the study period we could only recruit 29 patients who completed all 28 day follow up period. About the half of the patients in clinic A and three quarters in Clinic B were males (table 2). Table 2 also shows age stratification of the patients, mean values for the age, weight, height of the patients together with the mean parasite counts (geometric) and temperature at admission. The major presenting symptom was fever in 61 patients of the 62 patients (98.4%) and vomiting in the majority. All patients had been treated as outpatient cases and followed-up at the clinic, home or school. All patients who completed the follow-up had negative blood films on the third day of treatment (Day 2) and continued to be negative for the rest of the follow-up period of 28 days. No Side effects were recorded for the first line treatment while the second line treatment received complaints in 5 patients that included gastric disturbance, excessive sleepiness and one patient complained of dizziness. None of the patients withdrew because of severe side effects.

Table 1. Summary of the patients and the outcome of treatment lines

Drugs	AS/SP	Coartem
	N (%)	N (%)
Total suspected patients	277	645
Total positive for falciparum malaria	118 (42.6)	100 (15.5)
No. enrolled	62	29
No. lost to follow-up or withdrew	2 + 1	3
ACPR	59	26
Treatment failure:		
• ETF	0	0
• LCF	0	0
• LPF	0	0

ACPR, adequate clinical and parasitological response, ETF early treatment failure, LCF late clinical failure and LPF, late parasitological failure.

Table 2. Characteristics of the enrolled patients

	AS/SP cohort	Coartem cohort
Mean age in years ±SD	16.2 ±14.8	21.3 ± 13.7
< 5	6.4%	3.4%
5-15	58.1%	31.1%
Adults	35.5%	65.5%
Weight in Kg ±SD	39.13 ± 19.2	46.2 ± 17.1
Height in cm ±SD	146.8 ± 23.7	155.8 ± 26.3
Male patients	41.9%	72.4%
Parasite counts per μL {geometric mean (range)}	11495 (2000-100000)	8096 (2000-26000)
Mean temperature °C ±SD	38.25 ± 1.23	37.51 ± 0.63

Conclusion

Malaria treatment failure has rendered falciparum malaria a dangerous disease in the Sudan and many deaths were sadly encountered because of failing treatment. This study has shown that ACT is very efficacious and safe for second year in use. It has been known from previous studies that addition of artesunate to SP would improve its effectiveness [26,7]. That was the case in this study without adverse effects in contrary to another study carried out in eastern Sudan [7]. The effect of the combination therapy can be explained by the fact that artesunate will quickly kill most of the parasites leading to the rapid improvement of the patients [24]. AS/SP has quickly acquired reputation in the community by being quick and effective and started to get nicknames in the local languages. Coartem has shown similar efficacy in this study with minimal side effects. Coartem has been reported by the manufacturers and other reports to produce mild side effects including sleep disturbance, dizziness and gastrointestinal disturbance (Novartis Pharma Ltd, Beijing, China). A few patients from our study population had experienced sleepiness, dizziness and gastrointestinal disturbance, which subsided upon completion of treatment. Previous investigators have confirmed the efficacy of coartem [26]. Our results also confirmed that coartem is a successful second line of treatment. Our results will further recommend the preservation of this second line treatment until evidence of resistance appears for the first line, which is not the case now.

The high positive rate of malaria in clinic A does not reflect high prevalence of malaria in the area because only highly suspected patients were asked to participate. This was not the case in clinic B where similar prevalence to last year was found [31]. The low transmission rate had made the recruitment and follow up periods to be longer in clinic B. However, the number which is not exclusively high has been predetermined by the study protocol. It is interesting that the average age for the first line sample was 15 years that was clearly different from the average age of the second cohort, which is explained by the different locations of the health centres.

Another question is raised here whether resistance to a drug is permanent or people will come to enjoy the efficiency of chloroquine and others again. Experience in eastern Sudan has shown that chloroquine resistant parasites as well as the sensitive ones survive the long dry season as asymptomatic parasitemia and gametocytes [32]. The sensitive parasites are more in the beginning of the rainy seasons as an implication of the lack of the advantageous selective pressure to the resistant parasites. However these studies did not find evidence that resistance will be eliminated by the reduced drug usage in the contrary that resistance continued to rise [32]. However, there is accumulating evidence from other studies where chloroquine usage has been stopped for several years like in Malawi that sensitive parasites re-emergence in the community [4]. Malawi is the first country in Africa to switch from chloroquine to sulfadoxine-pyrimethamine as the first line of treatment of malaria since 1993 and five years later it was observed that in vitro testing of parasite isolates to show that 65% were sensitive, 31% borderline and only 3% were resistant [4]. Malawi case promises that if chloroquine usage could be reduced to acceptably low levels, countries may enjoy re-emergence of sensitive P. falciparum in Africa.

A third concern is that the production of ACT is limited by the availability of the artemisinins [32] and therefore other combinations have to be explored before we reach the situation that ACT production is optimized by synthesis and genetic engineering strategies in transgenic plants and yeast production [27]. Combinations of dapsone, atovaquone, chloroproguanil and chlorocycloguanil have been tested for this purpose and were found to act synergistically and effectively in an *in vitro* set up [33].

In this study the antimalarial drugs were provided free of charge and the issue of cost was not a matter. However, both first and second line medicines have been deployed to the private pharmacies with prohibitive prices of equivalent to $4 and $8, respectively. The national programme through the global fund is providing free treatment for positive blood smears. However, there is still a problem of accessibility and awareness in rural areas. Many sick patients may not visit public health facilities and others go directly to pharmacies or drug sellers. Then the cost matters. On the other hand many treating doctors refrain from prescribing these medicines partly because of the prices and partly because of lack of information. Because the drugs are made widely available in the private sector their use for malaria treatment in the Sudan needs regular monitoring from the national programme and its partners if success is to be the expected outcome. Previous experience has shown that price of treatment is the most important determinant of compliance and often families divide one person's dose for other members of the family and the outcome can be disastrous [25]. Studies in different parts of the world have shown that adherence to the proper dose of malaria therapy varies according to the efficiency of the treatment and the length of the time it has to be used. Problems arise when antimalarial treatment is used for several days [29]. Another problem in the Sudan is that AS/SP combination is provided in adult and children packages with artesunate being 50 mg or 100 mg tablet which may pose problems when the drug is self administered. It is unfortunate that two areas of the same country will choose different combinations as is the case of the south and northern Sudan. As people move freely between the two distinct regions of the country it would have been more appropriate to use the same ACT to prolong the life span of the treatment and have the other as a reserve. Finally, if we have to enjoy the promising outcome of this study the country and the Roll

Back Malaria initiative though have done much so far have to face the question of accessibility and prices and keep an open eye on such concerns.

Acknowledgements: This study was supported by a fund from the national malaria control programme. We are grateful to the National Health Insurance in the White Nile State who provided all the logistics needed. We thank our patients for participating in this follow-up study. We thank Elsir Wagie Alla, Aisha Musa, and Ali Omer for assistance.

References

[1] Staedke SG, Mpimbaza A, Kamya MR, Nzarubara BK, Dorsey G, Rosenthal P (2004). Combination treatment for uncomplicated falciparum malaria in Kampala, Uganda: randomised clinical trial. *Lancet;* 364:1950-57.

[2] Severini C, Menegon M, Sannella AR, Paglia MG et al (2006). Prevalence of pfcrt point mutations and level of chloroquine resistance in plasmodium falciparum isolates from Africa. *Infect. Genet. Evolution.* 6: 262-268.

[3] Valderramos SG, Fidock DA. (2006). Transporters involved in resistance to antimalarial drugs. *TRENDS Pharmacol Science;* doi:10.1016/j.tips.2006.09.005

[4] Laufer MK, Plowe CV. (2004). Withdrawing antimalarial drugs: impact on parasite resistance and implication for malaria treatment policies. *Drug Resistance Updates.* 7: 279-288.

[5] Omer AH. (1978). Response of Plasmodium falciparum in Sudan to oral chloroquine. *Am. J. Trop. Med. Hyg;* 27: 853-857.

[6] Bayoumi, R. A., Babiker, H. A., Ibrahim, S. M., Galib, H. W., Saeed, B. O., Khider, S., El Wasila, M. and Awad El Kariem, F. M. (1989). Chloroquine resistant *Plasmodium falciparum* in eastern Sudan. *Acta Tropica;* 46: 157-165

[7] Adam I, A-Elbasit IEA, Idris SM, Malik EM and Elbashir MI (2005). A comparison of the efficacy of artesuate plus sulfadoxine-pyrimethamine with that of sulfadoxine-pyrimethamine alone, in the treatment of uncomplicated *Plasmodium falciparum* malaria in eastern Sudan. *Annals Trop. Med. Parasitol;* 99(4): 1-7

[8] Tagelsir N, Ibrahim Z, Medani A, Salih O et al (2005). High frequency of Plasmodium falciparum PfCRT K76T and PfpghN86Y in patients clearing infection after chloroquine treatment in the Sudan. *Acta Tropica;* 97:19-25.

[9] Van den Broek IVF, Gatkol T, Owoko B, Nzila A, Ochong E, Keus K. (2003). Chloroquine, sulfadoxine-pyrimethamine and amodiaquine efficacy for the treatment of uncomplicated Plasmodium falciparum malaria in Upper Nile, South Sudan. *Trans. Roy Soc. Trop. Med. Hyg;* 97: 229-235.

[10] Stivanello E, Cavailler P, Cassano F, Omar SA, Kariuki D, Mwangi J, Piola P Guthmann J-P. (2004). Efficacy of chloroquine, sulphadoxine–pyrimethamine and amodiaquine for treatment of uncomplicated *Plasmodium falciparum* malaria in Kajo Keji county, Sudan. *Trop. Med. Int. Health;* 9(9): 975-980.

[11] Giha HA, Elbashir MI, A-Elbasit I, A-Elgadir TME, ElGhazali GE, Mackinnon M, Babiker HA. (2006). Drug resistance-virulence relationship in Plasmodium falciparum

causing severe malaria in an area of seasonal and unstable transmission. *Acta Tropica;* 97: 181-187.

[12] Walliker D, Hunt P, Babiker H, (2005). Fitness of drug-resistant malarial parasites. *Acta Tropica.* 94: 251-259.

[13] Kamya MR, Bakyaita NN, Talisuna AO, Were WM, Staedke SG (2002). Increasing antimalarial drug resistance in Uganda and revision of the national policy. *Trop. Med. Int.Health.*7(12): 1031-1041

[14] Checchi F, Piola P, Kosak C, Ardizzoni E, et al. (2004). Antimalarial efficacy of sulfadoxine-pyrimethamine, amodiaquine and a combination of chloroquine plus sulfadoxine-pyrimethamine in Bundi Bugyo, western Uganda. *Trop. Med. Int. Health;* 9(4): 445-450.

[15] Depoortere E, Guthmann J-P, Presse J, Sipilanyamble N, Nkandu E, Balkan S, de Pecoulas PE, Legros D. (2005). Efficacy and effectiveness of the combination of sulfadoxine/pyrimethamine and a 3-day course of artesunate for the treatment of uncomplicated falciparum malaria in a refugee settlement in Zambia. *Trop. Med. Int. Health.* 10(2): 139-145.

[16] Grandessoa F, Bachya C , Donamb I, Ntambic J, Ntambic J, Habimanac J, D'Alessandrod U, Maikerec J, Vanlerberghec V, Kerahb CH, Guthmann J-P. (2006). Efficacy of chloroquine, sulfadoxine—pyrimethamine and amodiaquine for treatment of uncomplicated *Plasmodium falciparum* malaria among children under five in Bongor and Koumra, Chad. *Trans. Roy. Soc. Trop. Med. Hyg;* 100: 419-429.

[17] Sowunmi A, Fehintola FA, Adedeji AA, Gbotosho GO, Tambo E, Oduola MJ (2005). Open randomized study of artesunate-amodiaquine vs. chloroquine-pyrimethamine-sulfadoxine for the treatment of uncomplicated Plasmodium falciparum malaria in Nigerian children. *Trop. Med. Int. Health.* 10(11): 1161-1170.

[18] Ouellette M. (2001). Biochemical and molecular mechanisms of drug resistance in parasites. *Trop. Med. Int. Health,* 6(11): 874-882.

[19] Nzila AM, Nduati E, Mberu EK, Sibley CH *et al* (2000). Molecular evidence of greater selective pressure for drug resistance exerted by the long-acting antifolate pyrimethamine/sulfadoxine compared with the shorter-acting chlorproguanil/dapsone on Kenyan *Plasmodium falciparum. J. Infect. Dis;* 181: 2023-2028

[20] Ibrahim, M., Awad El Kariem, F., Elhassan, I. M. and Mubarak, A. (1991). A case control study of *Plasmodium falciparum* malaria sensitive to chloroquine but resistant to sulfadoxine /pyrimethamine (Fansidar) in Sennar, Sudan. *Trans. Roy. Soc. Trop. Med. Hyg.* 85:466

[21] Price RN, Uhlemann A-C, Brockman A, McGready R et al (2004). Mefloquine resistance in plasmodium falciparum and increased pfmdr1 gene copy number. *Lancet.* 364: 438-447.

[22] Dorsey G, Njama D, Kamya MR, Cattamanachi A, et al (2002). Sulfadoxine/ pyrimethamine alone or with amodiaquine or artesunate for treatment of uncomplicated malaria: a longitudinal randomised trial. *Lancet.* 360: 2031-2038.

[23] Edwards G, Biagini G. (2006). Resisting resistance: dealing with the irrepressible problem of malaria. *Br. J. Clin. Pharmacol.* 61(6): 690-693.

[24] Olliaro PL, Taylor WR (2004). Developing artemisinin based drug combinations for the treatment of drug resistant faciparum malaria: a review. *J. Postgrad. Med;* 50(1): 40-44.

[25] Whitty CJM, Allan R, Wiseman V, Ochola S et al (2004). Averting a malria disaster in Africa: where does the buck stop? *Bull. World Health Organ.* 82(5): 381-384.

[26] International Artemisinin Study Group (2004). Artesunate combinations for treatment of malaria: meta-analysis. *Lancet;* 363:9-17.

[27] Golenser J, Waknine JH, Krugliak M, Hunt NH, Grau GE. (2006). Current perspectives on the mechanism of action of artemesinins. *Int. J. Parasitol.* doi:10.1016/j.ijpara.2006.07.011.

[28] Piola P, Fogg C, Bajunirwe F, Biraro S et al (2005). Supervised versus unsupervised intake of six-dose artemether-lumefantrine for treatment of acute, uncomplicated plasmodium falciparum malaria in Mbarar, Uganda: a randomized trial. *Lancet.* 365: 1467-1473.

[29] Yeung S, White NJ. (2005). How do patients use antimalarial drugs? A review of the evidence. *Trop. Med. Int. Health.* 10(2): 121-138.

[30] WHO. (2003). Assessment and monitoring of antimalarial drug efficacy for the treatment of uncomplicated *falciparum* malaria. Geneva. *WHO/HTM*/RBM/2003.5.

[31] Mohamed AO, Eltaib EH, Ahmed OA, Elamin SB, Malik EM. (2006). The efficacies of artesunate-sulfadoxine-pyrimethamine and artemether-lumefantrine in the treatment of uncomplicated. Plasmodium falciparum malaria, in an area of low transmission in central Sudan. *Ann. Trop. Med. Parasitol.* 100(1): 5-10.

[32] Babiker HA, Satti G, Ferguson H, Bayoumi R, Walliker D. (2005). Drug resistant Plasmodium falciparum in an area of seasonal transmission. Acta Tropica 94: 260-268.

[33] Nduati EW, Kamau EM. (2006). Multiple synergistic interactions between atovaquone and antifolates against Plasmodium falciparum in vitro: A rational basis for combination therapy. *Acta Tropica.* 97: 357-363.

[34] Mohammed AO, Attalla B, Bashir FMK, Ahmed F, El Hassan AM, Ibnauf G, Jiang W, Cavalli-Sforza LL, Karrar ZA, Ibrahim ME. (2006). Relationship of the sickle cell gene to the ethnic and geographic groups populating the Sudan. *Community Genet*; 9: 113-120.

In: Progress in Malaria Research
Editor: Lee O. Koning, pp. 205-210
ISBN: 978-1-60021-590-2

Chapter VII

Changes in Serum Lipid Profile in Adult Patients Presenting with Acute, Uncomplicated *Falciparum* Malaria Infection

I. H. Garba [* 1]***, G. A. Ubom*** [2] ***and T. D. Adelola*** [3]
[1,3] Industrial Chemistry Programme, School of Science,
Abubakar Tafawa Balewa University, P. M. B. 0248 Bauchi, Nigeria.
[2] Department of Biochemistry, Faculty of Medical Sciences,
University of Jos, P. M. B. 2048, Plateau Nigeria.

Abstract

The serum concentration of total lipids, β- / pre-β-lipoproteins and cholesterol were measured in fifty adult patients (25 males and females each), age range 18 – 35, presenting with acute, and uncomplicated *falciparum* malaria infection. Diagnosis was confirmed by microscopic examination of Giemsa-stained thin blood slides (parasite density = 1000 – 10,000 asexual forms / ml of blood). An age-matched group comprising of 20 healthy, malaria-negative adults were enrolled for comparative purposes. There was an insignificant increase in the serum concentration of total lipids in both the patient groups: (12.43 ± 4.61 g/l, males) and (13.77 ± 4.42 g/l, females) relative to the healthy individuals (9.84 ± 0.51 g/l) $p > 0.05$. β- and pre-β lipoprotein concentration was significantly elevated in the patients when compared to the healthy individuals: 7.58 ± 3.28 g/l (male patients), 7.60 ± 5.11 g/l (female patients) and 6.22 ± 2.40 g/l (healthy individuals), $p < 0.05$. Serum cholesterol was also significantly elevated in the malaria patients: 15.75 mmol/l (male patients), 12.08 ± 2.95 mmol/l (female patients) and 9.35 mmol/l (healthy individuals), $p < 0.05$. Uncontrolled haemolysis of both parasitized and unparasitized erythrocytes of all ages is one of the major determinants of the pathogenicity of human *falciparum* malaria infection. It leads to massive destruction of red blood cells, release of parasite-derived toxins and oxidant compounds responsible for

* Corresponding author: I. H. Garba; Tel: 0802-086-5276

the pathogenic outcomes observed in this endemic tropical disease. Since the erythrocyte membranes are predominantly lipid in composition, the release of such lipids following haemolysis can account for the observed perturbations in the serum lipid profile of patients presenting with this disease.

Key words: Malaria, *falciparum,* lipids, blood, erythrocytes.

Introduction

Malaria is a disease caused by the species of the obligate intracellular parasite of the genus plasmodium within the class sporozoa. The various species of the genus plasmodium are responsible for causing malaria infection depending on the host [1-2]. Among the numerous species of plasmodium so far identified, the following four are known to be responsible for causing human malaria infection: P. *vivax*, P. *malariae,* P. *ovale* and P. *falciparum* [3-4]. This disease stands out among the systemic infectious diseases of humans for many reasons; apart from the sheer scale of problems it causes [5]. Global figures for deaths from malaria range from 1.5 to 2.7 million annually, most of whom are children under 5 years of age and pregnant women [6-9]. Almost all these deaths are caused by falciparum malaria, which is the commonest African malaria. A child is estimated to die from malaria every 12 or so seconds. The mortality burden is on Sub-Saharan Africa, where more than 90 % of these deaths occur, before reaching the age of 5 years. Malaria is responsible globally for 500 million cases of clinical disease and presents a public health problem for 2.4 billion people, representing over 40 % of the world's population [10-11]. From an economic point of view, malaria is a costly disease. An estimated 1.8 billion US Dollars is spent annually on both direct costs such as lost productivity, time costs and other direct costs and losses. This is approximately equal to the entire gross domestic product (GDP) of some countries such as Malawi, Benin, or Togo [12]. This disease is associated with headache, muscular discomfort, weakness and malaise and as the untreated infection becomes synchronized, the fever becomes periodic with pyrexial spikes every one, two or three days, associated with chills or rigors [13]. If the disease progresses, the headache, limb pains and general malaise increases [14]. Anxiety and mental confusion are common at this stage. Fever becomes irregular without distinct periodicity. Hyperpyrexia, with temperatures well above 40 degrees centigrade is not uncommon [15] together with convulsion and consequent aspiration pneumonia [16]. The pulse and respiration rate are more rapid. Nausea, vomiting and diarrhoea increase in intensity with an associated pulmonary involvement, leading to cough. There is hepatomegaly and splenomegaly with slight jaundice [17]. Occasionally, *falciparum* malaria presents with encephalopathy and fever mimicking fulminant hepatic failure [18]. Additionally, a significant percentage of malaria patients present with thrombocytopenia, hyponatremia and liver dysfunction [19]. In this study we investigated the changes in the serum lipid profile of patients presenting with acute, uncomplicated *falciparum* malaria infection based on our hypothesis that merozoites-induced haemolysis of both infected and uninfected erythrocytes during *falciparum* malaria infection can lead to a significant perturbation in the serum lipid profile of such patients.

Patients and Methods

Study Locale

The southern and northern limits of Bauchi State, Nigeria, where the study was conducted are demarcated by latitudes 9°30' North and 10°30' North respectively. Its Western and Eastern limits are bounded by longitudes 8°45' East and 11°0' East respectively. Two thirds of the land area is in the south of latitude 11°15'.

Patients and Study Design

Patient selection and pre-qualification was done by simple random sampling of individuals presenting at the Bauchi Specialist Hospital Outpatient Department with a history of fever and malaise within a period of 1-7 days, and who were confirmed to be infected with the *falciparum* malaria parasite by microscopic examination of Giemsa stained thin blood slides. Exclusion criteria include patients with diabetes, myocardial infarction, leprosy, alcoholism, cancer and liver diseases. Based on the above criteria, 50 patients were found to be qualified for participation in the study. The qualified patients consisted of a group each of 25 adult males and females each within the age range of 18-35 years. A control group of 20 age-matched healthy adults were also enrolled for comparative purposes.

Serum Sample Collection and Preparation

Blood samples from each of the participants were collected between the hours of 9.00 a.m. and 11.00 a.m. by venepuncture of the antecubital vein into clean, sterile, plastic centrifuge tubes. The samples were centrifuged at 3000g for ten minutes after clotting. Sera was collected by aspiration using a Pasteur pipette and assayed within 24 hours.

Assays

Total serum lipid concentration was assayed using the sulphophosphovanillin method. Cholesterol was assayed using Ilca's Method. Serum β- and pre-β lipoprotein was assayed using Turbidimetric Method [20].

Statistical Analysis

Data was analyzed using the Statigraphics (Version 5.0) Statistical Software. Results are expressed as mean ± SEM. Mean serum total lipids, β- and pre-β lipoproteins, and cholesterol concentrations were analyzed using One-way Analysis of Variance (ANOVA). The method of Least Significant Difference (LSD) was used to determine the difference between the means. P values < 0.05 were considered significant.

Ethics

This work was conducted in accordance with the CIOMS / WHO International Guidelines for the Conduct of Research Involving Human Subjects [21].

Results

The changes in the pattern of serum lipid profile shown in table 1 indicate that total serum lipids increased by 26.32% in male patients and 39.93% in the female patients, $p < 0.05$. β- and pre-β lipoprotein increased by 21.86 % and 22.20% respectively in the male and female patients, $p < 0.05$. Serum cholesterol increased by 68.45% in the male patients and 29.20% in their female counterparts, $p < 0.05$. With the exception of cholesterol where the highest increase was observed in the male patients, the female patients have the highest increase in the other lipid fractions.

Table 1. Serum concentration of total lipids, β- and pre-β lipoprotein, and Cholesterol in *falciparum* malaria patients and healthy adults

Subjects	Total Lipids (g/l)	β- and pre-β lipoprotein (g/l)	Cholesterol (mmol/l)
Male patients	$12.43 \pm 4.61^*$	$7.58 \pm 3.28^*$	$15.75 \pm 4.06^*$
Female patient	$13.77 \pm 4.42^*$	$7.60 \pm 5.11^*$	$12.08 \pm 2.95^*$
Healthy adults	9.84 ± 0.51^a	6.22 ± 2.40^b	9.35 ± 1.79^c

Total lipids [* vs. ^{a} $p < 0.05$] β- and pre-β lipoprotein [* vs. ^{b} $p < 0.05$] Cholesterol [* vs. ^{c} $p < 0.05$].

Discussion

The key pathogenic events in *falciparum* malaria infection are invasion of the host hepatocytes by infective sporozoites and the merozoites invasion of the host red blood cells leading to the lyses of the red blood cells [22-23]. Among these events, merozoites-induced haemolysis can be said to be at the root of the changes in the pattern of serum lipid profile observed in this study. This is because the predominant class of macromolecules found in the membranes of erythrocytes are lipid in nature. Such lipids include triacylglycerols, lipoprotein complexes and cholesterol, which specifically plays an important role in cellular membrane organization, dynamics, function and sorting [24]. Therefore, lyses of the host red blood cells leads to the breakdown of the membranes and release of the membrane's components into the host circulation with an accompanying elevation in the concentration of various lipid fractions in serum. This can account for the observed increase in fluidity and oxidation of malarial lipoproteins earlier reported by Sibmooh and co-workers [25]. The haemolytic event in malaria infection has also been shown to be associated with the release of parasite-derived toxins and oxidant compounds [26]. The effect of these oxidant compounds on lipid fractions, particularly lipoproteins, can serve as the genesis of the oxidative stress associated with this disease, since Thiobarbituric Acid Reactive Substances (TBARS) which are major indicators of lipid peroxidation and cellular oxidative stress are found to be increased in malaria infection [27-28]. The results obtained in this study are in agreement with those reported by Das and co-workers [29], Davis et al. [30] and Mohanty et al. [31] and at variance with those obtained by Sibmooh et al. [25]. These variations are to be expected since malaria differs in its characteristics from country to country and even within the same country [6].

References

[1] Hoffman, SL; Crutcher, JM; Puri, SK; Ansari, AA; Villinger, F; Franke, ED; Singh, PP; Finkelman, F; Gately, MK; Dutta, GP; Sedegal, M. Sterile protection of monkeys against malaria after administration of interleukin-12. *National Medicine*, 1997, 3, 80 – 83

[2] Le Moyec , L; Ekwalanga , M; Eugene , M ; Bouanga, JC; Bauza, G; M'Bengue, A; Mazier, D; Gentilini, M. Brain metabolites in mice co-infected with plasmodium berghei- ANKA and LP-BM5 virus: Assessment by proton magnetic resonance spectroscopy. *Experimental Parasitology*, 1997, 85, 296-298

[3] Moody, AH; John, SM; Sudarsanam, A; Sitarram, U. Evaluation of Optimal, a dipstick test for the diagnosis of malaria. *Annals of Tropical Medicine and Parasitology*, 1998, 92, 621 – 22

[4] Sachs, J; Malaney P. The economic and social burden of malaria. *Nature*, 2002, 415, 680-685

[5] Clark, IA; Alleva, LM; Mills, AC; William, BC. Pathogenesis of malaria and other clinically similar conditions. *Clinical Microbiology Reviews*, 2004, 17, 509-539.

[6] Phillips, RS. Current status of malaria and potential for control. *Clinical Microbiology Reviews*, 2001, 14, 208-226.

[7] Schwartlander, B. Global burden of disease. *Lancet*, 1997, 50, 141-142.

[8] Starchier, D. How much malaria is there worldwide? *Parasitology Today*, 1989, 5, 39-40.

[9] World Health Organization. Investing in health research and development. Document TDR/Gen/96.1 Adhoc Committee of Health Research Relating to Future Intervention Options, World Health Organization, Geneva, Switzerland 1996.

[10] Malaria Foundation International: http://www.malaria.org.

[11] Amador, R; Patarroyo, ME. Malaria vaccines. *Journal of Clinical Immunology*, 1996, 16,183 – 189.

[12] Foster, S. Economics and its contribution to the fight against malaria. *Annals of Tropical Medicine and Parasitology*, 1998, 92, 391-398.

[13] White, NJ; Ho, M. The pathophysiology of malaria. *Advances in Parasitology*, 1992, 31, 83-166.

[14] Buyse, D; Van-Den-Ende, J; Vervoorti, T; Van-Den-Ende, E. Sleeping sickness as an import pathology following a stay in Zaire. *Acta Clinica Belgica*, 1996, 51, 409 – 411.

[15] Long, HY; Lell, B; Dutz, K; Kremsner, PG. Plasmodium *falciparum*: in vitro growth inhibition by fibrile temperatures. *Parasitology Research*, 2001, 87, 553 – 555.

[16] Bruce-Chwatt, LJ. Essential Malariology. Oxford: Oxford University Press; 1985.

[17] Srivastava, A; Khanduri, A; Lakhtakia, S; Pandey, R; Choudhuri, G. *Falciparum* malaria with acute renal failure. Tropical Gastroenterology, 1996, 17, 172 – 174.

[18] Abisheganaden, J; Rajasoorya, C; Tari, PK; Chaw, LS. Malaria: an audit of 56 cases admitted to a hospital. *Singapore Medical Journal*, 1996, 37, 153 – 156.

[19] Maegraith, B. Aspects of the pathogenesis of malaria. *Southwest Asian Journal of Tropical Medicine and Public Health*, 1981, 12, 251 – 267.

[20] Stroeve, EA; Makarova, VG. Laboratory manual for Biochemistry. Moscow: MIR Publishers; 1986.

[21] Council of International Organization of Medical Sciences / World Health Organization (CIOMS/WHO). International Ethical Guidelines for Biomedical Research Involving Human Subjects. Geneva, Switzerland, 1993.

[22] Clark, IA; Schofield, L. Pathogenesis of malaria. *Parasitology Today*, 2000, 16, 451-454.

[23] Miller, LH; Baruch, DI; Marsh, K; Doumbo, OK. The pathogenic basis of malaria. *Nature*, 2002, 415, 673 – 679.

[24] Bansal, D; Bhatti, HS; Sehgal, R. Role of cholesterol in parasitic infections. *Lipids in Health and Disease*, 2005, 4, 4-10.

[25] Sibmooh, N; Yamanont, P; Krusood, S; Leowattana, W; Brittenham, G; Looareesuwan, S; Udomsangpetch, R. Increased fluidity and oxidation of malarial lipoproteins: relation with severity and induction of endothelial expression of adhesion molecules. *Lipids in Health and Disease*, 2004, 3, 3-15.

[26] Williamson, KC; Fujioka, H; Aikawa, M; Kaslow, C. Stage-specific processing of pfs 230, a plasmodium *falciparum* transmission-blocking vaccine candidate. *Molecular Biochemistry and Parasitology*, 1996, 78, 161 – 169.

[27] Kulkarni, AG; Suryakar, AN; Sardeshmukh, AS; Rathi, DB. Studies on biochemical changes with special reference to oxidant and antioxidants in malaria patients. *Indian Journal of Clinical Biochemistry*, 2003; 18, 136-149.

[28] Nanda, R; Mishra, PK; Das, UK; Rout, SB; Mohapatra, PC; Panda, A. Evaluating role of oxidative stress in determining the pathogenesis of falciparum malaria induced acute renal failure. *Indian Journal of Clinical Biochemistry,* 2004; 19: 93-96.

[29] Das, BS; Thurnham, DI, Das, DB. Plasma α-tocopherol, retinol, and carotenoids in children with *falciparum* malaria. *American Journal of Clinical Nutrition*, 1996, 64, 94-100.

[30] Davis, TME; Sturm, M; Zhang, YR; Spancer, JL; Graham, RM; Li, GQ; Taylor, RR. Platelet-activating factor and lipid pattern in acute malaria. *Journal of Infection*, 1993, 26, 279-289.

[31] Mohanty, S; Mishra, SK; Das, BS; Satpathy, SK; Mohanty, D; Patnaik, JK; Bose, TK. Altered plasma lipid pattern in *falciparum* malaria. *Annals of Tropical Medicine and Parasitology*, 1992, 86, 601-606.

In: Progress in Malaria Research
Editor: Lee O. Koning, pp. 211-216
ISBN: 978-1-60021-590-2

Chapter VIII

Community Based Actions for Fighting Against Malaria

D. Kinde-Gazard*[*]*, D. Gbenou and R. Houngnihin
PNLP, 03 BP 1428 Cotonou, Benin

Abstract

Most of deaths due to malaria occur in sub-Saharan region of Africa mainly children under five years who die in the 48 first hours of the illness. The necessity to have a quick diagnosis, a precocious, adequate and accessible treatment at all levels of society becomes mandatory to the endemic countries. The main objective of this document is to contribute to the reduction of the mortality and the morbidity related to malaria by proposing a better definition of the policies and strategies for fighting against malaria by using community based actions. Specifically, it is (i) to determine and to capitalize all community based management experiences for fighting against malaria, (ii) to determine the mechanisms of inter and into sector development of partnership for both mobilization of financial resource and the coordination of the community activities at all area of the medical pyramid of a country, (iii) to define ways to strengthen the social appropriation and the community participation for fighting against malaria, to create an impact and to perpetuate a long-term actions (iv) to provide to actors and community partners, orientations that imply or likely to be implied the Community based management of activities. To reach the Millennium Objectives for Development 2015, the endemic countries will have to overcome the challenge of malaria control at each level from family to community so that this disease does not represent any more neither, a major public health problem, nor a factor of impoverishment of the populations.

[*] D. Kinde-Gazard: e-mail: kindegazard@yahoo.fr

Introduction

Malaria constitutes an important problem of public health in Africa. In the majority of countries, indeed, this disease represents the first cause of the recourse to the care in the medical formations and is in the forefront of the principal diseases in the communities. According to World Heath Organisation (WHO), malaria is responsible for 1, 5 to 2, 7 million annual deaths [1] and 90% of deaths occur in sub-Saharan region of Africa, mainly children under five years who dies in the 48 fists hours of illness. The necessity to have a quick diagnosis, a precocious, adequate and accessible treatment at all levels of society becomes mandatory to the endemic countries. The deep socio-economic upheavals, whose width is undoubtedly estimated, vary according to epidemiologic facieses of malaria in the area considered. This paper wants to contribute to the reduction of morbidity and mortality related to malaria by proposing a better definition of the policies and strategies based on the scaling up of the Community interventions for fighting against malaria. To achieve this goal, it is specifically to:

1 Determine and capitalize all the best Community experiences of fight against malaria;
2 To determine the mechanisms of inter and into sector development of partnership, for both the mobilization of financial resources and the coordination of the Community activities, at all area of the medical pyramid of a country;
3 To define ways to strengthen the social appropriation and the Community participation for fighting against malaria, to create an impact and to perpetuate a long-term actions;
4 To provide to actors and community partners, orientations that implied or likely to be implied the Community based management of activities.It is important to recall that this document develops approaches generic, likely to be adapted to realities and contexts of each country.

1. Best Experiments

They are perceived to be a whole of innovative, powerful and perennial activities, reproducible in socio-cultural economic and political context, adaptable in any context. As subjective as it can appear, the concept of "better experiments" or "better practices", is, in the view of methodology, to validate activities in a consensual way by all the actors involve, on selection criteria basis. These activities must be technically efficient, economically realizable, have a positive and measurable impact on the communities, and be based on national policy and the fundamental documents of the National Malaria Control Program. In Republic of Benin, after 5 years of implementation of the strategies and activities, the practices which are better in time and spaces summarize as follows:

1.1. Strengthening the Managerial Capacities of the National Malaria Control Program (NMCP)

The transformation of government's intentions into realities and to honour its commitments after the signing of Abuja Declaration [2], decentralized structures were set up in each district (construction of buildings, recruitment of medical doctors, nurses, midwifes, equipment and cars). The adoption of this approach avoids the virtualization of the activities.

1.2. Collaboration IMCI/RBM

This collaboration between "Integrated Management of Childhood Illness (IMCI)" and "Roll Back Malaria (RBM)" started in years 2000, with the development, the validation and the adoption of IMCI training modules A national consensus was reached on the management of malaria on the first level of care, following IMCI/RBM guidelines. The process of integration was based on approaches and strategies concerning the implementation of joint policies, prevention and treatment, operational research and monitoring/evaluation. The training and retraining of heath workers at all levels and the available resources constitute the greatest challenges.

1.3. Implication of NGOs

The community based malaria control activities, executed with support from national NGOs, target the promotion of insecticide treated materials as well as the development and follow up of community based approaches to malaria prevention. These activities essentially consist of pilot phase and nation wide implementation phase. Thirty five NGOs were recruited to strengthen malaria control activities through: (i) conducting "Information Education Communication, (IEC) sessions for the communities. (ii) closed collaboration with women's association, school authorities, paramedical staff and other organized structures at the local level. Seventy animators from community radio stations' were trained to deliver through their radio, messages on the prevention and the treatment of malaria. The follow-up/evaluation of the activities of NGOs and community radio is very essential.

1.4. Involvement of the Teachers and the Pupils

Pupils taken individually or as a group and they teachers, serve as agents for the dissemination of information. The training started in 1999 with 40 teachers. It extended to more than 300 teachers per year. Their mission was to summarize what they had learnt in the teaching of their students. The successes of this approach include the increasing awareness amongst the school setting, who have understood the importance of keeping one's surroundings clean and of sleeping under a insecticide treated bed net. Anti-malarial clubs have been created to diagnose and treat uncomplicated cases of malaria in schools.

1.5. Outreach Strategy for Free Impregnation of Insecticide Treated Materials

The objectives of this initiative are to: i) increase the coverage of insecticide treated bed nets (ITN) at household level, ii) help communities to develop the habit of malaria prevention. The operation was very laboured intensive and expensive. However, there was a massive response from the people, especially the poorest family.

The determination of the best practices in the long term allows experience sharing as well between individual experts as between networks of organizations and institutions, in the way for fighting against malaria.

2. Management of Roll Back Malaria Partnership

In the RBM initiative context, several strategies of partnership were developed: - Collaboration was into sector (between Ministry of Health's structure: the Community IMCI, traditional health workers, the immunization, the Reproductive Health, the Integrated Monitoring/Evaluation) and inter sector (between the Ministry of health and the other Ministries: Agriculture, Education, Environment, Finances, Promotion of the woman, Institutions of research). The creation of an informal group, named "Facilitators Group" formalized by a ministerial order is today a framework for management of this partnership. The "Facilitators Group", contributes to better coordination of actions, better information sharing with and amongst partners increase in resources, creation of an enable environment for fighting against malaria. But the collaboration with the other ministries is not developed and the participation of the private sector is very weak. All partners involved in the implementation of the NMCP action plan must help whole heartedly to attain the set objectives by making sure that the activities of partners are integrated in the NMCP action plan, and by including the partners' actions in the NMCP annual report on malaria control activities. A RBM partnership must function on all the levels: strategic, operational and Community

3. Social Appropriation and Participation of Community

Firstly, any Community intervention consists in carrying out a baseline malaria data in the community. The baseline malaria data collecting consisted for investigating the various socio-cultural knowledge, attitude, beliefs and practices (KAP) about malaria: clinical signs, cause, recognition, treatment, and prevention. KAP investigation led NMCP to develop training materials of IEC (Information Communication Education) for Behaviour Change Communication (BCC). The production and distribution of IEC materials adapted to realities of the communities, was used for training the mothers of under fives years children or child keepers. The training required 3 levels of intervention: - the briefing of health workers (doctor, male nurse, midwives); - the social mobilization - the sanitary education of the communities and the pregnant women. It is carried out through a public campaign (discussion under the tree in village) with all the mothers/child keepers, women in age to procreate, pregnant women of each village or district. The effectiveness of home treatment depends upon heath education about malaria for early diagnosis, prompt appropriate and treatment. Caregivers should be taught to recognize signs of severe malaria for which they must immediately bring a child to nearest heath facility. Intermittent Preventive Treatment (IPT) with Sulfadoxine-Pyrimethamine shown to be effective to prevent malaria in the pregnant woman. As regards for vector control, the actions converged towards the use of the materials treated with insecticides, the education and the management of the environment. The Community based interventions and activities are often limited to their area. The results of activities and the actors are not known. It is necessary to develop monitoring/evaluation mechanisms for perpetuation of Community based for fighting against malaria.

4. Orientation System

The interventions have as a finality to provide to actors and community partners, orientations that imply or likely to be implied the community based management of activities, to support the community notification of the cases of malaria in the Benin. With this intention, it will be an important thing for designing a minimum package of activities (MPA) for fighting against malaria and for ensuring the training of the Community Workers on this MPA. This minimum package of activities must take into account the recording of the data and information at community basis, concerning the cases of clinical malaria/fever [3], of death in the children of less than 5 years and the pregnant women, the availability of the drugs, the impregnated mosquito bed net and the data carriers. The notification of these data must be systematic and monthly, and the transmission of the data cumulated at community level must be done towards the intermediary and national levels every quarter.

Conclusion

Malaria leads to poverty.

To reach the Millennium Objectives for Development 2015, the endemic countries will have to overcome the challenge of malaria control at each level from family to community so that this disease does represent any more neither, a major public health problem, nor a factor of impoverishment of the populations.

Reference

[1] Roll Back Malaria, www.rbm.who.int

[2] OMS/CDS/RBM, 2000, Sommet africain sur l'initiative *"Faire Reculer le Paludisme"*,72 p

[3] Massougbodji A, Zohoun Th, Odjo J, Sadeler BC; Fièvre et paludisme à Cotonou en République Populaire du Bénin; *Médecine d'Afrique Noire* : 1989,36 (4) :314-317

Index

2

A

B

C

D

E

F

G

H

I

J

K

L

N

O

P

Q

R

S